NORTHEAST MEDICINAL PLANTS

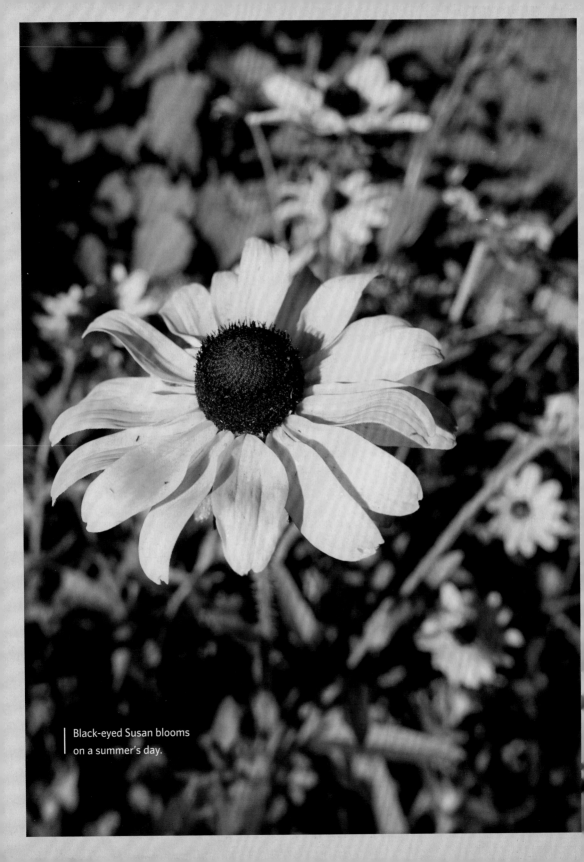

Black-eyed Susan blooms
on a summer's day.

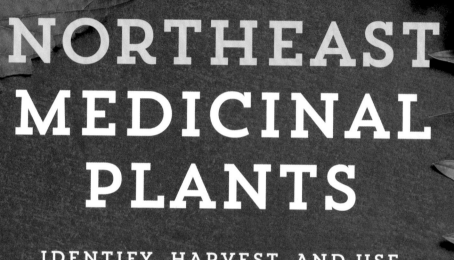

NORTHEAST MEDICINAL PLANTS

IDENTIFY, HARVEST, AND USE
❧ 111 WILD HERBS ❧
FOR HEALTH AND WELLNESS

LIZ NEVES

Copyright © 2020 by Liz Neves. All rights reserved.
Photography credits appear on page 403. Drawings by Alan Bryan.

Published in 2020 by Timber Press, Inc., a subsidiary of Workman Publishing Co.,
a subsidiary of Hachette Book Group, Inc.
1290 Avenue of the Americas
New York, NY 10104

timberpress.com

Printed in China on responsibly sourced paper
Third printing 2022

Text and cover design by Adrianna Sutton

ISBN 978-1-60469-913-5
A catalog record for this book is available from the Library of Congress.

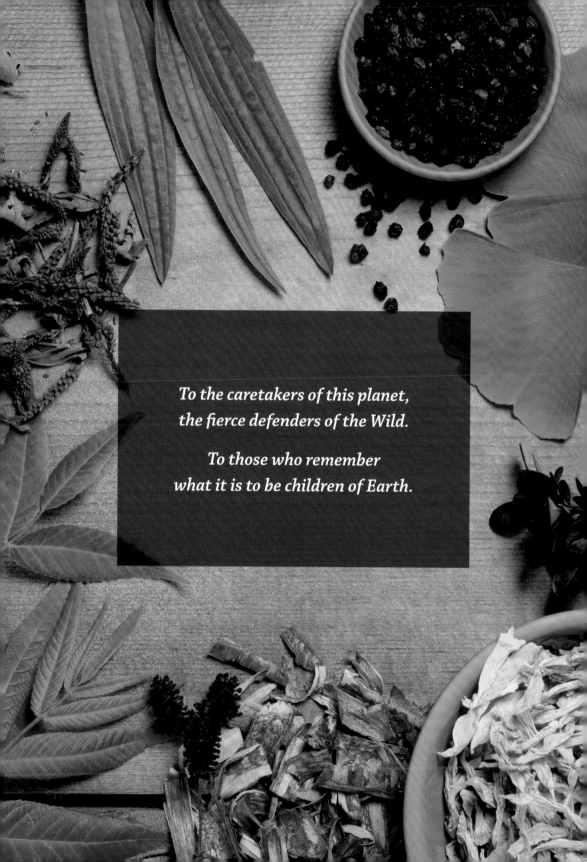

To the caretakers of this planet,
the fierce defenders of the Wild.

To those who remember
what it is to be children of Earth.

CONTENTS

WILD MEDICINAL PLANTS OF THE NORTHEAST • 98

Old growth pine branches touch the sky. Eastern white pine is known as the Tree of Peace by the Haudenosaunee Confederacy, with the five needles of each leaf grouping representing the original five nations (Mohawks, Oneidas, Onondagas, Cayugas, and Senecas).

PREFACE

Nothing is ever really lost, it's just forgotten.

I n high school I heard the wild calling. My school offered an opportunity to backpack in the Adirondack Mountains for a week. I don't know what compelled me to do it. In all my 15 years I had never been on a camping trip like this before. I distinctly recall packing the borrowed thermals the school provided, weighing out bags of pasta and oatmeal and distributing it among our packs.

In the days leading up to the trip, the five of us students practiced belaying on the school's ropes course, guided by our two teachers. On our way to the mountains we stopped at the Delaware Water Gap, just about 30 minutes northwest of my hometown, to practice more climbing and rappelling skills. Then we were off, 5 hours or so into the heart of the Adirondack high peaks region.

At the time, I appreciated nature, but did not sense the deep inseparable connection we have to Earth. *When did we start thinking we were separate from nature?* Like many people in the Western world, the idea that

nature was "somewhere out there" was well conditioned in me. Little I knew of the treasures that the wild gifts to the spirit. I did not grasp the immense healing that simply being surrounded by plants could have, let alone know the direct healing properties of these plants.

It was a difficult adventure, not without its rewards—mainly the thrill of reaching those spectacular unparalleled open mountaintop views. We hiked several miles a day with full packs. Up and down elevations that challenged us physically and mentally. On one of the last days of our trip, it felt like

> The following information is reference to supplement
> the knowledge you've already acquired about these
> plants.
>
> SASSAFRAS
> (Sassafras albidum)
>
> Sassafras is very common throughout our southern
> forest. It is usually a small shrubby tree, although
> it occasionally grows up to 80' high and 3' in
> diameter, with a deeply furrowed bark and short,
> stout, contorted branches. During the growing season,
> sassafras can be best identified by its three
> different leaves. One is oval and entirely margined,
> another is mitten-shaped, and the third is
> three-lobed; that is, the mitten has two thumbs. In
> the late fall and winter, sassafras can be identified
> .... and half-round leaf scar. The

A very simple field guide from my youth.

a great accomplishment to reach the highest peak at an elevation of 5343 feet, Mount Marcy, known as Tewawe'éstha in Kanien'ke-há:ka (Mohawk) or Tahawus meaning "cloud-splitter" in Algonquin.

Unfortunately for my feet, I had the wrong kind of boots. The impact of downhill hiking with a pack on my back brought heel blisters and cost me two toenails. Though painful to endure, it was a small price to pay for the lessons I learned and the seeds that were planted on that journey.

We each had a "solo night" away from the camp and without food. We were told we could eat clovers, but what I never wondered was, what are clovers doing on a mountain-top? I nibbled many clovers that evening under my makeshift poncho tent. I can assure you they aren't filling. And I wrote in the little photocopied survival guide journal our teachers provided. I still have that journal. Inside is the tiniest field guide to medicinal and edible plants I've ever seen. Eastern white pine, jewelweed, poison ivy, sassafras, violet.

Fast forward 27 years—after college, an abandoned advertising career, becoming a mother, and about 10 years of herbal and spiritual exploration—and here I am, writing about those very same plants in this book.

Retelling this story now, as a mother, I see it with fresh eyes. I see that sowing the seeds of plant medicine and other forms of earth wisdom in children is critical to ensuring that humans thrive on this planet alongside their green, winged, finned, and furry relations. Even if they don't pursue a path of plant medicine right away it'll be a thread in their life's fabric, and they will come back to it in some way. If we forget, we can remember. We can always return to the wise ways.

It is my hope that in connecting you with wild medicinal plants that we will all come to a greater appreciation of the natural world, understand our place in it, and become impassioned keepers of the land, protectors of wild spaces.

Let's remember, together.

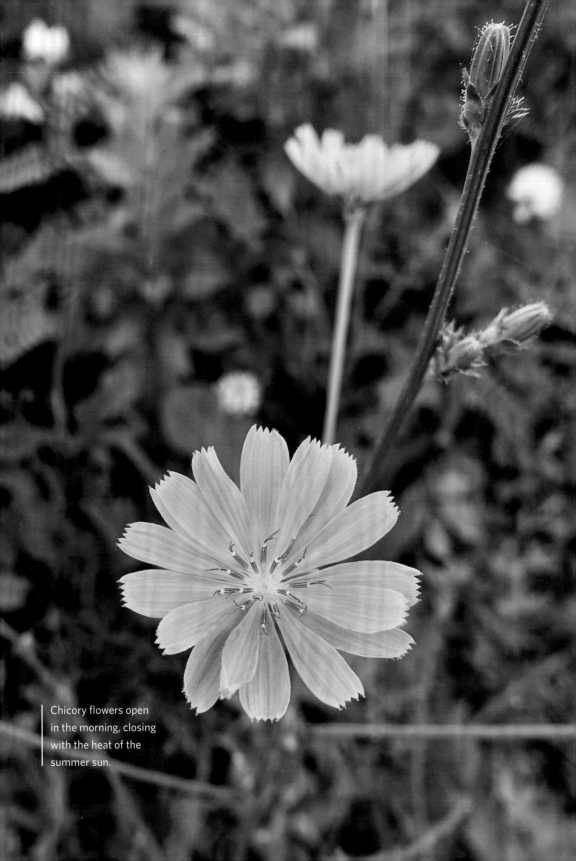

Chicory flowers open in the morning, closing with the heat of the summer sun.

HOW TO USE
THIS BOOK

The northeastern United States and southeastern Canada contain a rich abundance of medicine plants. I've selected 111 of the most versatile and plentiful that are present in a good chunk of the region. Through directly experiencing the plants, you will come to find your particular relationship with them. You may discover new ways of partnering with the plants that I have not included here, or that anyone has written about for that matter. The beauty of learning how to collaborate with medicinal plants is that it is a lifetime journey full of discovery.

PLANT NAMES

There are at least two ways to call a plant by its name. One is to use the common name; let's take dandelion, for example. Many people around the world know this plant's name as dandelion. However, if you live in France, you might call the plant *dent de lion* (for "lion's tooth," referring to the shape of the leaves) or *pissenlit* (for "wet the bed" because it's a diuretic). In England you might call the gone-to-seed flower of this plant "clocks"— legend has it, the amount of times required to blow the seeds loose from the flowerhead tells the time of day. In Hindi, this plant is called "Kukraundha," but so is blumea (*Blumea lacera*). Wait, what's that name in parentheses? And why are two plants given the same common name? This is where the challenge of common names arises. How do we know which plant we are talking about when more than one plant is named that way or when one plant has multiple common names? Enter, the scientific name!

Scientific names are based on a taxonomic system of grouping plants and other living creatures into categories of other related living things. The taxonomic system that we use today is based on the work of Carolus Linnaeus (aka Carl von Linné). Although our modern way of categorizing living beings is a bit different from Linnaeus's, the basic concept is intact. Just like life on Earth, scientific systems are ever-evolving. Plants are currently named, like all life forms, by these categories: domain, kingdom, phylum, class, order, family, genus, and species.

It's these last two, genus and species, that are usually put in parentheses or italicized after a plant's common name. In our example, we would express this as: dandelion (*Taraxacum officinale*). *Taraxacum* is the genus and *officinale* is the species. There are other *Taraxacum* species in the world, but there's no other like *officinale*. Except maybe a subspecies or varietal. You'd see that expressed

as *Taraxacum officinale* ssp. *officinale* or *Taraxacum officinale* var. *officinale*, respectively.

This genus and species part of the name is also sometimes referred to as the botanical or "latinized" name because, in most cases, the name is derived from a Latin or Ancient Greek root. The names often tell us something about the history of the plant, the way it looks, where it grows, who named it, and if it has been used medicinally in the past.

There are a couple of stories as to how the name *Taraxacum* originated. One version is that Al-Razi, tenth-century Persian physician and polymath, called the plant "tarashaquq" or "tarkhashqun," the same word for chicory and endive, two plants related to dandelion. It's also possibly derived from the Greek words *taraxos*, meaning "disorder" and *akos*

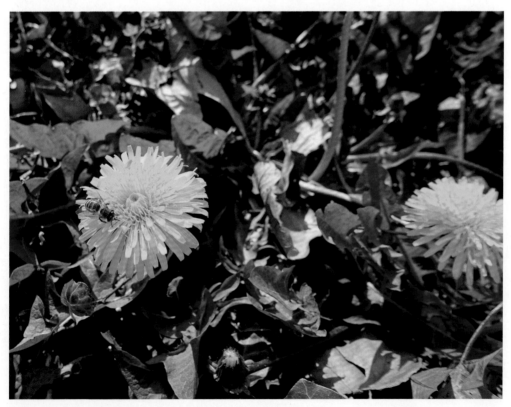

What's in a name? That which we call a dandelion by any other word would taste as bitter.

meaning "order." We do know that the word *officinale* tells us that this plant has been classified as an officinal medicinal plant, or an herb that has a history of medicinal use. Using the Greek derivation story, we get a pretty cool mnemonic device: dandelion is a plant that's long been used to bring order to disorder in the human body. Neat!

The beauty of this system is that there is a universal language for naming plants. No matter what the common name of a plant is in your region, when we use the scientific name, we know exactly which plant we're talking about.

One more thing about names, at least for the purpose of this book. In some cases, I've included a plant's family name. Still thinking about dandelion here, its family is Asteraceae (formerly Compositae), also known as the aster or sunflower family. In time, as you get to know the plant families, this becomes a really helpful identification tool. Plants in the same family, like siblings or cousins, share many of the same traits. Dandelions, like their Asteraceae relations, have an inflorescence that is a composite of smaller flowers. When you see a flower that becomes a big puff of seed fluff when it goes to seed, it's likely you have an aster family plant.

PARTS USED

Here's where you will find the parts of the plant that are utilized as medicine, based on traditional uses and personal experience. Some plants have multiple medicinal parts, like dandelion—roots, leaves, and flowers. Echinacea falls into this category, too. One reason it helps to know which parts to use is because sometimes, the leaves and flowers are just as efficacious as the roots, so we don't have to uproot and take the life of the plant.

Other plants may have parts that are more medicinally active than some of its other parts, like the rhizome of wild sarsaparilla, which is more active than the leaves. Still other plants have medicinal parts and potentially poisonous parts. Poke roots and berries, depending on who you talk to, are the medicinal parts of the plant *Phytolacca americana*. The mature stems and leaves are not so great to ingest. Best to compost them.

For some plants you'll use the entire aboveground or aerial portion of the plant, like chickweed, cleavers, or the aerial parts in flower, like self-heal and yarrow. When the parts are listed individually, harvest each part individually before, during, or after flowering, at different times of the year as indicated in the "Where, When, and How to Wildcraft" section. I've specified flowering tops as the parts used in cases where using the top portion of the plant in flower is ideal, such as with boneset, goldenrod, and motherwort.

There isn't always consensus on which plant parts are used and there may be cultural, regional, or personal variations. Perhaps someone does have a use for wild sarsaparilla leaves. I just don't know it yet.

HOW TO IDENTIFY

This section features some of the key identifying characteristics of the plants. Wherever possible, I use simple language to describe the plants without too much technical terminology.

If you are new to plant identification, looking out at a field of green in a meadow or forest may be a bit daunting. At first, all of the leaves and branches seem to intertwine in a mass of indistinguishable green and brown bits. I promise with time and practice you'll start recognizing plants from several feet away without a problem. You'll start to see the plants the way you would spot a friend's face in a crowd.

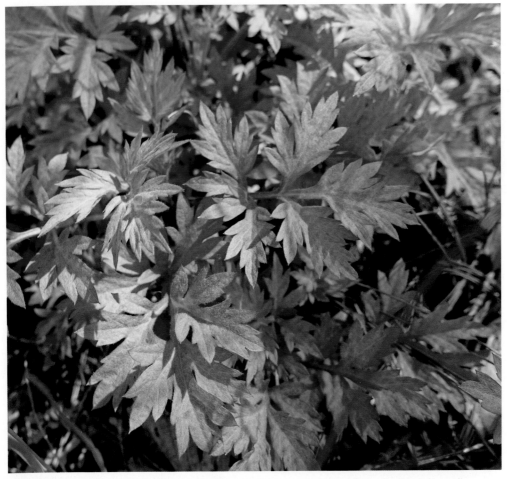

Mugwort emerges in spring, starting low to the ground. By summer's end it may be 6 or 7 feet tall.

A good rule of thumb for plant identification is to know at least three distinguishing features of a given plant. Take mugwort for instance:

The simple leaves are deeply divided with pointed lobes

The leaves have downy white undersides

The plant has a unique fragrance, somewhat spicy and earthy

Some questions to ask when identifying plants:

Is it herbaceous or woody?

Is the branching pattern opposite or alternate?

Are the leaves simple or compound? Toothed or smooth edged?

How many petals does the flower have?

Does the plant have a distinctive scent?

Are there any poisonous lookalikes?

A MAD Cap Bucking Horse

There are fewer opposite branching woody plants than there are alternate branching ones. So to assist you in identifying those few opposite branching plants, here is a fun mnemonic device:

- A for *Adoxaceae*, which includes elder and viburnums
- MAD for *Maple, Ash, Dogwood*
- Cap for *Cap*rifoliaceae or the honeysuckle family
- Bucking for *Buck*eye
- Horse for *Horse*chestnut

Another important part of identification is knowing the plant throughout the seasons and through its growth cycles. Mugwort, for instance, looks dramatically different in spring than it does in late summer. In the spring, it appears as gray-green leaves emerging from the soil on tender stems; by summer's end its stem is woody, its leaves are darker on the surface and hardier, it is in flower, and it reaches heights of 6 or 7 feet.

Some field guides categorize plants by flower color. Well what do you do if the plant you're looking for is not in flower? This book will give you an idea of basic plant features in different seasons. You'll learn when the plant flowers, when it fruits, and when it goes to seed. I also recommend acquiring a field guide with a dichotomous key, such as *Newcomb's Wildflower Guide*. A dichotomous key provides choices based on observable characteristics. Ideally, following the correct choices will lead you to the identity of the plant. See the resources section for helpful plant identification websites, too.

You might also notice where I've distinguished a plant as "introduced" or "native." *What's that all about?* The short story is that, before Europeans arrived on this continent there were certain flora present that we now call native. When Europeans began to colonize the land, they brought with them food and medicine plants they deemed valuable. Over time, plants from around the world were introduced to this land, creating a variety of plant life that did not exist here before colonization.

The interesting thing about this unplanned experiment of wild horticulture is that the plants that were once considered desirable are now vilified with language such as invasive, noxious, and opportunistic. It is true that the landscape has dramatically changed and that some garden escapees seem to be crowding out valued native plants. And it's true that native plants are becoming endangered. But is that the fault of the plants that were introduced, the ones we call weeds?

To quote Ralph Waldo Emerson, "What is a weed? A plant whose virtues have not yet been discovered." The very idea of a weed is a human invention, a matter of perception. It is humans who introduced the plants, humans who destroy habitat, humans who decide to poison or not to poison plants. It is a choice for us to understand the plants through a different lens and make peace. It is a choice to put our focus on what matters: caring for the land, healing our wounds, and caring for each other.

PLANT MORPHOLOGY

Here are some important identifying characteristics of the plants in this book.

LEAF SHAPES

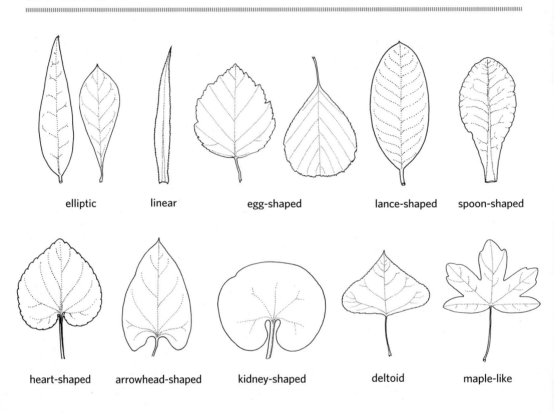

elliptic

linear

egg-shaped

lance-shaped

spoon-shaped

heart-shaped

arrowhead-shaped

kidney-shaped

deltoid

maple-like

COMPOUND LEAF TYPES

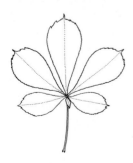

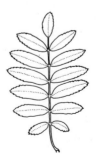

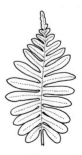

palmate compound

pinnate compound

pinnate lobed

LEAF MARGINS

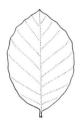
smooth-edged

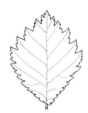
double-toothed

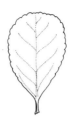
scalloped

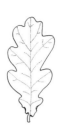
lobed

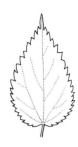
toothed

LEAF ARRANGEMENTS

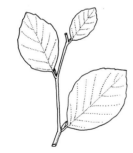
alternate

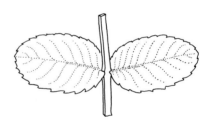
opposite

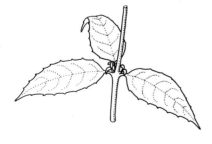
whorled

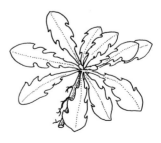
basal

FLOWER PARTS

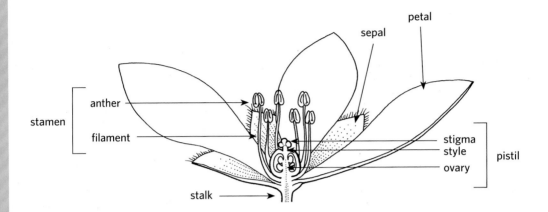

COMPOSITE FLOWER PARTS

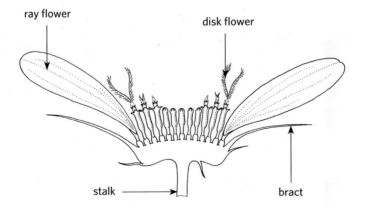

WHERE, WHEN, AND HOW TO WILDCRAFT

What is the Northeast? The predominating geopolitical worldview refers to this part of the world as northeastern North America, an area comprised of eleven U.S. states (Connecticut, Delaware, Maine, Massachusetts, Maryland, New Hampshire, New Jersey, New York, Pennsylvania, Rhode Island, and Vermont) and five Canadian provinces (Québec, Nova Scotia, New Brunswick, Prince Edward Island, and Newfoundland and Labrador). I'm adding southern Ontario to this mix as well.

From an indigenous standpoint, we are on Turtle Island.

Through an ecological perspective, we are in the northern temperate forests, comprising a blend of intermingling ecoregions, categorized according to their geological history and ecosystem dynamics.

Knowing the specific habitat of plants from the ecological perspective is a fundamental part of plant identification. It also helps to know where plants tend to grow so that you can find them. In this section you'll get to know the plants' preferences for

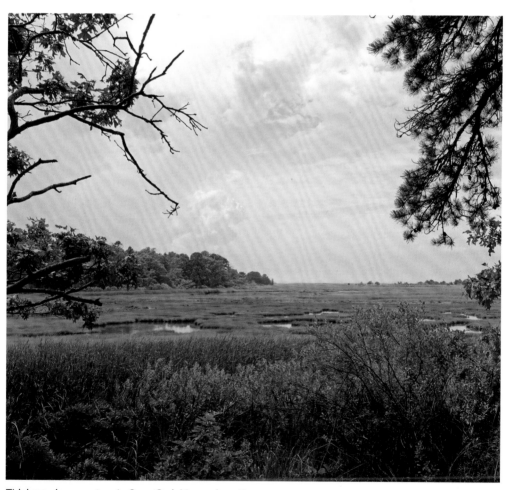

Tidal marsh ecosystem in Cape Cod, Massachusetts.

specific niches in the ecosystem. Eastern cottonwood, alder, and willow, for example, live in a wetland habitat. Introduced plants like chicory, dandelion, and plantain tend to grow in areas that are disturbed by human activity. This includes lawns, cracks in the sidewalk, edges of roadways and paths, public parks, and abandoned lots.

I used two main resources in acquiring some of the information provided in this section, the USDA PLANTS database and the Native Plant Trust's Go Botany website. Once you enter the scientific or common name of the plant, the USDA PLANTS database has zoomable distribution maps showing where it grows in most of North America. In addition to a dichotomous key, Go Botany provides maps showing county data from the Biota of North America Program (BONAP) plant atlas, information on plant habitat, as well as excellent color photographs of plants.

In this section you'll discover the best time to harvest particular plants and their parts. Roots are generally harvested in early spring or fall when the rest of the plant has either yet to send up shoots or has died back for the season and the energy of the plant is stored in the roots. Some leaves are gathered in spring when they are young and tender, while others can be harvested throughout the growing season. Still others, like evergreen leaves and needles, can be collected year-round.

You'll also get a general sense of how to wildcraft certain plants. Sometimes all you'll need is your two hands and something to catch leaves, flowers, or fruit in. Other harvests require special tools and more exertion. Roots call us to dig, sometimes deeply with shovel, trowel, knife, or digging stick. Sometimes we only need to dig a few inches below the soil with our hands. For bark, you'll prune branches with pruning shears or a pruning saw, or gather freshly fallen limbs or twigs off the ground following a storm.

MEDICINAL USES

Here I highlight some of the key uses of particular plants, based on my own experience, that of friends and teachers, of herbalists whose perspectives I admire, and of the people who've tended this land for thousands of years and know the plants in their bones. I would not have been able to write this book without the knowledge passed down by these fellow humans.

Aside from common medicinal uses, I've woven in information about the energetics of plants and how these attributes restore balance to health. If there are any signatures that would hint at the plant's medicinal uses, I've included those as well. You can read more about plant energetics in "Working with Plant Medicine." The vibrational medicine of flowers in the form of flower essences is also included for some plants. Learn more about this form of emotional-spiritual medicine in "Making Your Own Medicine."

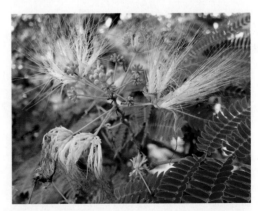

Mimosa's soft blossoms comprised of several silky stamens are reflective of the plant's ability to calm frazzled nerves.

The Doctrine of Signatures

Plants speak to us in ways we can comprehend, ways that tell us of their medicine, if we learn their language. Paracelsus, sixteenth-century physician-alchemist-astrologer, dubbed this language the "doctrine of signatures," though it is a universal concept that predates him. A major aspect of this system of "reading" the plants is that their color, shape, and growing patterns correspond to energies and systems of the body. By observing these patterns, we can translate them to heal imbalance. Here are just a handful of examples that reflect this idea.

- Red is associated with blood, as are plants that can prick you and make you bleed, such as hawthorn, raspberry, and rose.

- Yellow is linked with bile, the liver, kidneys, urine, and the solar plexus energy center (chakra). Plants that reflect this signature are dandelion, elecampane, goldenrod, and yellow dock.

- Plants with fine hairs or parts that resemble nerves correspond with the nervous system, such as mimosa, mullein, pine, and borage.

Take time to sit with the plants where they grow in the wild and let their signatures reveal themselves to you. In time you'll develop your own understanding of their unique language.

 PRECAUTIONS

Here you'll find out whether a plant has any safety precautions. Taking herbal medicine following recommended dosages and methods of administration is generally a very safe practice. However, some herbs are not suitable for every body or every context. This section highlights common contraindications, potential toxicity, possible untoward effects, and dosage safety.

FUTURE HARVESTS

Wildcrafting with respect for the land and the plants is vital for their survival, and ours. In this section you'll find out how to carefully harvest, potentially propagate, and protect plants for the future. For the most part, the plants I included in this book are abundant in the northeastern United States, and in the neighboring Canadian provinces of Ontario and Québec. There are a few exceptions to this rule. If a plant is at risk in a part of the range, you'll see it noted in this section. I cross-referenced between conservation website NatureServe, the USDA PLANTS database, and Go Botany to determine conservation status of the plants included in this book.

HERBAL PREPARATIONS

The act of making and taking herbal medicine is as individual as we are. As such, the preparation and dosage suggestions provided in this section are not definitive. Check the "Herbal Medicine Dosages" section (page 68) for dosage adjustments, particularly for children and elders. Try the recommended methods of preparation and then experiment by following your own hunches. The best way to learn is through trying it yourself. So go for it!

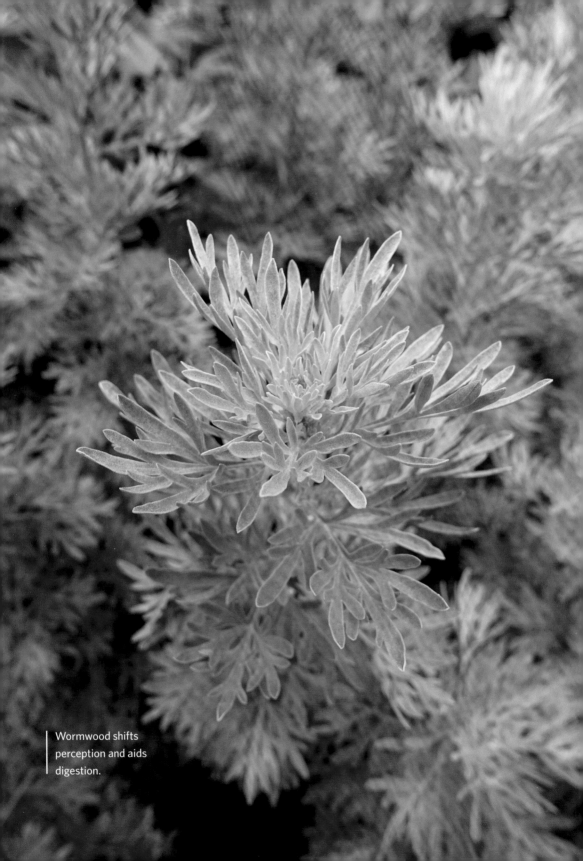

Wormwood shifts
perception and aids
digestion.

WILDCRAFTING BASICS

Our ancient human ancestors relied entirely on the natural world around them for all of their needs. Sourcing materials for shelter and clothing, foraging food, and wildcrafting medicine from the wild was the only way of life. There were no pharmacies, supermarkets, or even farms (up until the agricultural revolution around 12,000 years ago). Humans provided for their needs this way for thousands and thousands of years.

Despite the departure from these old wild ways, for many modern humans a rekindling is occurring. Those of us who have forgotten are beginning to recognize that the idea that we are separate from the natural world—a world that we are inextricably part of—is destructive and unhealthy. Many, like you dear reader, are remembering our connection to life. We are remembering our relationship to the plants, these overlooked members of our community. We are waking up to the magic of their healing power. Returning to the wild plants, relying on them for food and medicine, can heal our bodies, minds, and souls. We are remembering, too, that in our hearts, we are wild.

We've inherited a landscape of fragmented forest, plain, marsh, and coastal ecosystems. Since Europeans reached these shores, rapid and massive deforestation has ensued to the detriment of plant and animal life. Like the fragmented wilderness, our lives have also been broken and thrown off balance. We suffer from a wide array of cultural, environmental, and personal diseases: racial, gender, and class inequality; ecological degradation; loss of biodiversity; increased rates of incarceration, asthma, diabetes, and infant

> "Never take the first plant you find, as it might be the last—and you want that first one to speak well of you to the others of her kind."
>
> —*Braiding Sweetgrass*, by Robin Wall Kimmerer

mortality. Restoring ecosystems, daylighting streams, planting trees, encouraging wild growth, and immersing ourselves in this wildness is not only possible, it's necessary for healing these deep wounds. Tending the wild places on Earth and in our hearts brings us alive again. It restores our sense of belonging to something greater than ourselves.

Let's come back to the earth together. We can start by learning the reciprocal relationship of wildcrafting medicinal plants.

SEVEN STEPS TO WILDCRAFTING WITH SEVEN GENERATIONS IN MIND

The following seven steps to wildcrafting are inspired by the "Honorable Harvest" described in Robin Wall Kimmerer's *Braiding Sweetgrass*. It is a way of honoring the plants and the land that is aligned with traditional ecological knowledge (TEK), including the sustainable harvesting practices of the First Peoples of these lands. It is centered on the recognition that plants are our kin and that it is their right to give us what we need, rather than us deeming what we feel we need to take.

1. Set an intention

2. Ask permission

3. Know the plant well

4. Make an offering

5. Be fully present

6. Use and share the medicine

7. Become a wild gardener

Set an Intention

Before you even approach the plants, start an inquiry with yourself. Why are you seeking medicine? Do you need the help of the plants? What is your *intention* for gathering medicine? Slowing down to listen to the answers helps us witness our ingrained conquering and overconsumptive impulse. That feeling that we must have something to fill an empty hole, to feed the hungry ghosts. If our intentions are purely needs-based, if we really need the medicine, nature abides.

As you go to sleep at night, ask for guidance in your dreams. You might be surprised by what you see, hear, and feel. Write down your dreams and sit with their potential meanings. In time, the plants will start speaking with you in both day and night dreams.

Pay attention, also, to synchronicities in your day-to-day life. Notice if someone mentions a plant that you feel connected with, one that you are considering gathering medicine from. Maybe you'll see a picture of the plant or read the name somewhere. At the root of the word "coincidence" is *coincidere*, Latin for "to agree." Think of these coincidences as an agreement that it is okay to proceed to the next step.

Ask Permission

Before you put your pruners to the branch, take a step back. Go back to your intention. Tell your intention to the plant you are about to take from and listen.

Now turn your intention into a question. May I?

Listen again.

The "yes" comes in many forms. A gentle breeze may sway the branches, a bird may begin singing, the sun may suddenly burst forth from behind the clouds. Sometimes you'll hear a voice as if the plant is speaking to you directly. Or you'll get a tingling sensation at the back of your neck. Often, it's an inner knowing. This is a practice, and it may take time to discern yes from no.

There have been times I've received a definite "no" to later find out that a place had been sprayed with herbicides. One time I was gathering linden blossoms and I heard an inner "no." It turned out there was a man hiding in the tree leering at me. I thanked the tree for her wisdom and went elsewhere to harvest.

There may be plants you return to year after year. If you can, visit those plants often, even when it isn't the season to harvest. Tell them your intentions for partnering with them. Get specific. With these intentional, repetitive visits, you will develop a rapport with the plant. It'll also serve as a meditation to ground you in your reasons for harvesting in the first place.

The other part of this step is asking the landowner for permission. Say you spy a beautiful mimosa tree, its blossoms waving to you from afar. You feel compelled to go nearer, except, there's a fence between you and the tree. There is also a house. In our age of texting, we may have forgotten the simple art of knocking on someone's door. It's a thing we used to do, once-upon-a-time before we all carried cell phones 24/7. You can knock. If someone answers, tell them your intentions and ask permission. If they don't answer, leave them a note with your phone number and maybe they'll call you back. If they don't, it's okay. There will be other mimosa trees.

If you are on public lands, know the rules. In New York City parks, it is illegal for anyone except parks employees to carry gardening tools. In some state parks, it's okay to gather

How the Plants Speak to Us

Lest you think you won't be able to hear what the plants have to say, I'll share a story. A friend and fellow plant lover relayed this to me about her experience with yarrow.

"Last night I scraped my hand with a fork in the community garden. After a moment, it started to bleed. Although I had never used yarrow intentionally, I instinctually reached for some nearby yarrow leaves and put it on my cuts. I was astonished by my instinct to do something I had never done, without consciously thinking. It was like the plant spoke to me. I was also astonished by the results—which were amazing. The blood stopped and the cut seemed to close up. The healing after 12 hours was remarkable, like what I would expect after 2–3 days."

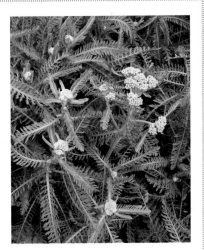

Yarrow is an excellent herb to carry in a first-aid kit for stanching bleeding and healing wounds.

berries for trail snacks, but not to remove other plant materials. These kinds of rules change with changing administrations and vary from one location to another. In 2016, the National Park Service changed the rules to allow indigenous people registered in federally recognized tribes to gather plants for medicine and other traditional crafts.

Respect boundaries, especially where the habitat is easily disturbed by human activities. It just takes one misstep to uproot a plant in sandy soil.

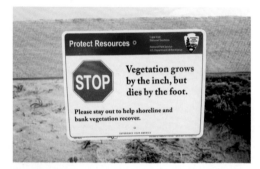

Respect fragile ecosystems, such as dunes and wetlands.

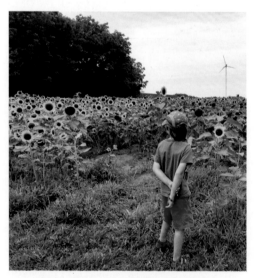

If you don't have permission to harvest from private land, you can still enjoy the beauty of what's growing there without taking.

Know the Plant Well

What does it mean to know a plant? We relate to the world around us with a myriad of senses. To get familiar with something or someone we may use our sight, hearing, taste, smell, touch, intuition, proprioception, and other senses. We may use logic or our rational mind to decipher what something is as well. Using all of our faculties, we can begin to embody the knowledge of plants and their medicine. Like getting to know a person, let's start with an introduction.

Introduce yourself. When you are first starting out on this journey, I suggest getting to know one plant at a time. Take a meandering walk in a meadow or the woods. In time you may feel called toward a certain plant. Approach and introduce yourself. You can speak your name aloud or say it in your mind. Sit with that plant. As long as you know it isn't poisonous to touch, reach out and touch it. (It's not very likely that it would be poisonous to touch; however, check the "Poisonous Plants" section just in case.) Feel the texture of the leaves and the stems. Take in the overall appearance of the plant. Notice its physical features. Then sit down near the plant and let your gaze soften and your heart space open. Allow your visual perception to absorb what is in front of you. Notice if you feel anything or if any impressions arise. Bring a journal with you to write down anything that comes to mind.

Once you've sat with the plant for a while, consult a field guide to determine which plant you've been called to. Refer to this book or any herbal guide you like to see if any of your impressions sync up with the traditional uses of the plant. It's likely they will. If they don't, it doesn't mean your feelings were wrong. If you feel like you need external confirmation, it may come in time. Be patient and let it unfold.

GOOD TO KNOW: POISONOUS PLANTS

It is said that all plants have medicine, even the toxic ones, and what determines their toxicity is a matter of dose and intent. While this blanket statement may be true for most herbs, there are some plants that you wouldn't want to even consider touching, let alone ingesting. In the Northeast these poisonous-to-touch plants fall into two families, the carrot (Apiaceae) family and the cashew (Anacardiaceae) family.

In the carrot family, two plants you would not want to mess with are poison hemlock (*Conium maculatum*) and water hemlock (*Cicuta maculata*). While the taproot of wild parsnip (*Pastinaca sativa*) can be cooked and eaten, the juice in its leaves can cause severe skin burns and blisters when activated by sunlight. Cow parsnip (*Heracleum maximum*) roots and leaves are edible and medicinal, but its leaves and stems also contain phototoxic sap. A poisonous relative that also causes severe skin damage is giant hogweed (*H. mantegazzianum*).

In the cashew family, it's a good idea to be able to identify poison ivy (*Toxicodendron radicans*) and poison sumac (*T. vernix*), too, as the majority of the population react to the urushiol present on their leaves and stems. These poisonous plants teach us how to pay attention to our surroundings. In lieu of carelessly traipsing through forested areas, becoming tuned into plants like poison ivy becomes an exercise in mindfulness.

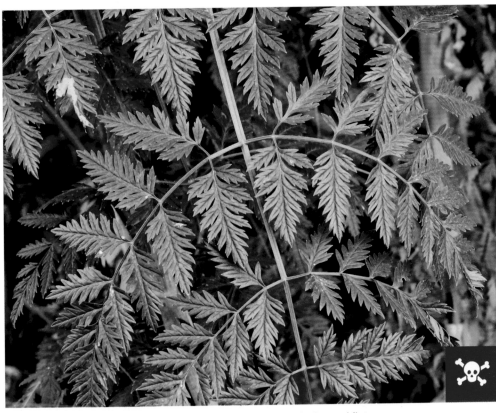

The leaves of poison hemlock are distinctively dark green, triangular, and flat.

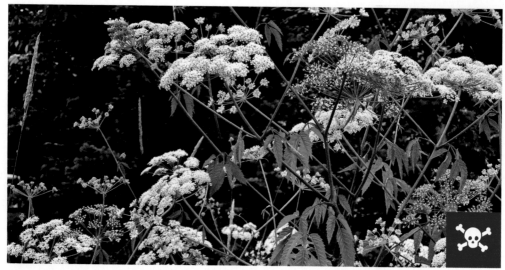

Water hemlock has pinnate compound leaves, sometimes doubly so. The leaflets feature lateral veins that end at the notches, rather than the tips of the teeth.

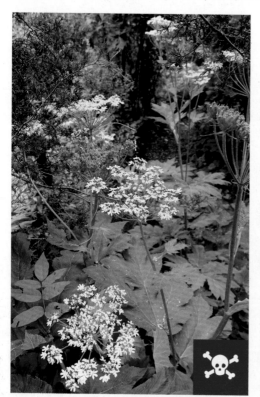

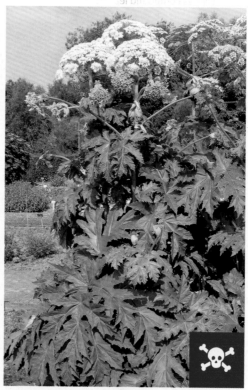

The broad-toothed leaves and umbel of white flowers of cow parsnip are large compared with other carrot family plants.

Just as the name suggests, giant hogweed is a giant. It looks similar to cow parsnip but it's twice the size and its leaves have deeper lobes.

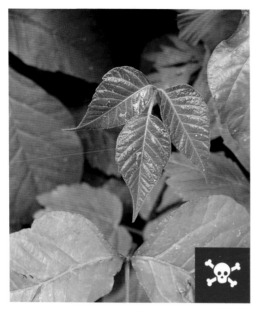

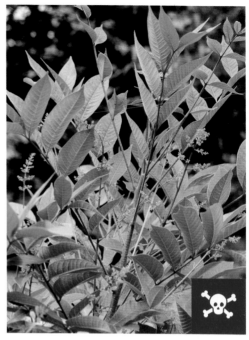

Poison ivy has compound leaves with three distinctive leaflets. Look closely, but don't touch—do you see how the margins of each leaflet are unique? Some are smooth, some are wavy, and some have rounded teeth.

Poison sumac has smooth stems and its leaflets have smooth margins, distinguishing it from other sumacs (*Rhus* spp.).

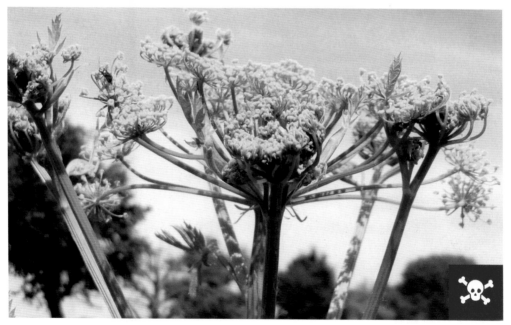

Wild parsnip dons tiny yellow flowers in flat umbels 3–8 inches across. Wear gloves if harvesting the edible root, as the leaves and stems are phototoxic.

Now that you have positively identified the plant and confirmed that it isn't poisonous, go back to it. Say hello and, after a mindful pause, pick a leaf. Smell it. Place it on your tongue. Let it sit there for a while. Feel the energy that it emits. Chew. Notice how the flavors develop in your mouth. What else do you notice? Has your mood or energy level changed? If you are comfortable, close your eyes and just feel. Write down any sensations or insights in your journal.

Once you feel comfortable with this one plant, you can start making new friends. What I like about this method of learning

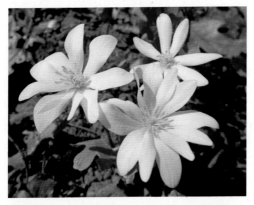

Bloodroot is an ephemeral spring beauty that's at risk in New York and Rhode Island.

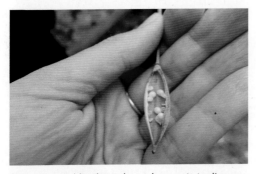

Slow-growing bloodroot depends on ants to disperse its seeds; the elaiosomes (fatty substances) on bloodroot seeds are an important food source for these insects. This relationship is known as myrmecochory.

one plant at a time is that, while it may seem slower than reading books or listening to lectures, the knowledge becomes embodied. It's a deeper way of knowing the plants that is very rewarding.

Keying out species. If you are a more logical-minded individual or used to learning from books, you may feel compelled to start here before introducing yourself directly to the plants. That's okay, though I strongly recommend telling your left brain to take a rest, just for the sake of experimentation—and deeper connection. When we sit in the presence of the plants, we embody their wisdom, developing a true relationship with them. We shake off the reductionist thinking that is conditioned in us. It's also way more playful, fulfilling, and fun this way.

After you've introduced yourself to the plants, you can geek out on their botany. Grab your field guide and dig in! A field guide with a dichotomous key or the Go Botany website are great resources. Take this book along, too. Keying out the unique botanical features of each plant will be a great advantage to your success as a wildcrafter. You'll gain confidence as you begin to recognize the patterns in nature. Instead of seeing a field of green, a quilt of distinctive plants will begin to emerge. In time, you won't need the field guides so much.

Learn about conservation status. We are in the midst of the sixth great extinction where irresponsible human activity is contributing to the loss of biodiversity around the planet. Clearcutting, mountaintop removal, filling in wetlands, and other forms of ecological destruction spell habitat loss for animals and plants alike. In our region, several medicinal plants are affected by careless land management and overharvesting. Below are some of the plants that I chose not to profile in this book, because they are at-risk in our region. Use your discretion when harvesting these plants in the wild. Check the conservation status in your region by cross-referencing NatureServe, the USDA PLANTS database, and your state or province's plant conservation database.

black cohosh (*Actaea racemosa*)

bloodroot (*Sanguinaria canadensis*)

blue cohosh (*Caulophyllum thalictroides*)

butterfly weed (*Asclepias tuberosa*)

eastern prickly pear (*Opuntia humifusa*)

gentian (*Gentiana* spp.)

ghost pipe (*Monotropa uniflora*)

ironweed (*Vernonia* spp.)

northern white cedar (*Thuja occidentalis*)

purplestem angelica (*Angelica atropurpurea*)

slippery elm (*Ulmus rubra*)

trillium (*Trillium* spp.)

uva-ursi (*Arctostaphylos uva-ursi*)

wild ginger (*Asarum canadense*)

wild indigo (*Baptisia tinctoria*)

wild yam (*Dioscorea villosa*)

Do not harvest the following plants from the wild as they are endangered throughout the region:

American ginseng (*Panax quinquefolius*)

false unicorn root (*Chamaelirium luteum*)

goldenseal (*Hydrastis canadensis*)

lady's slipper (*Cypripedium* spp.)

unicorn root (*Aletris farinosa*)

Despite their scarcity, there are still ways you can work with these endangered plants. If you are lucky enough to find them, make a no-pick flower essence (see page 54) or meditate with them, calling on the spirit of

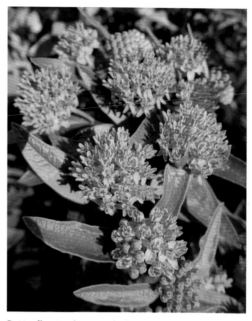

Butterfly weed is at-risk throughout the Northeast.

the plants. If you have access to a forest garden, obtain seed or rootstock from a native plant nursery to encourage a comeback of at-risk plants.

Know the land, too. Many of the plants you'll encounter are good at taking up heavy metals and other contaminants from the soil. While this can be beneficial to the ecosystem, ingesting these plants is harmful to your body's ecosystem. It's important to know the land use history where you plan to wildcraft to find out if the soil or water is contaminated with industrial pollutants.

Avoid collecting plants downhill from or downstream of conventional farming operations, golf courses, cemeteries, or industrial sites that use chemicals. Likewise, avoid harvesting from your neighbor's lawn, unless you are certain they do not use chemical fertilizers, herbicides, or pesticides.

Avoid collecting plants too close to the roadside. If the land along the road slopes downward, harvest about 100 feet away from the road. If the land is level with the road, you can move a little closer, about 50 feet from the road. If the land adjacent to the road is at an upward incline, your harvesting safety zone can be even closer, about 10–20 feet from the road. There are some exceptions to the rules, mainly in the form of fruit. There's a mulberry tree on my block in Brooklyn that I regularly gather berries from, and this practice is generally considered safe. However, I would not gather the leaves or any other part of this tree for medicine.

Make an Offering

Good neighbors give back, especially if they are taking something. The gifts you offer the plants can be very personal. I often sing as an offering, give a bit of my hair, or sprinkle dried flowers like lavender and rose. You may want to leave a little honey as is done in Celtic traditions. You may also wish to research the offerings and rituals of your ancestors, or the ancestors of the land that you inhabit. Whatever you decide to give, make sure it's compostable.

Another way to give back is by thinking of ways to help the plants thrive. Spread their seeds, give them water if it has been dry, and take extra care in how you handle the plant when you harvest.

Be Fully Present

Before you harvest, take a few breaths and center your awareness and attention. You may choose to sit in meditation for a brief moment. Here is a simple meditation for connecting with the energy of the earth and sky in your heart that I use to ground myself in the present moment.

Stand or sit directly on the earth. Your eyes can be open or closed. Center your attention on your body. As you breathe in and out notice any tension and breathe into it. Let the tension melt off you and release into the earth. Now bring your attention to your heart center and breathe into that space. With every in and out breath, send your heart energy downward, through your body and into the earth. Your heart attention goes deeper and deeper into the earth with every breath. It connects with the soil and all of the life in the soil. It touches the roots of the plants around you and all over the world. Your heart energy dives deeper into the rocky layers, then the molten layers of the planet, until it reaches the core. This dynamic center of the earth is said to spin in opposition to the upper layers, creating the electromagnetic field. Tap into that energy and when you are ready, breathe the energy up through all the layers of the earth and into your heart. Rest in the connection between your own heart's electromagnetic field and that of the earth. When you are ready, begin to bring that energy up from your heart, through the crown of your head and into the space above you. Let your awareness soar above the treetops, flying where the birds catch thermal currents. Your heart energy reaches the upper limits of Earth's atmosphere and then reaches out and into the solar system, past the moon, the sun, and all of the known planets. Let your awareness go even further, out of the Milky Way into neighboring galaxies and the farthest reaches of known space. Touch on the energy beyond what we know, to the place from which the universe was born. Now breathe the energy from that place back down through all of the layers of space, into Earth's atmosphere, down through the crown of your head, and into your heart. Let the energy of earth and sky mingle in your heart. Take a few deep breaths here. Bring your awareness back to your intention.

Use and Share the Medicine

For the sake of the plants, and for the health of the creatures who share this planet with us, take only what you truly need, what you have time to process, and what you can process in a timely manner.

Taking what you need. Go back to your intention. Who and what is this medicine for? It may be that you are stocking your apothecary with just-in-case herbs or you may have a specific person or condition in mind. In either case, it may take a few seasons of practice to get the hang of how much to gather. If you end up with an abundance of medicine, share with family and friends.

Processing time. It can be easy to get overly excited and ambitious when you come across a plentiful amount of plant material, like a smattering of just-fallen pine branches. Before you take those branches home, consider the amount of time it'll take to strip the outer bark, separate the inner bark, put it up in tincture, and then later decant and bottle it. For other plants, it may simply be a matter of bundling the herbs and hanging them to dry, if you intend to use them later. Know which instance applies and budget the appropriate time and materials in that case for your own sanity and to prevent waste.

Timeliness of processing. Knowing whether the plant materials you've gathered need to be processed right away is just as important as knowing how much time it will take to process them. Let's say you've brought home a basket full of dandelion blossoms. If you don't get to them right away, all of those golden bee-fodder flowers will turn into a big basket of seed fluff. You could refrigerate them for a day or two to preserve them a bit longer, but don't wait more than that.

Become a Wild Gardener

Plants predate us by millions of years. So, when we step into their realm, we enter as children. And the plants like to play. They pull us closer with their scent and beauty. They sway in swirls of wind, entrancing us with their dance. Lured by their fruit, we gather it up, eating as much as we can pick, at least all that has been left to us by the birds. Along with the birds, chipmunks, and bears, we redistribute the seeds in the soil. We blow dandelion seeds to the wind. The plants beckon us to be wild gardeners.

There is a misconception that, in order to save the natural world, we need to leave

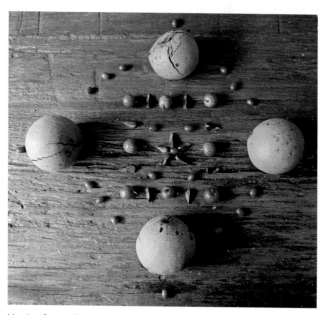

Having fun with a modest harvest of black walnut, spicebush fruit, hawthorn berries, and beech nuts.

it alone. Quite the opposite is true. We need to love it deeply and touch it daily. We are here for each other, like a good community or family. We evolved together and are woven together in the fabric of life. In order to be a good supportive family, we need to help plants proliferate. If we are concerned about invasive introduced plants crowding out endangered native species, we can harvest, and in most cases, utilize the invasive plants as food or medicine. When a native plant goes to seed, we can collect those seeds to plant later or directly sow them in the soil. If we know a plant is endangered, we can cultivate it in a forest garden to encourage its future. Two good resources to consult are Plant Native (for a list of nurseries in your area) and Prairie Nursery, which has a good stock of medicinal native plants. If you don't have access to land and still feel strongly called to work with the medicine of these endangered plants, find a reputable herbal medicine-maker who uses sustainably farmed plants in their preparations.

HOW TO WILDCRAFT

How to harvest depends on what you aim to collect. For leaves, buds, flowers, fruit, and seeds you'll need little more than your hands and a receptacle in which to amass your medicinal treasures. Whichever plant part you're after, here are some basic guidelines for harvesting, along with which tools would be most helpful for the job.

Leaves and Buds

In many cases, deciduous leaves are gathered by hand in spring when they first emerge. Other leaves, like oak, can be gathered from spring through fall. Collecting evergreen leaves year-round is acceptable, though spring is still considered the prime time to gather.

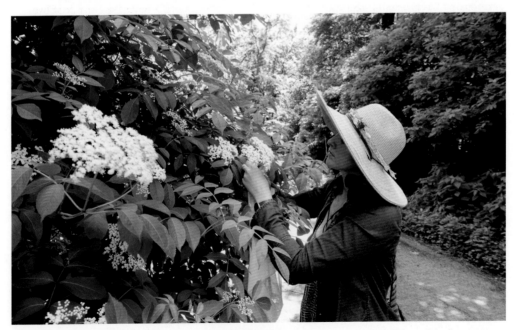

Sometimes all you need are your hands and something to collect your harvest in. When elderflowers are ready to collect, the umbels easily separate from the branch with a gentle coaxing back and forth at the node where opposite compound leaves meet.

Consider, if you are harvesting leaves and buds from trees or shrubs, how the plant will appear without that foliage. Think about what the plant needs to photosynthesize, selecting from shaded areas a bit closer to the trunk rather than in the sun. Whenever possible, collect leaves and buds from recently fallen branches. A good time to go out looking for tree medicine is right after a storm or windy day. If gathering directly from the tree, graze over it choosing one leaf or bud here and there, not taking too many in any one section. Do not take terminal buds from a tree, in other words the buds at the ends of a branch.

When wildcrafting herbaceous plants, that is, plants that are not woody, sometimes picking a leaf here and there off the stem is suitable. Oftentimes, however, you'll gather the top portion of the plant. This is usually true of plants in the mint and aster families. For plants like catnip, motherwort, and boneset, I like to gather about the top third of the plant in flower.

Flowers, Fruit, and Seeds

Graze over flowers, fruit, and seeds, leaving plenty for the birds, bees, and other wild creatures who depend on them for food. You'll want to use two hands for picking, so it's useful to have a container you can strap to your body for efficient collecting. There are special foraging baskets on the market, or you could use a wicker fishing creel with a hole in the lid, or simply strap a bucket to your waist. I usually have a stash of cloth produce bags in my backpack for impromptu wildcrafting sessions. I either tie them to

a belt or secure them with a carbineer to my backpack for stowing my cache. Another option is to place a small bucket in the bottom of a sling bag that you wear across your body or over the back of your neck. It can be a fun creative experiment to find the method that works best for you.

Twigs, Bark, Sap, and Resin

Wind can be a good friend to the wildcrafter. After a storm or gusty day, if I am able, I head out looking for fallen branches. Usually a branch or two offers plenty of material to keep me busy for an afternoon stripping off bark and setting it up to dry or tincturing it.

If you aren't able to find fallen branches, carefully prune small branches with shears or a pruning saw. Take a step back and examine the overall habit of the tree or shrub. Look first for suckers, watersprouts, intersecting branches, secondary branches, or branches that grow inward toward the trunk of the tree or shrub. If a branch is thin enough, about 1 inch in diameter or less, you can use pruning shears to lop it off. If the branch is thicker than 1 inch, use the three-cut method to avoid damaging the tree.

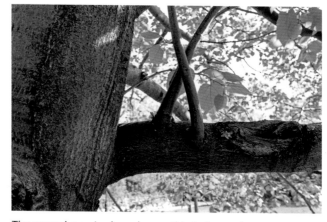

The upward-growing branches on this linden are known as watersprouts. They block light and air flow, so pruning them can benefit the tree as well as provide a sustainable harvest.

If you are cutting a twig back to a primary branch, get as close to that primary branch as possible. If you are trimming a shrub mid-branch, cut back to the nearest bud.

Do not gather bark by girdling the trunk, this will starve the roots of nutrients and effectively kill the tree.

Tree sap can be collected by tapping (see page 238 for instructions). Harvest resin from evergreens like pine and spruce by gently scraping it from the bark where a natural or pruning wound occurs. The resin is there to seal the wound on the tree, so leave enough behind for the tree's benefit.

The Three-Cut Method

Measure about 3 inches out on the branch from where the base of the branch meets the trunk (branch collar), and make a small notch cut up from the bottom of the branch about halfway into the branch. Make a second cut about 1–2 inches from the first cut, on the side closest to the branch's end, this time from the top of the branch downward. Continue cutting all the way down and through the branch. Removing the end of the branch this way takes the weight off the branch so that when you make your final cut at the end of the branch collar, you'll avoid tearing the bark. Cut the stub from the top of the branch downward at an angle to the branch collar.

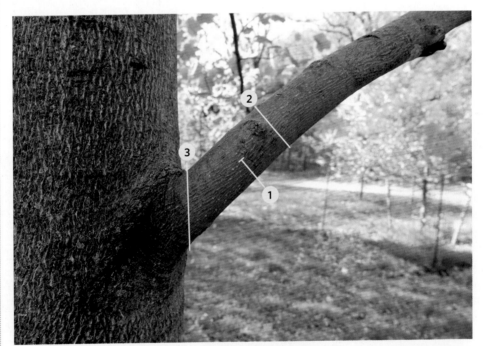

Use the three-cut method for pruning to prevent damage to the tree: 1) cut about halfway into the branch from the bottom, 2) make a second cut slightly further out on the branch, 3) remove the stub by cutting just outside of the branch bark collar so that the tree can heal properly.

Equipment for Wildcrafting

When I go out to wildcraft, often I just have a knife and a bag to carry my harvest, though sometimes I need a bit more assistance. Here is a suggested list of gear for those times.

- offerings for the plants
- bag, pouch, basket, or bucket for gathering
- pruning shears
- pruning saw
- hand trowel
- hori-hori knife

- pocketknife
- scissors
- digging fork
- digging stick
- brush for cleaning off roots
- hand lens or loupe

- field guides
- appropriate clothing (sunhat, layers, gloves)
- sunscreen
- bug spray

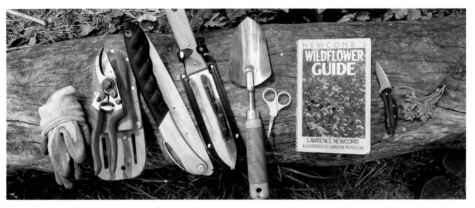

Some of the gear that can come in handy on a wildcrafting outing. From left to right: gardening gloves, pruning shears, pruning saw, hori-hori knife, hand trowel, baby nail scissors, field guide, pocketknife, and some maple flowers to nibble.

Roots

Consider that, in the case of herbaceous plants, when you remove the root you are taking the life of the plant. If you know the aerial parts are just as efficacious, leave the roots be.

Roots often require more effort to harvest than their aerial counterparts. Shallow roots, like those of wild sarsaparilla, may only involve hands to unearth and a knife or pruning shears to cut them from the rest of the root system. Deep taproots, like burdock, ask for a little more sweat and muscle. For taproots, dig a circumference a few inches from the crown of the plant, where the aboveground parts meet the soil. Loosen the soil with a garden fork or digging stick. Continue circumnavigating the crown and root until the soil is really loose. Wedge the shovel or digging stick into the earth adjoining the root and lift up a few times to help release the grip of the root from the soil. Gently tap off the excess soil and cover the hole you made with the surrounding earth. Use a brush to remove any remaining dirt from the root, keeping as much in situ as possible.

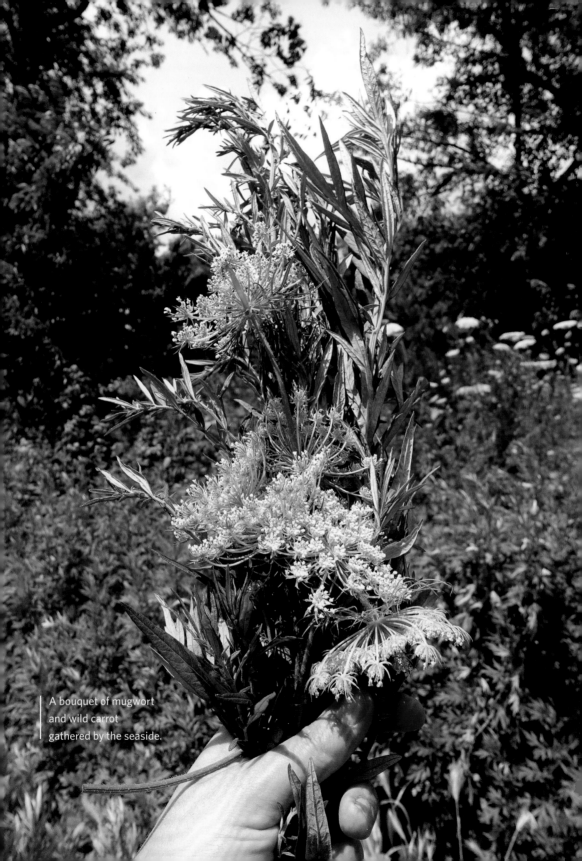

A bouquet of mugwort
and wild carrot
gathered by the seaside.

MAKING YOUR OWN MEDICINE

So you've gone out and wildcrafted some beautiful medicinal leaves, flowers, roots, fruit, or seeds. Now what? Well, naturally you've got to do something with your harvest. At the very least you can dry the plant materials if you gathered them for infusions or decoctions. However, some plant parts are best set up fresh, and you'll want to know some basic methods for preserving and administering the herbs.

MEDICINE MAKING SUPPLIES

It's a good idea to have a kitchen apothecary stocked with basic processing and storage equipment. The good news is that you likely already have some of these supplies on hand, or if not, you can easily improvise some of them.

- glass jars with tight-fitting lids
- amber glass bottles and jars for storage
- small funnel
- mesh strainer
- stainless steel pot
- bucket
- glass measuring cups
- mixing tools (spoons, knives, chopsticks, etc.)
- tongs
- sharp knives
- scissors
- kitchen scale
- mortar and pestle, suribachi, or electric seed grinder
- tincture press
- paper bags (for drying)
- screen (for drying)
- string or twine (for bundling herbs)
- dehydrator or oven with dehydrate setting
- muslin or cheesecloth
- labels

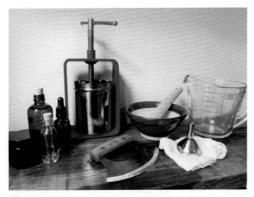

Besides plant materials, the other main component you'll need to make medicine is menstruum—the solvent used to extract medicinal compounds from plants. Here are some common choices for menstruum:

- vinegar
- spirits (vodka, rum, brandy, etc.)
- honey
- vegetable glycerin
- oils
- butters (cocoa, shea, mango, etc.)
- wax (beeswax, candelilla wax, carnauba wax)

Some of the equipment you might want to have on hand for processing herbs into medicine.

Solubility of Constituents

Before you set off to make your tincture or oil, it's helpful to know whether that plant actually lends itself well to a particular menstruum. With a little research—and sometimes taste testing—you can determine whether the plant you are working with contains alkaloids, resins, or other plant constituents to extract. Here's a basic gist of which plant chemicals extract into which media and some examples of herbs that contain those constituents.

CONSTITUENT TYPE	EXAMPLES	MEDIA
alkaloids	barberry, lobelia, red root	alcohol, water, vinegar
essential oils	chamomile, lemon balm, mint	alcohol, oil, water (slightly), vegetable glycerin (slightly)
flavonoids	ginkgo, hawthorn, Japanese knotweed	water, alcohol, glycerin
glycosides	elderflower, rose family plants	water, alcohol
minerals, trace elements	burdock root, horsetail, stinging nettle leaf	water, vinegar
mucilage	mallow root, mullein, plantain	water (cool), alcohol (somewhat)
polysaccharides	burdock root, larch, wild sarsaparilla	water, alcohol
resins	eastern cottonwood buds, pine, sweetgum	alcohol, oil (heated)
saponins	American spikenard, chickweed, wild sarsaparilla	water, alcohol
tannins	oak, wild geranium, witch hazel	water, vegetable glycerin
vitamins	dandelion, rosehips, spruce	water, except for A, D, E, K, which are fat soluble

MEDICINE MAKING METHODS

Few things in life are more satisfying than transforming raw plant material into efficacious, and often really enjoyable, medicine. Here are some of the fundamental methods for preparing plant medicines. These are by no means definitive or exhaustive instructions. You may find other herbalists who describe different ways of making medicine, or you may discover your own way of processing the plants that works for you. That's the cool thing about herbalism. It is very customizable and individualized. Don't be afraid to experiment and sometimes fail. Even the most-seasoned herbalist has a good story about herbal experiments gone awry. Start by making small batches of herbal preparations and as you find the methods that work best for you, scale up.

Herbal Water Extracts

It's probably safe to say you've had a cup of tea before. But what exactly is tea? To be quite literal about it, the word "tea" refers specifically to the plant *Camellia sinensis*, the leaves of which we use to make black, green, and white tea. Despite that, most folks, including herbalists who are particular about precise terminology, use the word "tea" pretty loosely to describe any beverage made by infusing or decocting plant parts. Tisane is another word you might see describing these herbal beverages.

Whatever you call it, there are two main ways of preparing herbs in water: infusion and decoction. Basically, infusions are just what they sound like: plant parts infused in water, either hot or cold. Leaves, flowers, and fruit are typically prepared as hot infusions. If you are looking to extract mucilage, say, from mallow roots, cold infusions are the best bet. In general, roots, bark, and seeds are prepared as decoctions, which is a fancy way to say gently simmer the herbs in water.

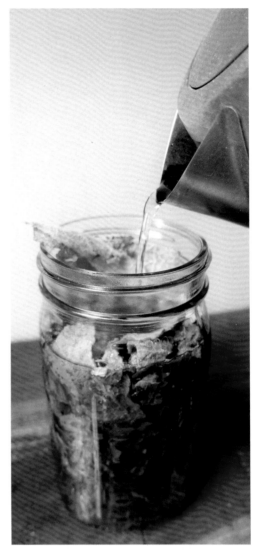

Making effective herbal medicine can be as simple as brewing a single plant infusion, like this mullein leaf.

Hot infusions. Add a handful of dried herbs to a heatproof container, such as a mason jar. Pour 1 quart (32 ounces) of boiling water over the leaves. If you're into more precise measurements, weigh out 1 ounce of herb to 32 ounces of water (by volume). Dried herbs provide a more concentrated infusion, with less water content and lots of broken-down cellular structure, as well as surface area. If you're using fresh herbs, fill the jar. Cover and steep for 20 minutes to several hours. Some plants and their parts are better steeped in smaller quantities and for less time. Experiment with quantities and steep times and eventually you'll know what tastes right to you. Usually I like to steep herbs overnight in a long infusion. It's a simple, effective way to get a strong tea that you can then strain off in the morning and sip all day long. If you have any left, you can refrigerate it for the next day and then if you still have some left the following day, use it as a bath tea or hair rinse.

A Matter of Spirits

Before getting into the process of tincturing, let's first consider the spirits. Not in a metaphysical sense, per se. I mean the kind of spirits you might drink as a social lubricant. First, there's the consideration of alcohol by volume (ABV) content. Throughout the herbal preparation boxes in this book, you'll note that the alcohol to water ratio for each of the herbs varies. This is dependent on which chemical constituents you aim to extract (alkaloids, glycosides, etc.). Refer back to "Solubility of Constituents" on page 42 to get a general sense of which herbs contain which constituents and which of those are alcohol soluble.

Plants containing resins, for example, require 95–100% alcohol to extract them. Other herbal preparations call for a little more water to extract additional constituents, like the tannins in witch hazel, for instance. Most spirits are available in the 40–75% range or in the higher range like 95%. So, what if you want something between that range, say at 80%? Simply get some of the higher-proof stuff and add the amount of distilled or filtered water needed to reduce the alcohol percentage. Yes, you might have to break out the calculator and do some squinting and brain squeezing like I do, but it's worth the effort in order to make the most out of the precious plant material you have.

Here's how you do it. You have a bottle of 95% alcohol and want to reduce it to 80% alcohol and your total liquid measurement for tincturing is 1000 milliliters. First divide 80% by 95% and then multiply by 100 to determine the amount of 95% alcohol you'll be using. In other words: $80/95 \times 100 = 84\%$. And 84% of 1000 milliliters is 840 milliliters. Now add the amount of water needed to come up to 1000 milliliters, that's 160 milliliters. Phew! Time for a drink.

The other thing you'll want to consider is the taste and energetics imbued by the tincturing alcohol. All alcohol is both

Cold infusions. Why make a cold infusion? Some plant chemicals extract more readily into cold water, particularly aromatic essential oils and mucilage. There's nothing as refreshing and uplifting as a fresh cold lemon balm infusion (aromatic essential oils) or as coating and soothing as the slimy goodness of a mallow root infusion (mucilage). As with hot infusions, if you use fresh herbs, pack the jar and if you have dried plant material, use the 1:32 rule.

Decoctions. You can use the 1:32 rule or the folk method of a handful. Add the roots, bark, or seeds to a quart of cold water and simmer gently for 20 minutes or more. The longer you simmer, the stronger the decoction, in general. Turn off the heat and let the decoction continue to steep for another 10 minutes or more. Roots and bark are generous and sometimes you can strain off the decoction and then add more water for a second, albeit weaker, batch.

heating and cooling, depending on how you look at it. The initial energy is warming and dispersing to the periphery. However, after the effect wears off, the dispersal of energy cools the body. There's also the issue of taste, and this can be as simple as choosing a spirit you find pleasurable to imbibe. Personally, I enjoy mezcal, so I use it a lot for tincturing, especially for herbs that stimulate

dreaming since it is also a "dreaming spirit." Most herbalists use either straight-up vodka or ethanol watered down to the desired amount, since these are both neutral, clear spirits with no additives.

Here is a look at the alcohol by volume (ABV) content, base ingredients, and taste and energetics of some of the most common spirits.

SPIRIT	ABV	BASE INGREDIENTS	TASTE AND ENERGETICS
ethanol	95%	grains, sugar	neutral
vodka	40% or higher	grains, starches	neutral
rum	40-70%	sugar	warm, sweet
bourbon, rye	40%	grains	warm, sweet
whiskey	40%	grains	warm, dry
gin	37.5-50%	juniper and other herbs	herbaceous
brandy	35-60%	grapes, apples	warm, sweet
tequila	32-60%	agave	sweet
mezcal	32-60%	agave	warm, sweet, smoky
wine	9-16%	usually grapes	warm, sweet, sour

Tincturing

Tincturing is a way of making medicine that extracts plant compounds into a concentrated form. The menstruum, or solvent, most often used for this process is alcohol. After the initial maceration phase, tinctures are a very convenient way to take plant medicine. You can easily stow tincture bottles in a bag or backpack and use tinctures on the go without having to brew an infusion or decoction.

There are two basic methods to making tinctures. If you aren't big on following recipes to a T, or you just want to keep it simple, this folk or simpler's method is for you:

1. If using fresh plant material, chop or tear up the herb and place it in a clean jar that has a tight-fitting lid. You may wish to sing, hum, or pray as you process the medicine. If you are using dried herbs, use about one-quarter the amount you would use of fresh herb. You can crush seeds and fruit in a mortar and pestle or with the whack of a mallet or knife.

2. Pour in your spirit of choice, ideally one that is at least 40% alcohol by volume so that the tincture preserves well. Fill the jar to the top, making sure the herbs are covered completely.

3. Cover the jar with the lid and label the jar with the contents and date. If you feel called, hold the jar to your heart and whisper an intention to the medicine. Ask the plant for guidance and healing.

4. Put the jar in a place where you will see it daily. Shake the jar whenever you can to mix up the medicine and help the maceration process.

5. After 4–6 weeks, decant your medicine through a fine-mesh strainer or cheesecloth into a glass container, such as a measuring cup. Squeeze all the goodness out of the herbs. A tincture press makes it easier to get more medicine out of the herbs, yielding at least a few ounces more than squeezing with bare hands could do. Once you've extracted all the liquid from the herbs, compost the marc (the solid part that's left over). Pour the tincture into dark glass dropper bottles and label them. I like to add the plant's common name, scientific name, alcohol percentage, date infused, and date decocted, as well as any planetary aspects that coincide with those dates (e.g., full moon in Aries). The shelf life of tinctures is at least several years when stored in a cool, dry, dark place.

Ways to Use Tinctures

You can take tinctures directly in the mouth by the drop, though I usually recommend taking the tincture in a little bit of water to improve absorbability and reduce the burning sensation of the alcohol. Another way to use tinctures is to apply them topically as a liniment, usually for muscle aches and joint pain, or add them to salves and lotions for wound-healing or skin-toning benefit.

If precision is more your thing, then you'll generally want to follow this herb to alcohol ratio for tinctures—1:2 for fresh herbs and 1:5 for dried herbs. (You might see some exceptions to this rule in this book, such as with peach pits and wild lettuce latex, which are both 1:4 fresh.) In this ratio, the "1" represents the amount of herb measured in weight while the "2" or "5" represents the amount of menstruum in volume.

1. Grab a scale and start weighing your herbs. An easy place to start is 100 grams.

2. Based on the weight of your herbs, figure out the corresponding volume of alcohol. In this case, if you're using fresh herbs it would be 200 milliliters of alcohol. If dried, then 500 milliliters of alcohol.

3. Add the herbs to an appropriately sized jar based on the volume of alcohol.

4. Pour the measured-out alcohol over the herbs, stirring if needed to ensure none of the herbs are floating on top. Cap and label with the date and ingredients.

5. Let the mixture macerate for 6 weeks. Strain through a fine-mesh sieve or cheesecloth into a measuring cup. Squeeze the heck out of the herbs (yes, that's very scientific) or use a tincture press. Using a funnel, pour the tincture into dark glass dropper bottles. Label with the common and scientific names of the herb, percent alcohol, and dates the tincture was infused and decanted.

Succus

A succus is basically an alcohol-preserved herbal juice. This method works well for plants that are best used fresh, such as chickweed or beggarticks. To make a succus, juice fresh plant material in a juicer or blender. If using a blender, add a splash of water and then strain the juice through a nutmilk bag, food mill, or fine-mesh sieve. Once you have your juice then add enough alcohol to preserve it. The finished product should contain at least 25% alcohol. I like to store the succus in the freezer, just in case.

Glycerites

A glycerite functions just like an alcoholic tincture, but it's made with vegetable glycerin instead of alcohol. Vegetable glycerin is bacteriostatic, meaning it halts the proliferation of bacteria. It's added to tinctures with high tannin content to keep the contents incorporated, preventing the tannins from binding and clumping. It's also used as a humectant in moisturizing skincare products. Glycerites are a good choice for crafting children's medicine and for folks who cannot use alcohol. Here are two ways to prepare glycerites. The cold maceration method is great if you have time to let the herbs infuse and the canning method is helpful if you need the glycerite right away.

For the cold maceration method:

1. If using fresh herbs, fill a jar two-thirds of the way with fresh chopped or torn plant material using the folk method (or use a 1:2 herb to menstruum ratio for a more scientific method). If using dried herbs, fill a jar one-quarter of the way with dried herbs (or follow a 1:5 herb to menstruum ratio).

2. Mix 3 parts vegetable glycerin with 1 part distilled water in a separate container. Pour this mixture into the jar with the herbs. Stir to ensure everything is incorporated and to remove any big air bubbles. Cover and label.

3. Shake the jar daily for 4–6 weeks, then decant through a fine-mesh strainer or cheesecloth. Bottle in dark glass dropper bottles and label. Glycerites keep for about 1–2 years when stored in a cool, dry place.

For the canning method:

1. Fill a canning jar to the top with fresh chopped herbs.

2. Mix 3 parts vegetable glycerin with 1 part distilled water in a separate container. Pour this mixture over the herbs and stir together.

3. Cover the jar tightly with a canning lid. Place the jar in a boiling water bath or canner and process for 15 minutes.

4. Remove the jar and let it cool. Then strain the herbs through a fine-mesh sieve or cheesecloth. Bottle in dark glass dropper bottles and label. Glycerites keep for about 1–2 years when stored in a cool, dry place.

Herbal-Infused Honey

One of my favorite ways to enjoy herbs is by infusing them in honey. Every year I look forward to elderflower season so that I can infuse the blossoms in that delightful amber liquid. Infused honey works best with aromatic herbs, like rose petals, mint, and elecampane root. Honey is antibacterial, antitussive, and wound healing in itself, so consider combining honey with herbs that match these actions for a deliciously effective medicine.

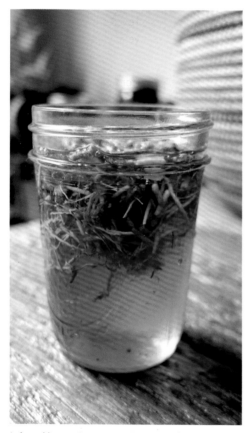

Infused honey is a yummy way to take medicine that also imparts the benefits of this precious golden substance.

1. Choose high-quality, raw honey from a local apiary for your health and for the health of the bees.

2. Fill a jar with fresh chopped herbs. If you are using dried herbs, fill the jar about one-third of the way.

3. Pour in enough honey to fill the jar. Stir well to incorporate the herbs and honey and to eliminate any large air bubbles. Tiny air bubbles are normal, but larger bubbles could create an environment for mold. Cover the jar with a tight-fitting lid and label with the date and ingredients. Let infuse for a few days up to 4 weeks. Taste the honey periodically to determine if it's to your liking. Store infused honeys in a cool, dry place or refrigerate to extend shelf life, which is 6–12 months.

4. It's up to you if you want to strain the herbs out; I usually leave them in. The benefit of straining the honey is that it may extend the shelf life. If you plan on straining the herbs, gently warm the jar in a bowl of warm water first to make the honey more pourable. Remember to relabel the jar you store your strained, infused honey in.

5. Enjoy by the spoonful, or for a sweet herbal tea, add 1 tablespoon of infused honey to a cup of hot water. Here's another idea: drizzle some of this delicious medicine on toast or yogurt or add it to salad dressing.

Herbal-Infused Vinegar

Vinegar infusions or extracts, also known as aceta, are another form of tincturing using, you guessed it, vinegar. Like glycerites, vinegar tinctures are a good form of medicine for those who cannot take alcoholic tinctures. Unlike vegetable glycerin, vinegar is really good at extracting alkaloids and minerals. Sometimes vinegar is added to tinctures during the macerating process to enhance the alkaloid content.

Like infused honey, infused vinegar makes a great food-as-medicine condiment. I like to add a spoonful of infused vinegar with a bit of honey to sparkling water for a refreshing kombucha-like drink. Sometimes I add a splash to smoothies for a little kick. Infused vinegar also makes a great base for salad dressings.

Most herbalists use raw, unfiltered apple cider vinegar. You could also infuse herbs in red or white wine vinegars or homemade vinegar made with apple scraps or grapes, provided you've tested the pH and it is below 4.

1. Just like alcohol-based tinctures, you can use the folk method or scientific one. So, either fill your jar with fresh chopped herbs or use a 1:2 ratio of herbs (by weight in grams) to vinegar (by volume in milliliters). For dried herbs, fill the jar one-quarter of the way or use a 1:5 ratio.

2. Cover the herbs in the jar with vinegar and screw on the cap. Use a non-corrosive top such as a plastic lid—mason jar manufacturers sell these—or place a layer of waxed paper between the metal cap and the macerating herbs. Label the mixture with the contents and date.

3. Let steep for 4–6 weeks. Shake the jar when you remember and say a prayer or blessing giving thanks to the plants for this medicine. After the infusion period you can leave the herb material in or strain it out, depending on how you'll use it. It'll last longer if you strain it. Shelf life is about 6–12 months at room temperature. Store in a cool, dry place out of direct sunlight.

Oxymels

Now you have your vinegar and you have your honey. What happens when you put them together? You get an oxymel! *Oxy* is ancient Greek for acid and *mel* means honey. Oxymels are another delicious way to take what might be not-so-great-tasting medicine. A good example of an oxymel is the pungent antimicrobial classic fire cider made famous by Rosemary Gladstar.

You can keep it simple by using just one herb or blend a bunch together for a complex medicinal treat. If you want to, you can add a previously infused honey and a previously infused vinegar together to craft something entirely new. There are no set rules to making an oxymel, so experiment to your likings. Here's one way to do it.

1. Mix equal parts apple cider vinegar and honey. You like things sourer? Use more vinegar. Sweeter? Add more honey.

2. Fill a jar to the top with fresh herbs or one-quarter of the way with dried herbs.

3. Pour the vinegar-honey mixture over the herbs. Cap, label, and shake the jar vigorously to incorporate the ingredients. Give the jar an occasional shake every day or so. After about a week, taste the mixture. If you want it stronger, let it continue infusing for 2–6 weeks.

4. Strain, rebottle in a dark glass bottle, and relabel. Store in a cool, dry place for up to 1 year. Enjoy the oxymel by the spoonful, or add it to sparkling water, juice, or smoothies.

Herbal Elixirs

By the alchemical definition, an elixir is a substance capable of changing base materials into gold. The elixir of life, like the philosopher's stone, is said to grant one immortality. While herbal elixirs are pretty magical in their own right, and sometimes have an air of esotericism about them, I can't promise they'll help you live forever. Still, taking them can invoke a mystical experience, if they're made with that intention. And crafting an elixir, or any herbal medicine for that matter, can be a sacred creative endeavor.

From a practical standpoint, the process of making an elixir is the same as for an oxymel, only you replace vinegar with alcohol. Elixirs fall into the ambiguous territory between the kingdom of medicine and the pleasurable realm of cocktails. Bitters blends and Italian digestivi like amaro, both crafted to improve digestion and assimilation, could be made using the elixir method of blending. So, if you like to mix the occasional grown-up beverage with the bonus of medicinal benefits, read on.

1. Mix equal parts raw honey and alcohol of choice (see "A Matter of Spirits" on page 44 if you need inspiration). Brandy is a popular choice for elixirs, but any spirit with at least 40% ABV will work.

2. Fill a jar to the top with fresh herbs or one-quarter of the way with dried herbs.

3. Pour the honey-alcohol mixture over the herbs. Cap, label, and shake the jar vigorously to incorporate the ingredients. Give the jar an occasional shake every day or so. Let steep for 4–6 weeks or longer, depending on your taste preferences.

4. Strain, rebottle in a dark glass bottle, and relabel. Store in a cool, dry place. Take elixirs on the tongue by the drop, add to a little water by the dropperful, or splash into sparkling water or cocktails.

Herbal Syrups

Syrups are a convenient, versatile, and sweet way to take your medicine. You can take syrups straight up, add them to sparkling water, smoothies, and cocktails, or use as a topping for breakfast porridge and pancakes.

1. To craft a syrup, first make a strong decoction. Add about ¼ cup of dried herbs or up to 1 cup of fresh plant material to 1 quart of water or unsweetened fruit juice. You can also use a combination of fresh and dried herbs, depending on what you have on hand. Cover and gently simmer for 20–30 minutes. Turn off heat and let steep, covered, for an additional 10 minutes. Strain.

2. Add the liquid back to the pot and reduce by half by gently steaming (barely simmering) the decoction, uncovered.

3. Once the liquid is reduced, turn off the heat and while it's still hot, add an equal amount of honey, maple syrup, or vegetable glycerin. Stir to combine. Of these, vegetable glycerin is the most shelf-stable. If using honey or maple syrup, you may wish to mix equal parts sweetener and brandy to further preserve the syrup.

4. Store herbal syrups in dark glass bottles in the fridge for up to 6 months.

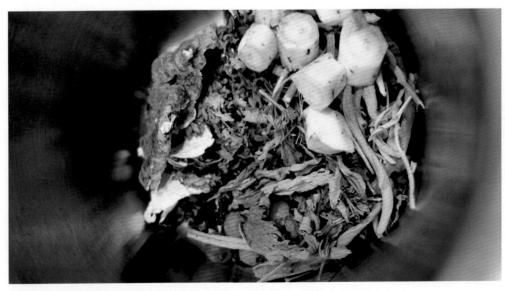

Fresh and dried herbs on their way to becoming a nourishing syrup.

Lozenges

Knowing how to craft an herbal syrup gets you one step closer to making portable lozenges or cough drops. For making lozenges, you'll want to use honey or granulated sugar as the sweetener in your herbal syrup. (Granulated sugar may be preferred as it is easier to work with and less likely to scorch than honey.) Add the syrup you made—one that consists of equal parts reduced decoction to sweetener—to a pot and warm the mixture, stirring frequently. Simmer slowly and gently for a few minutes until it reaches the hard crack stage on a candy thermometer (295–309°F) or until you can drop some into a bowl of cold water and it forms semi-hard drops. Once it reaches this stage, immediately pour the mixture into silicone molds, onto a silicone mat, or onto parchment paper to harden. Once hardened, you can dust the lozenges with powdered marshmallow root or other powdered herbs to prevent sticking. Wrap in small pieces of waxed paper and store in an airtight container.

Electuaries

Electuaries are yet another example of how pleasurable herbal medicine can be. All you need is a bowl, spoon, honey, and powdered herbs. Combine the ingredients to your desired consistency. Electuaries can be made thin and spoonable or thick and rollable. For a thin, spoonable electuary, use a higher honey to herb powder ratio. For a thick electuary, use more herb powder. Thick electuaries can be rolled into balls to use as lozenges or pills.

Here's a simple immune-boosting tonic electuary. Combine equal parts hawthorn berry, elderberry, stinging nettle, rosehip, and chickweed powders. Add honey little by little to your desired consistency. Take 1–3 teaspoons daily. You can eat it straight up or sprinkle it over oatmeal, granola, or yogurt.

Flower Essences

The morning dew of flowers has been prized for centuries for its healing powers. In the 1930s, English physician Dr. Edward Bach developed a way to replicate the healing effect of flower dew. The end product he created is known as a flower essence. Flower essences are a diluted infusion of freshly picked flowers used to heal emotional or spiritual imbalances. They capture the vibrational essence of the flowers to assist in shifting subtle energies of the body, mind, and spirit.

Dr. Bach created 38 flower essences from English wildflowers, all of which are still produced today. Several companies around the world make flower essences from a wide variety of flora. And you can, too.

What you'll need:

Tweezers
Scissors
Small glass bowl
Spring water
Small funnel
Brandy, vinegar, or vegetable glycerin
Dark glass bottles for storage

Like wildcrafting medicine, crafting flower essences requires intention and reflection. Take a walk outside on a spring or summer morning and notice which flowers you are drawn to. Approach the plant and introduce yourself. Sit down for a bit and listen. Pay attention to the flower and its form and notice how it makes you feel. You may want to write down any impressions that come. Tell the plant your intention and ask if you can make an essence with its flowers.

The following are two basic ways to prepare flower essences. In both cases, the flowers can be infused under the morning sun on a mostly cloudless day or the full moon on a clear night.

Picked flower essence. Fill a small glass bowl with spring water, then harvest the flowers. Some folks who prepare flower essences use their hands, and others believe that it's best not to add your energy to the flowers. If you are in the latter camp, bring along some tweezers and scissors to pick your flowers. You'll only need a few flowers, maybe three to five. In the case of larger flowers, like sunflowers, you'll only need one. Place them face up in the water, as best as possible, then place the bowl in the sun. Let the flowers infuse like this for 3–5 hours. Yes, this exercise takes patience! Spend the time meditating, praying, singing, journaling, drawing, or painting. If you are making a lunar infusion, you may want to take the bowl with you and place it just outside your home or in a window that receives lunar light. Or plan the essence making for a camping trip where you can leave the bowl outside undisturbed.

No-pick flower essence. If you are drawn to flowers from an endangered plant, use this method. Fill a glass bowl with spring water and instead of picking the flowers, place the bowl below the plant. You may wish to use a clear quartz crystal to direct the energy of the flowers to the bowl. Leave the bowl in place for 3–5 hours. Meditate, get creative, or just take a rest while the flowers infuse.

For both methods, once the flowers are done infusing, pick them out and give them back to the earth. Pour the essence you've made into a measuring cup and add equal parts brandy, vinegar, or vegetable glycerin to preserve it. This is the mother tincture. To create the stock tincture, add 2 drops of this essence to a 1-ounce dropper bottle with equal parts spring water and brandy, vinegar, or vegetable glycerin.

I love to work with flower essences when I'm feeling stuck, when I'm working through a challenging time, and to enhance meditation and dreaming practices. Take a few drops of the essence on the tongue or in a glass of water; add to room or body sprays; or blend into oil, salve, or lotion to massage into the body.

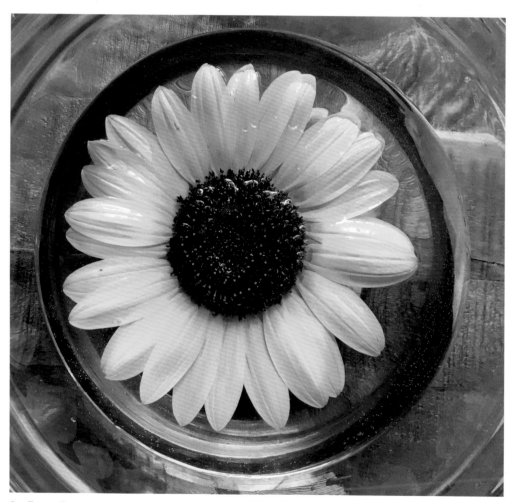

Sunflower flower essence helps us orient to the sun, boosting confidence and belief in ourselves.

Herbal-Infused Oils

When you infuse oil with herbs you create a rich topical treatment for the skin. You can use the oil directly on wounds, bites, or skin irritation. It can also penetrate deeper into the body to relieve sore muscles, stiff joints, or abdominal distress when massaged into the affected part. Herbal-infused oil serves as a base for salves, lip balms, lotions, and crèmes as well.

A great range of topical and culinary oils are available on the market. How do you choose which one to infuse? Many herbalists turn to olive oil since it is so ubiquitous, it has a nice feel, it benefits the skin, and it's less likely than nut and seed oils to go rancid. Here, along with olive oil, are some other options, along with key characteristics that will lend unique qualities to your finished product.

apricot kernel—neutral, light, quickly absorbable

avocado—deeply nourishing, moisturizing

castor—drawing, protective, thick, shiny

coconut—cooling, drying, cleansing

jojoba—closest to sebum in texture

meadowfoam seed—antioxidant, shiny, good for lip balm

olive—nourishing, antioxidant, shelf-stable

rosehip seed—antioxidant, emollient, absorbable

sesame—grounding, warming

sweet almond—emollient, easily absorbable

sunflower—nourishing, softening

You can infuse oil via a heat- or slow-infuse method. The heat-infuse method works great for dried plant materials, including powdered and cut and sifted herbs. (If choosing powder, you'll need a coffee filter or cheesecloth to strain out the powdered material.) The slow-infuse method works best with fresh or very aromatic dried plant material. You may wish to let very moist plant material dry or wilt a bit for a few hours or overnight before infusing.

External Herbal Applications

There are just as many methods of applying herbs externally as there are ways to take herbal medicine internally. Our largest organ, the skin, is a wonderful porous barrier that protects our insides, represents our inner health, and reflects our life experiences. When we apply herbs to the exterior of our bodies, it benefits both the skin and what lies beneath. Infused oils, salves, lotions or crèmes, poultices, compresses, baths, and steams are all ways of absorbing herbal medicine through our outsides to help heal our internal landscape.

For the heat-infuse method:

1. Fill a heatproof container (e.g., glass measuring cup or mason jar) about one-quarter to one-third full with dried plant material. Top off with oil.

2. Place the container in a pot filled with water and gently warm the oil and herb mixture, stirring occasionally. The water should be just steaming. Continue warming the oil for several hours. Refill the pot with water as needed. Turn off and continue as needed, too. I like to do this for 2–3 days, turning it off if I leave the house and when I go to sleep. If you have a slow cooker to dedicate to this, you can either fill it directly with herbs and oil or fill the pot with enough water to cover a canning jar filled with herbs and oil. Then you can let the warming process continue at a low temperature for several days.

3. Strain the oil. To filter out sediment, strain again through cheesecloth or a coffee filter. Bottle in dark glass bottles or jars and label. Store in a cool, dry, dark place for up to 2 years.

For the slow-infuse method:

1. Fill a jar completely with chopped herbs if using fresh, or one-quarter of the way if using dried.

2. Top off the jar with oil. Fresh material tends to go moldy, especially if any of the herb is peeking out of the oil. To prevent this, cover the top of the jar with cheesecloth and secure with the rim of a canning lid or rubber band. This will allow any moisture to escape and prevent molding.

3. Place in a warm, sunny spot for 4–6 weeks. Check the oil regularly for mold. If mold forms on top, your oil is still salvageable, as the spoilage is most often isolated to the exposed portion of herbs. Simply remove the moldy material from the top of the mixture.

4. Strain the oil through cheesecloth. If there is any sediment or spoilage (appearing as dark globs of oil), filter again through cheesecloth or a coffee filter. Store in dark glass bottles or jars in a cool, dry, dark place for up to 2 years.

Salves

Salve—also known as balm, ointment, or unguent—is a wonderful medium for stabilizing herbal-infused oils, making them more transportable, less messy, and easier to apply than just straight up oil. The basic method is to melt beeswax, carnauba wax, or candelilla wax, and then add infused oil. Beeswax is available as blocks or pastilles or pellets. You can shave the beeswax ahead of time or what I like to do is melt a beeswax block down and pour it into silicone ice cube trays for easy-to-grab, premeasured beeswax (my tray yields ½-ounce-sized cubes). Candelilla and carnauba wax are usually sold in shaving or pellet form. As always, obtain the waxes from a reputable, sustainable source. Blending tinctures or essential oils into your salve to add further medicinal benefits is an option to consider.

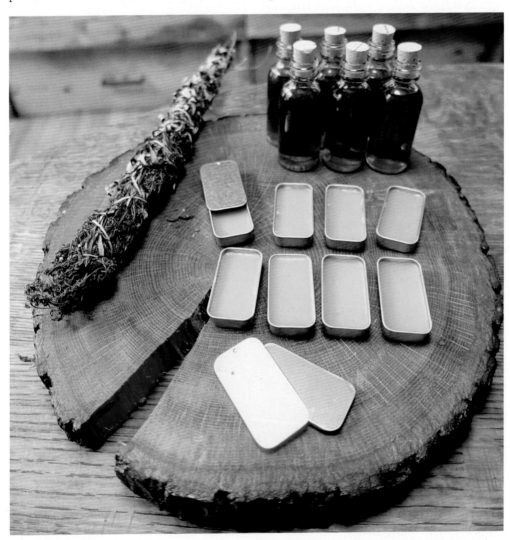

Some plants lend themselves well to many forms of medicine. Mugwort can be transformed into an oil, salve, tincture, infusion, vinegar, honey, elixir, oxymel, and more.

To make a salve:

1. Measure out 4 parts oil to 1 part beeswax, carnauba wax, or candelilla wax (by volume). Increase the amount of oil up to 8:1 if you prefer a softer salve. Gently melt the wax in a double boiler or a heatproof glass measuring cup in a pot of water on low heat. The water in the pot should be just steaming.

2. Add the oil to the melted wax and stir. It will form swirly clouds of wax that will melt fairly quickly into the oil. Gently heat until the wax is completely melted.

3. Take the mixture off the heat and continue to stir as it cools. It will take several minutes for the mixture to cool and solidify. Add essential oils or tinctures at this stage if you like. If adding essential oil, use about 10 drops per ounce of carrier oil. For tinctures, add 20–40 drops per ounce of oil. I also like to add a bit of vitamin E oil to preserve the salve and for added antioxidant effects.

4. While it's still warm enough to pour, do so into tins or dark glass jars. Cover, label, and enjoy. The shelf life varies depending on how the salve is stored and used, anywhere from 6 months to 2 years. If you see mold or the salve smells off, it's time to discard and make a new batch.

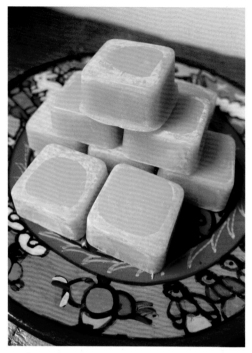

Ready-to-use premeasured beeswax cubes for salve and lotion making.

Lotions and Crèmes

You know the saying "prevention is the best medicine"? That's how I like to think about lotions and crèmes. Applying moisturizing lotion daily protects and strengthens the skin, helping to prevent sunburn and nicks like papercuts. It's also a sensual act of self-care that keeps the skin supple and healthy.

What's the difference between a lotion and a crème? It's a matter of water content. Crème contains less water than lotion, so it's literally creamier. (Think of crème as lotion's thicker cousin.) Here is a simple lotion recipe that you can alter to your preferences. Reduce the water content by half for a creamier crème concoction.

What you'll need:

1 part herbal-infused oil

1 part distilled water

$\frac{1}{16}$ part beeswax, carnauba wax, or candelilla wax

Essential oils (optional)

Immersion mixer, hand mixer, or standing blender

Glass or metal bowl

Spatula

Storage jars

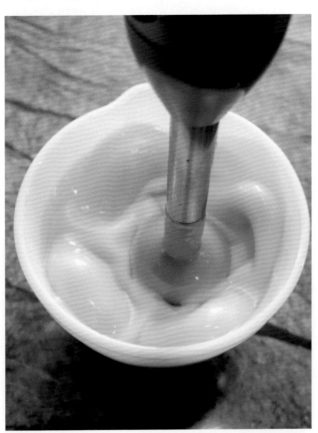

Oil and water do mix! Witnessing the process of emulsification is a magical aspect of blending your own lotion from scratch.

1. Gently heat the wax and oil in a double boiler or a heatproof glass measuring cup in a pot of water. Stir until incorporated.

2. Remove the wax-oil mixture from the pot. While the wax-oil mixture cools slightly, pour the distilled water into a clean measuring cup and gently warm. (I like to heat the distilled water in the still-warm water of the double boiler.) Emulsification in the next step goes more smoothly if the oil and water are a similar temperature.

3. Pour the wax-oil mixture into a mixing bowl or the pitcher of a standing blender. I highly recommend having a dedicated tool for the job, as you wouldn't want food in your lotion (it would spoil it) or lotion in your food (it might not taste great). If you don't have access to any of these electronic contraptions, you can also hand whip the lotion with a whisk. It takes a bit longer, but it works.

4. Start blending the wax-oil mixture and slowly pour in the water. When the mixture looks uniform, stop blending. Gently stir in the essential oils, if using, and pour into jars while it is still warm. Label your concoction. Feel free to get creative with the name. There's nothing like homemade lotion, so you'll likely use it up before it goes bad, which would be around 6-12 months.

Poultices

A poultice, also once known as a fomentation, is an application of fresh or reconstituted dried plant material placed directly on a part of the body that is affected by pain, injury, or illness. There are a few different ways of preparing and applying poultices. This can be as simple as making a spit poultice to put on a mosquito bite or something a bit more involved, like covering swollen joints with layers of mashed-up herbs. Here are the basic methods:

Spit poultice. This method comes in handy when you are outside, say enjoying a hike or a picnic, and you get a bee sting, bug bite, or scrape. Common plants like plantain, chickweed, yarrow, and dock leaf make great spit poultice material. Find a clean leaf, or clean it quickly with some water, then chew up a large piece of it. Apply the chewed-up plant material to the affected area. Replace every 10 minutes or so until the pain and irritation subside.

Standard poultice. Using a bowl with a wooden spoon or a mortar and pestle, mash up fresh or dried plant material with a splash of hot water. Another option is to blend it in a food processor. You can also make a paste with powdered herbs in the same way. Let cool to a comfortable temperature. If the affliction is hot and inflamed, a cool poultice may be more appropriate than a hot one. If the aim is to open the pores and draw something out, a hot poultice is more fitting. Place the mashed herb on the affected area. Replace every 30–90 minutes until symptoms subside.

Compresses

A compress is similar to a poultice, but instead of directly applying the plant material, you'll place a soaked cloth on the affected area. Like poultices, you can adjust the temperature according to your needs. You can make a compress using herbal infusions, decoctions, tinctures or a combination of these preparations. Start by infusing or decocting dried herbs. Strain off the liquid, reserving some in a separate bowl or jar. Dip a cloth into the liquid. If you are using a tincture, pour or squeeze droppers full onto the cloth. Place the cloth on the affected area and replace every 20–45 minutes until you feel relief. You can secure the compress with a bandage if you need to be mobile.

Here are some herbs that work well as compresses, along with conditions they can help:

chamomile—stomachache, headache, burn, hyperactivity

chickweed—bleeding injury, insect bites or stings

rose—eye infection, sunburn, rash, irritation, headache, heat exhaustion

yarrow—bleeding injury, wounds, bruises

Herbal Baths

Immersing yourself in a bath is the ultimate in self-care. On a physical level, herbal baths can heal the skin; reduce fever; and relieve soft tissue injury, muscle aches, and joint pain. Baths are also incredibly restorative to the emotional and spiritual self. The simplest way to enjoy an herbal bath is to make a strong infusion, draw a bath, then strain the infusion directly into the tub. Many herbs are suited for this purpose. Some of my favorite bath herbs include rose, yarrow, mugwort, birch, oak, and comfrey.

When you don't want to commit to a full body bath, footbaths are a great option.

They're also helpful for those who cannot take herbs internally, such as elder folk. Feet are very receptive to treatment with herbs; soaking feet in a small tub infused with herbs is restorative to the whole body and spirit. A warm footbath is an excellent way to bring warmth and circulation to the feet and body. A cool or cold footbath is a great remedy for inflammation due to external heat. When I was pregnant, at the end of a hot summer day I would put my feet in an ice-cold footbath infused with chamomile and rose. This treatment brought down the swelling in my feet and ankles, restored my energy levels, and readied me for sleep.

Sitz baths are, just as the name suggests, for sitting in—sitz comes from the German word *sitzen*, meaning "to sit." Special basins that are fitted to the toilet seat are made just for this purpose. Sitz baths provide a healing bath for the delicate tissues of the anus, rectum, labia, vagina, and testes. Herbal infusions are added directly to the bath vessel to aid in healing conditions such as hemorrhoids, postpartum tearing, and testicular pain. For hemorrhoids, use astringent herbs such as plantain, witch hazel, and blackberry leaf or root. To relieve postpartum tenderness, reduce bleeding, and prevent infection of vaginal tears, make a decoction with astringent and antimicrobial herbs including barberry root, echinacea, raspberry leaf, wild geranium root, and shepherd's purse. Anti-inflammatory and pain-relieving herbs such as honeysuckle, plantain, peach, birch, crampbark, and bull thistle can bring relief to testicular pain.

Herbal Steams

An herbal steam is a simple treatment for the skin and respiratory tract that can also evoke the feeling of a luxurious spa therapy. Rose, chamomile, and elderflower make a lovely

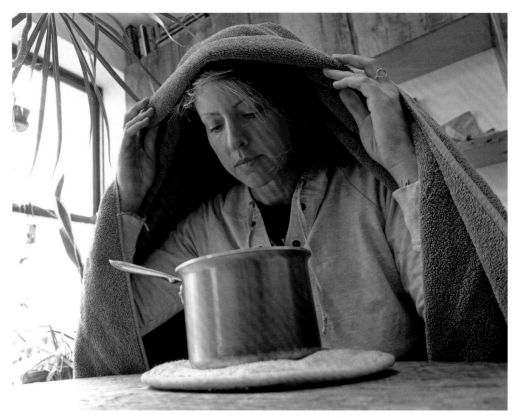

Herbal steams open up the airways to improve respiration, while opening and clearing the pores of the skin.

sensual steam for improving facial tone. Decongestant herbs such as pine, spruce, ground ivy, mint, and New England aster are excellent for clearing the sinuses and relieving coughs.

To make an herbal steam, gently simmer a handful of herbs in a small pot or saucepan with filtered water. Cover and let simmer for 5–10 minutes. Turn off the heat. Bring the pot to a steady, heatproof surface, like a table, where you can pull up a chair and sit comfortably. Carefully feel the temperature of the steam before placing your face over it. When the temperature is right, place your face over the steam and drape a towel over the top of your head, creating a tent over the pot. Enjoy the sensation of the steam and the aroma of the herbs opening your pores and nasal passages.

Vaginal steams, also known as v-steams or yoni steams, have also become more popular in recent years as a way to heal women's reproductive imbalances and as a mode of self-care. The preparation is basically the same as with a facial steam except for the set up. There are special chairs designed for v-steams. Or you can use two chairs to support your body and place the pot of steaming herbs on a few blocks or a small secure stool between the chairs and underneath you. Be extra careful to let the simmered herbs cool to a moderate temperature before sitting over the pot. Drape a towel over your lap to seal in the warmth.

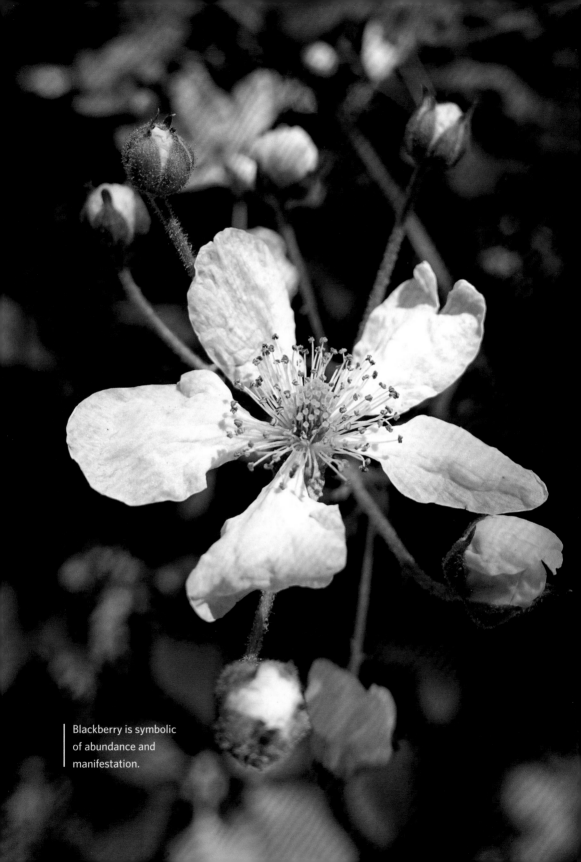

Blackberry is symbolic
of abundance and
manifestation.

WORKING WITH PLANT MEDICINE

Working with plants as medicine invites us to slow down from our modern lightning pace. It calls us to shift our perspective from the status quo of conventional allopathic medicine and quick-fix culture. While some herbs have immediate effects, sometimes markedly so, many herbal remedies require patience to notice their effects. It can take equal parts experimentation, curiosity, creating new habits, and adjusting expectations. I assure you that whatever effort you put into this paradigm of healing is extremely rewarding and totally worth it.

PATHS ARE MANY

Acquiring herbal knowledge is a very personal journey and the avenues to learning are many. Herbalists may study in a formal certification program, or they may learn from an elder in their family. Some herbalists I know have been guided almost exclusively by intuition, dreams, and visions. Still others are self- and plant-taught through experimentation and field research. Most piece together learnings from many or all of these sources.

Whichever road you take to discover this time-honored tradition, you'll come to learn pretty quickly that herbs are not one-size-fits-all remedies. Every human body is different as is their unique relationship to the herbs. Herbal medicine requires us to pay attention to individual quirks and needs. The practice of herbal medicine can also recondition us away from the propensity to treat symptoms and conditions to instead consider the whole person.

The way you approach herbalism is also as unique as your experiences and passions. One of my favorite ways to relate to and practice with herbs is through dreamwork. Sometimes the herb that my body needs comes through in dreams. Sometimes I ask in dreams which herb would be beneficial for someone I'm helping. I also love to work with plants that stimulate lucid dreaming and dream recall.

There are as many systems or healing paradigms that entail working with plant medicine as there are languages spoken, perhaps even more. What many of them share, in essence, is the perspective that the primal elements—earth, air, fire, and water—or some variation of them, are reflected in our state of health and embodied in the herbs and the way they influence our body, mind, and spirit. For the sake of brevity and because it is the system that I am most familiar with, I'll give a very broad overview of some basic concepts from the Western herbalism lens.

WESTERN HERBALISM

What is today known as Western herbalism has a long and winding past that would fill tomes. We can trace its roots from these colonial shores back to Europe; from ancient Rome back to ancient Greece; and before that to Kemet, the place we now call Egypt. Yes, Western herbalism's roots are in Africa. While for at least 2000 years we have associated Western herbalism with Euro-descendant people, the basis for this system, like all of our origins, traces back to the motherland of Africa. I am not a historian and it would be difficult to cover all of the changes and adaptations that

have occurred over the years to this system of practicing medicine in this book. We'll look at some of the basic concepts that have arisen over time, some old and some newish (like 200-years-old new) that still apply today.

Constitution

Our personal constitution refers to our baseline state of being in terms of health, strength, and vitality. It is influenced by what we've inherited from our ancestors, our historical and ongoing personal experiences, and our lifestyle factors or habits. Our histories and our current realities are reflected in the environmental characteristics of our bodies.

In a simplistic sense, like the natural environment we inhabit, each of us embody tendencies toward specific temperature, moisture, and tissue states. Determining your constitution starts with noticing, observing, and getting to know your patterns of balance and imbalance.

The Six Tissue States

This system for understanding disease and how to restore a healthy balance was developed at the turn of the nineteenth century by Dr. Joseph M. Thurston, an American physiomedicalist influenced by fellow plant medicine doctor Samuel Thomson. It is inspired by Native American healing traditions, as well as Greek and Kemetic medicine. We can thank Matthew Wood for framing these states in a modern vernacular. In his book *The Earthwise Herbal Repertory* he also includes this framework neatly juxtaposed within the Ayurvedic system.

Tastes or Flavor Dynamics

The following describe some of the flavor traits of herbs and their associated actions. The first five (sweet, salty, sour, bitter, pungent) are known as the primary tastes and

TREATING TISSUE STATES WITH BALANCING HERBS

TISSUE STATE	ELEMENTAL IMBALANCE	BALANCING HERBAL ENERGETICS	HERB EXAMPLES
heat/excitation	excess fire	cooling, calming	elder, honeysuckle, lemon balm, rose
cold/depression	deficient fire	warming, stimulating	mugwort, shepherd's purse, sunflower, wild bergamot
damp/stagnation	excess water	astringent or drying, dispersive	barberry, burdock root, red clover, yellow dock
dry/atrophy	deficient water	moistening	American spikenard, burdock root, common mallow, mullein
damp/relaxation	deficient earth	astringent, toning, nourishing	black walnut leaf, cinquefoil, Saint John's wort, stinging nettle
wind/tension	excess air	relaxing	agrimony, chamomile, hops, wild lettuce

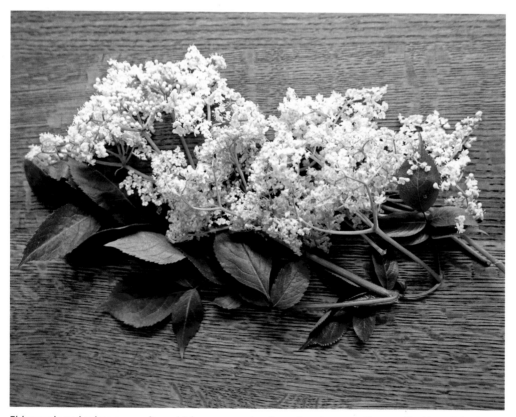

Elder cools and calms excess fire, which can present as fever, burning sensations, or flushing of the face.

the rest are common taste impressions or sensations. None of these are mutually exclusive and one herb may elicit multiple flavors and sensations.

sweet—nourishing, harmonizing, moistening

salty—grounding, strengthening, alkalinizing

sour—cooling, cleansing, toning

bitter—clearing, assimilating, drying

pungent/spicy—warming, stimulating, penetrating

aromatic—moves heat to exterior

acrid—dispersing, penetrating

astringent—tightening, toning, drying

demulcent—moistening, coating

HERBAL MEDICINE DOSAGES

The dosages provided in this book and on the packaging of commercially distributed herbal preparations are given as a general guideline based on a typical adult person of average weight (around 150 pounds) and health. But just as each herb is unique, so are all of us humans. How we respond to the medicine varies, based on our own particular makeup. Some of the major factors to consider when calculating dosage are age, weight, and metabolism. There are a few ways to adjust dosing to suit children. Generally, these guidelines refer to those under the age of 18.

Young's rule—Add 12 to the child's age then divide the child's age by this total. For example, for a 4-year-old: 4 divided by 16 (4+12) = .25, or ¼ of the adult dosage.

Clark's rule—Take the child's weight in pounds and divide by 150 pounds and then multiply it by the adult dosage. For example, for a child weighing 35 pounds: 35 divided by 150 = .23. If the adult dose is 30 drops every 4 hours, then multiply .23 × 30 drops, which equals 7 drops every 4 hours.

Often, elder folk tend to weigh less than younger people. Use Clark's rule for people

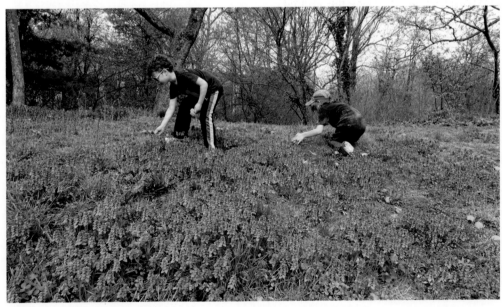

Children are enthusiastic participants in the gathering and preparing of herbal medicine.

who weigh less than 150 pounds. The same rule can be applied for those weighing more than 150 pounds.

SAFETY FACTORS

On the whole, most medicinal herbs are very safe and at the very least, unlikely to cause death. The most common concern in relation to herb safety is the potential for herb-drug interactions. Some pharmaceutical medications do not mix well with herbs. For example, it is not a good idea to take blood-thinning agents with blood-thinning herbs. Some herbs have multiple contraindications, such as Saint John's wort, which should not be taken concomitantly with a wide range of prescription medications. If you are taking any pharmaceutical medications—or are just uncertain about the safety of an herb or whether it is right for you—it's wise to consult with an herbalist, naturopath, or other health professional who is familiar with herbal medicine.

While many herbs can safely be taken in typical therapeutic doses, like around 30 drops or more of tincture, some herbs are safest and most effective in small doses. Another way to express this is to say they have a narrow therapeutic index. One medicinal plant that commonly grows in the Northeast with a narrow therapeutic index is poke (*Phytolacca americana*). The dose for poke root tincture is 1–5 drops. Anything more than that will cause an unpleasant and potentially dangerous reaction in the form of strong evacuation of the bowels and severe vomiting. It's important to know these low-dose herbs well and pay heed to their recommended dosages and associated precautions.

Pregnancy and Breastfeeding

In the first trimester, it is advised to use as little herbal intervention as possible unless there is just cause, such as threatened miscarriage or nausea and vomiting of pregnancy (NVP). Throughout pregnancy, regular intake of nutritive herbs such as stinging nettle, raspberry leaf, and rosehips is generally considered safe. Some herbs are safe to use at the end of the third trimester to prepare the body for labor and delivery, including crampbark, motherwort, and partridgeberry.

Here are some of the herbs to avoid throughout pregnancy:

- emmenagogic or uterine-stimulating herbs (e.g., mugwort, yarrow)
- stimulating laxative herbs (e.g., buckthorn, rhubarb, senna)
- herbs with high amounts of volatile oils (e.g., peppermint, oregano, thyme in therapeutic doses; as a seasoning in food these are okay)
- herbs with potentially harmful alkaloids (e.g., barberry, borage, coltsfoot, comfrey)
- herbs known to be teratogenic or harmful to the developing embryo (e.g., peach pit, black cherry bark)

After birth, many herbs can be safely added back in to a nursing mother's herbal repertoire. Keep in mind that some herbal constituents may be transferred to the breastmilk. The herbs to avoid during this time are those with potentially harmful alkaloids and herbs with strong purgative actions. Also avoid therapeutic amounts of the following herbs during breastfeeding, unless weaning is the goal: black walnut, garden sage, and parsley.

Herbs that improve breastmilk production include hops, raspberry leaf, red clover, and stinging nettle. Breastfeeding provides an opportunity to gently deliver herbs to the nursing baby. Herbs like chamomile, lemon balm, and catnip can both soothe a mother's nerves and ease the sensitive digestion of the little one.

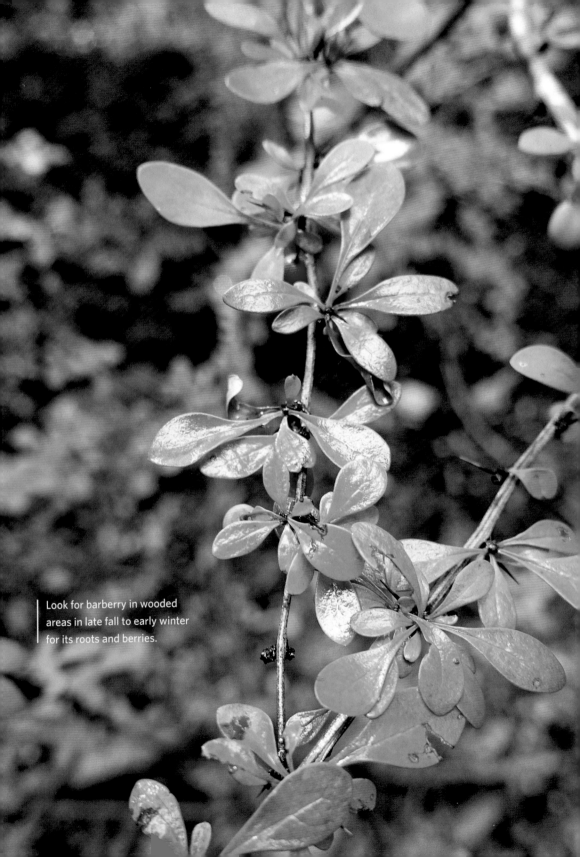

Look for barberry in wooded areas in late fall to early winter for its roots and berries.

WILDCRAFTING SEASON BY SEASON

How fortunate we are to live in a region where we experience so much change throughout the seasons. It's a joy to experience the gradual yet dramatic shifts that occur here in the Northeast—from the ice and snow and openness of bare trees in winter to the bright days and fresh leaves and blooms of spring. If you're not the type who enjoys the extremes of the seasons, like the sweltering summer heat or the darkness of winter, I hope in time you'll come to see the beauty of these periods through the lens of the plants. Perhaps you'll look forward to the brambleberries despite the sweat dripping down your back, or the sap flow of late winter even though you're still bundled in cumbersome layers of clothing.

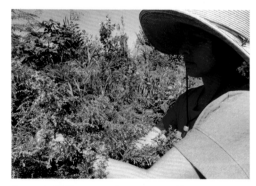

An early fall harvest of mugwort in flower.

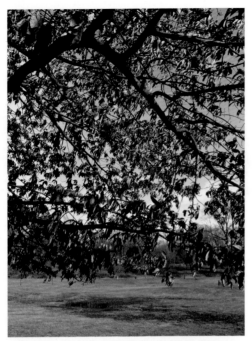

Walking the land throughout the seasons familiarizes us with the plants' cycles and awakens us to the diversity of plants around us. You'll begin to make mental maps of where your favorite plants are and get a sense of which plants provide the best harvest and about when that would be each year. It may be useful to keep a journal, or to take photographs that display the date taken, so that you'll have a general sense of when the plants leaf, flower, fruit, and set seed.

Something you'll notice is how climate variation from one year to the next affects plant emergence. Take note of which tree flowers bloom first—red maple (*Acer rubrum*) is a likely bet. Or if you're in New York City like me, then it's usually cornelian cherry (*Cornus mas*). Based on your yearly observations you'll get an idea of whether, for instance, the dandelions will start to bloom in March because of a mild winter, or April due to a long and late snow cover.

The rattling sound of dried oak leaves in winter provides a soundtrack for meditating with the land. Like our immense inner worlds, the herbs available in winter can be hidden from view. Roots tucked into the soil and syrup made from last spring's sap flow nourish and sustain us with their earthy sweetness. Evergreen leaves of conifers provide vitamin C and help us through cold and flu season with their antimicrobial and expectorant properties.

A really cool phenomena of these seasonal changes is that what the land provides at a given time of year corresponds directly with what our bodies need then. For example, chickweed and cleavers emerge in spring, just when we need to cleanse the blood and

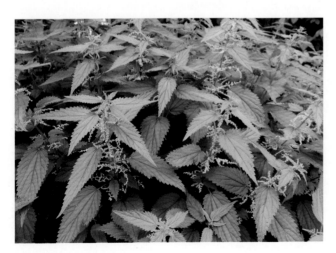

Stinging nettle in late spring. The returning light and warmth of spring brings renewal to the land and our hearts. New growth emerges—buds, branch tips, tender young leaves, and ephemeral blossoms. These plants cleanse our bodies and help us shed the stagnation of the still, winter months. Spring tonic herbs also give our bodies an immune boost to cope with the coming onslaught of seasonal allergies.

move lymphatic fluids after the dark, cold months of winter. Nourishing roots are ready to harvest in fall when we need to prepare our bodies for the reduction of fresh fruits and vegetables in the more barren months. When we live in rhythm with the seasons as our ancestors did, we sync up with a way of life that's deeply in tune with the earth. This connection to natural cycles turns out to be a more sustainable way to live, too. We rely less on the packaged and shipped mono-culture crops available all year long in the supermarket and more on the nourishment of the wild land we lovingly tend. And what's more, through the changing currents of light and temperature, of bud and leaf and fruit, we enrich our lives with a ritual honoring of the land. We celebrate the elder blossoms in spring for making syrups and elixirs and the goldenrod in summer for infused oil and tea.

The following table is a general guide to which plants will be emerging when and where. There may be variation, depending on your altitude and latitude as well as yearly climate fluctuations. You'll notice some of the plants are listed in multiple habitat sections, since, like us, certain plant species like to inhabit a variety of environs.

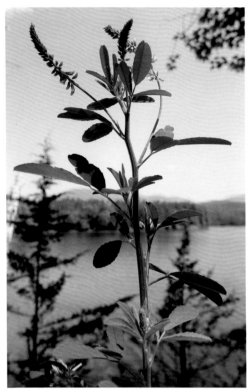

The smell of sweet clover is synonymous with summer. Expansive, hot summer is a time of abundance. Deep green foliage, flowers, and fruit cool and hydrate our bodies, heal wounds from outdoor adventures, and ease sore muscles after exerting ourselves during this active time of year.

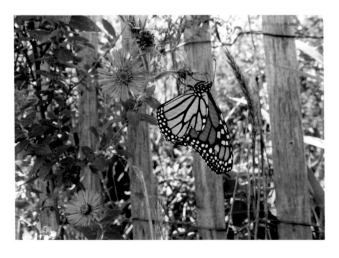

A monarch butterfly gathering nectar from New England aster before migrating south in fall. In autumn, plants set seed to prepare for the coming time of spiraling inward and incubating in preparation for rebirth. This is the time to dig roots, harvest remaining fruit and seeds, and prepare or preserve them for the coming cold and darkness.

	EARLY WINTER	LATE WINTER	EARLY SPRING	MIDSPRING
WOODLANDS AND PARTIALLY SHADED PLACES				
American spikenard rhizomes				
barberry bark, roots	●	●	●	●
barberry fruit	●			
beech leaves (green)				●
beech leaves (marcescent)	●	●		
beech nuts				
blackberry flowers				
blackberry fruit				
blackberry leaves				●
black cherry bark				
black cherry flowers				
black cherry fruit				
black walnut leaves				●
black walnut nut hulls, nuts				
coltsfoot flowers, stalks			●	
coltsfoot leaves				
crampbark bark, twigs				●
crampbark fruit				
eastern redcedar cones	●	●		
eastern redcedar leaves, twigs	●	●	●	●
elderberries				
elderflowers				
elder leaves, twigs				●
English ivy leaves	●	●	●	●
field garlic bulbs, leaves	●	●	●	●
garlic mustard flowers			●	●
garlic mustard leaves			●	●
garlic mustard roots			●	●

LATE SPRING
EARLY SUMMER
MIDSUMMER
LATE SUMMER
EARLY FALL
MIDFALL
LATE FALL

WOODLANDS AND PARTIALLY SHADED PLACES (continued)	EARLY WINTER	LATE WINTER	EARLY SPRING	MIDSPRING
garlic mustard seeds				
goldenrod flowering tops				
goutweed leaves				●
goutweed roots				●
hawthorn flowers				●
hawthorn fruit				
hawthorn leaves, thorns				●
Japanese honeysuckle flowers				
Japanese honeysuckle leaves, stems	●			
jewelweed aerial parts				
larch bark, needles			●	●
linden flowers				
linden leaves				●
maple bark, sap	●			
maple leaves				●
mint aerial parts				
motherwort flowering tops				
mulberry fruit				
mulberry leaves, root bark, twigs				●
oak bark, leaves			●	●
oak flowers			●	●
oak nuts (acorns)				
partridgeberry fruit				
partridgeberry leaves, stems	●	●	●	●
periwinkle flowers				●
periwinkle leaves, stems	●	●	●	●
pine bark, needles, twigs	●	●	●	●
pine pitch			●	●
pine pollen				

LATE SPRING	EARLY SUMMER	MIDSUMMER	LATE SUMMER	EARLY FALL	MIDFALL	LATE FALL

WOODLANDS AND PARTIALLY SHADED PLACES (continued)	EARLY WINTER	LATE WINTER	EARLY SPRING	MIDSPRIN
pipsissewa flowers				
pipsissewa leaves	■	■	■	■
prickly ash bark			■	■
prickly ash fruit				
ragweed flowers				
ragweed leaves				
raspberry flowers				■
raspberry fruit				
raspberry leaves				■
raspberry roots			■	■
red root leaves				
red root root bark			■	
rose flowers				
rose hips	■			
rose leaves, prickles, stems				■
rose roots				
sassafras leaves				■
sassafras root bark			■	■
Solomon's seal flowers				■
Solomon's seal rhizomes				
spicebush fruit				
spicebush leaves, twigs				
spruce bark, tips, twigs			■	■
spruce needles, resin	■	■	■	■
stinging nettle leaves			■	■
stinging nettle roots				
stinging nettle seeds				
sweetgum fruit, leaves, twigs				
sweetgum resin, twigs		■	■	

LATE SPRING
EARLY SUMMER
MIDSUMMER
LATE SUMMER
EARLY FALL
MIDFALL
LATE FALL

WOODLANDS AND PARTIALLY SHADED PLACES (continued)	EARLY WINTER	LATE WINTER	EARLY SPRING	MIDSPRING
tulip poplar inner bark, branch tips, twigs		■	■	■
tulip poplar branch tips, flowers, leaves, twigs				■
violet flowers				■
violet leaves			■	■
wild geranium flowers, leaves				■
wild geranium leaves, rhizomes			■	
wild grape flowers				
wild grape fruit, seeds				
wild grape leaves				
wild lettuce aerial parts in flower, latex, roots, stems				
wild lettuce leaves				
wild sarsaparilla rhizomes				
wild strawberry flowers			■	■
wild strawberry fruit				
wild strawberry leaves				
wintergreen fruit	■	■	■	
wintergreen leaves	■	■	■	■
witch hazel bark, twigs			■	
witch hazel flowers				
witch hazel leaves				■
OPEN MEADOWS, DISTURBED SOILS, SUNNY AREAS, AND THE EDGES OF SUNNY AREAS				
agrimony burs				
agrimony flowers				
agrimony leaves				
barberry bark, roots	■	■	■	■
barberry fruit	■			
beech leaves (green)				■
beech leaves (marcescent)	■	■		

LATE SPRING	EARLY SUMMER	MIDSUMMER	LATE SUMMER	EARLY FALL	MIDFALL	LATE FALL

OPEN MEADOWS, DISTURBED SOILS, SUNNY AREAS, AND THE EDGES OF SUNNY AREAS (continued)	EARLY WINTER	LATE WINTER	EARLY SPRING	MIDSPRING
beech nuts				
blackberry flowers				
blackberry fruit				
blackberry leaves				▓
blackberry roots			▓	▓
black-eyed Susan flowers				
black-eyed Susan leaves				
black-eyed Susan roots				
black walnut leaves				▓
black walnut nut hulls, nuts				
blue skullcap aerial parts in flower				
blue skullcap leaves				
blue vervain flowering tops, leaves				
boneset flowering tops, leaves				
borage leaves				
borage flowers				
bull thistle flowers				
bull thistle leaves				
bull thistle roots	▓	▓	▓	
burdock leaves				
burdock roots	▓	▓	▓	▓
burdock seeds				
catnip flowering tops				
catnip leaves				
chickweed aerial parts			▓	▓
chicory flowers				
chicory leaves			▓	▓
chicory roots			▓	
cinquefoil flowers, leaves				▓

LATE SPRING	EARLY SUMMER	MIDSUMMER	LATE SUMMER	EARLY FALL	MIDFALL	LATE FALL

OPEN MEADOWS, DISTURBED SOILS, SUNNY AREAS, AND THE EDGES OF SUNNY AREAS (continued)	EARLY WINTER	LATE WINTER	EARLY SPRING	MIDSPRING
cinquefoil roots				
cleavers aerial parts			▓	
comfrey flowers				
comfrey leaves				
comfrey roots				
common mallow flowers				
common mallow fruit				
common mallow leaves				
common mallow roots				
dandelion flowers, leaves			▓	
dandelion roots				
echinacea flowers				
echinacea leaves				
echinacea roots				
elderberries				
elderflowers				
elder leaves, twigs				▓
elecampane flowers				
elecampane roots				
English ivy leaves	▓	▓	▓	▓
evening primrose flowers				
evening primrose leaves				▓
evening primrose roots				
evening primrose seeds				
feverfew flowers, leaves				
forsythia flowers			▓	
forsythia fruit (green)				
forsythia fruit (ripe)				
garlic mustard flowers			▓	

LATE SPRING	EARLY SUMMER	MIDSUMMER	LATE SUMMER	EARLY FALL	MIDFALL	LATE FALL

OPEN MEADOWS, DISTURBED SOILS, SUNNY AREAS, AND THE EDGES OF SUNNY AREAS (continued)	EARLY WINTER	LATE WINTER	EARLY SPRING	MIDSPRING
garlic mustard leaves			■	
garlic mustard roots			■	
garlic mustard seeds				
German chamomile flowers				
ginkgo leaves (green)				
ginkgo leaves (yellow)				
ginkgo seeds				
goldenrod flowering tops				
ground ivy aerial parts in flower				■
ground ivy leaves			■	
hops strobiles				
Japanese honeysuckle flowers				
Japanese honeysuckle leaves, stems	■			
Japanese knotweed rhizomes			■	
Japanese knotweed shoots				■
lemon balm flowering tops				
lemon balm leaves				
lobelia aerial parts				
meadowsweet flowers, leaves				
mimosa bark				
mimosa flowers				
mint aerial parts				
motherwort flowering tops				
mugwort flowering tops				
mugwort leaves				■
mulberry fruit				
mulberry leaves				■
mulberry root bark, twigs				■
mullein flowers, stalks				

LATE SPRING
EARLY SUMMER
MIDSUMMER
LATE SUMMER
EARLY FALL
MIDFALL
LATE FALL

|---|---|---|---|---|
mullein leaves				■
mullein roots	■	■		
New England aster flowers, leaves				
peach flowers, twigs			■	
peach fruit, pits				
peach leaves				
plantain leaves				■
plantain roots			■	
plantain seeds				
poke fruit				
poke roots			■	
raspberry flowers				■
raspberry fruit				
raspberry leaves				■
raspberry roots			■	
red clover flowering tops				
red root leaves			■	
red root root bark			■	
Saint John's wort flowering tops				
self-heal aerial parts in flower				
shepherd's purse aerial parts in flower			■	
spotted Joe Pye weed flowers, leaves, stems				
spotted Joe Pye weed roots				
sumac bark			■	
sumac fruit				
sumac leaves				■
sunflower flowers, leaves				
sunflower seeds				
sweet clover flowering tops				

LATE SPRING
EARLY SUMMER
MIDSUMMER
LATE SUMMER
EARLY FALL
MIDFALL
LATE FALL

OPEN MEADOWS, DISTURBED SOILS, SUNNY AREAS, AND THE EDGES OF SUNNY AREAS (continued)	EARLY WINTER	LATE WINTER	EARLY SPRING	MIDSPRING
sweetfern leaves				
teasel flowers				
teasel roots				
valerian flowering tops, leaves				
valerian roots				
white horehound flowering tops				
wild bergamot flowers, stems				
wild bergamot leaves				
wild carrot flowers, seeds				
wild carrot leaves			■	■
wild carrot roots		■	■	
wild lettuce aerial parts in flower, latex, roots, stems				
wild lettuce leaves				
wild strawberry flowers			■	■
wild strawberry fruit				
wild strawberry leaves				
yarrow aerial parts in flower				
yarrow leaves				
yellow dock leaves			■	■
yellow dock roots		■	■	
yellow dock seeds	■			
WETLANDS, RIVERBANKS, LAKESIDES, BOGS/MARSHES				
alder bark	■	■		
alder leaf buds, catkins, twigs			■	■
alder leaves				■
beggarticks flowers, leaves				
beggarticks roots				
birch bark, catkins, leaf buds, sap		■	■	

WETLANDS, RIVERBANKS, LAKESIDES, BOGS/ MARSHES (continued)	EARLY WINTER	LATE WINTER	EARLY SPRING	MIDSPRING
birch catkins, leaves, twigs			■	
blue flag iris flowers				
blue flag iris rhizomes				
blue skullcap aerial parts in flower				
blue skullcap leaves				
blue vervain flowering tops, leaves				
boneset flowering tops, leaves				
coltsfoot flowers, stalks			■	
coltsfoot leaves				
crampbark bark, twigs				■
crampbark fruit				
cranberry fruit	■			
eastern cottonwood leaf buds, twigs		■		
goldenrod flowering tops				
horsetail aerial parts				■
Japanese knotweed rhizomes			■	
Japanese knotweed shoots				■
jewelweed aerial parts				
mugwort flowering tops				
mugwort leaves				■
spotted Joe Pye weed flowers, leaves, stems				
spotted Joe Pye weed roots				
sweet clover flowering tops				
sweet flag rhizomes			■	
sweetgum fruit, leaves, twigs				
sweetgum resin, twigs		■	■	
white water lily flowers				
white water lily rhizomes				
wild grape flowers				

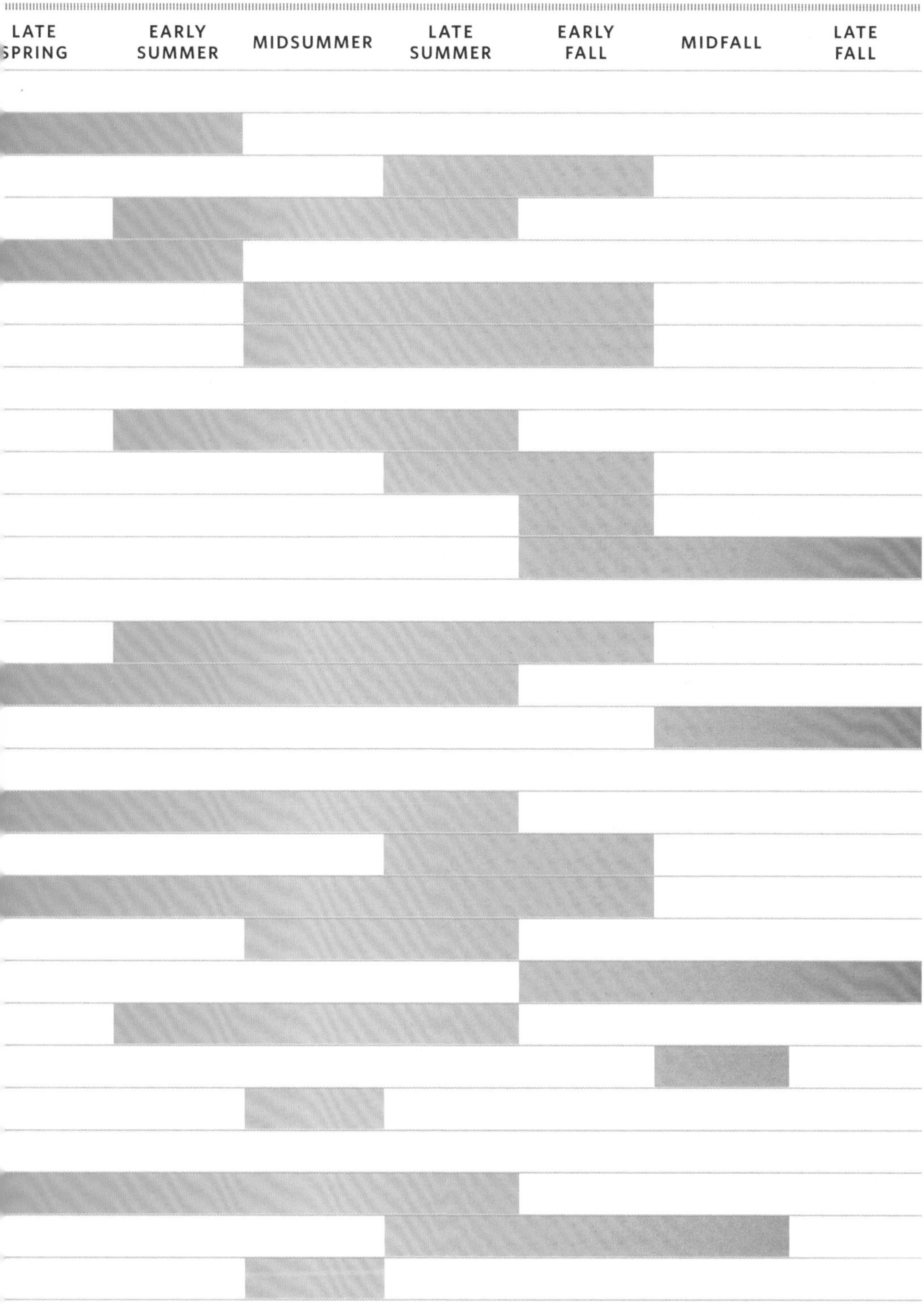
LATE SPRING
EARLY SUMMER
MIDSUMMER
LATE SUMMER
EARLY FALL
MIDFALL
LATE FALL

WETLANDS, RIVERBANKS, LAKESIDES, BOGS/ MARSHES (continued)	EARLY WINTER	LATE WINTER	EARLY SPRING	MIDSPRIN
wild grape fruit, seeds				
wild grape leaves				
willow bark		▓	▓	
willow catkins			▓	
willow leaves				▓
yellow dock leaves			▓	
yellow dock roots		▓	▓	
yellow dock seeds	▓			
SEASHORE AND COASTAL AREAS				
blackberry flowers				
blackberry fruit				
blackberry leaves				▓
blackberry root bark			▓	
boneset flowering tops, leaves				
eastern redcedar cones	▓	▓		
eastern redcedar leaves, twigs	▓	▓	▓	▓
elderberries				
elderflowers				
elder leaves, twigs				▓
evening primrose flowers				
evening primrose leaves				▓
evening primrose roots				
evening primrose seeds				
goldenrod flowering tops				
Japanese honeysuckle flowers				
Japanese honeysuckle leaves, stems	▓			
mimosa bark				
mimosa flowers				
mugwort flowering tops				

LATE SPRING	EARLY SUMMER	MIDSUMMER	LATE SUMMER	EARLY FALL	MIDFALL	LATE FALL

SEASHORE AND COASTAL AREAS (continued)	EARLY WINTER	LATE WINTER	EARLY SPRING	MIDSPR…
mugwort leaves				■
pine bark, needles, twigs	■	■		
pine pitch			■	
pine pollen				
raspberry flowers				■
raspberry fruit				
raspberry leaves				■
raspberry roots			■	■
rose flowers				
rose hips	■			
rose leaves, prickles, stems				■
rose roots				■
sweetfern leaves				
wild carrot flowers, seeds				
wild carrot leaves			■	■
wild carrot roots		■	■	
wild geranium flowers, leaves				■
wild geranium leaves, rhizomes			■	
yellow dock leaves			■	■
yellow dock roots		■	■	
yellow dock seeds	■			

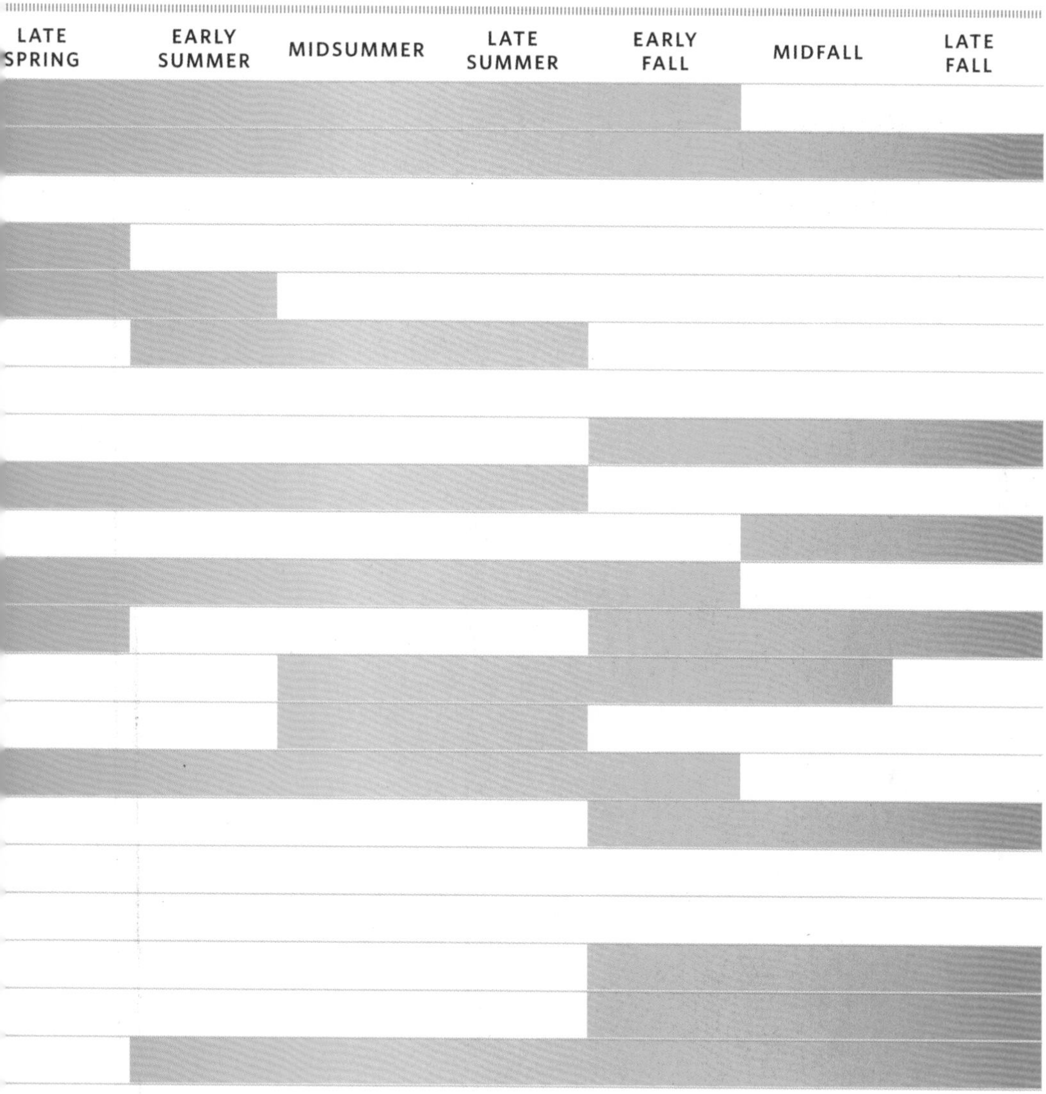
LATE SPRING
EARLY SUMMER
MIDSUMMER
LATE SUMMER
EARLY FALL
MIDFALL
LATE FALL

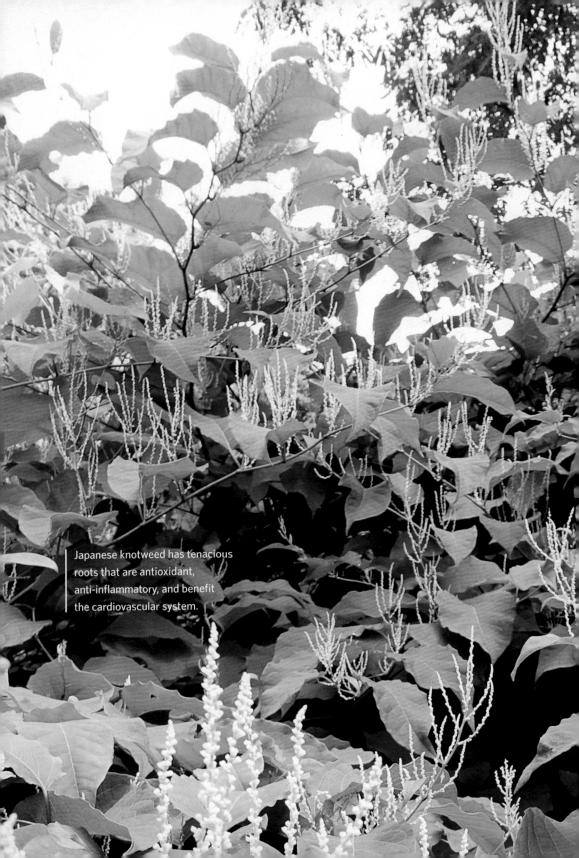

Japanese knotweed has tenacious roots that are antioxidant, anti-inflammatory, and benefit the cardiovascular system.

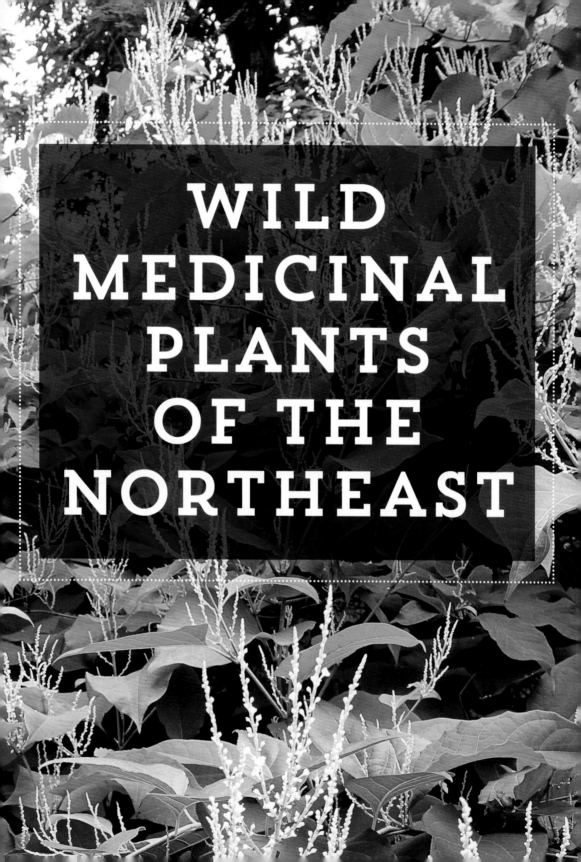

WILD MEDICINAL PLANTS OF THE NORTHEAST

agrimony

Agrimonia species

tall hairy agrimony (*A. gryposepala*), woodland agrimony (*A. striata*),
soft grooveburr (*A. pubescens*), churchsteeples (*A. eupatoria*)

PARTS USED burs, flowers, leaves

Agrimony, a mildly sweet, bitter, and astringent herb in the rose family, brings both relaxation and regulation to the urinary system. It is also traditionally used to treat diarrhea and vomiting.

How to Identify

Agrimony is a perennial herbaceous plant in the rose family. Tall hairy agrimony can grow to 5 feet while roadside agrimony and the European species known as churchsteeples tend to be shorter, up to about 3 feet.

The leaves of agrimony are toothed and pinnately compound with an odd number of leaflets (three to nine), which are reminiscent of strawberry leaflets but more numerous.

Smaller leaflets are interspersed between larger ones, especially closer to the leaf stalk. Terminal leaflets tend to be the largest. Leaves and stems, especially the undersides, are downy.

Small, fragrant, yellow, five-petaled flowers grow alternately up a long, slender spike. The fruit is a small bristly bur that clings readily to clothing. The root is long, black, woody, and sweetly scented.

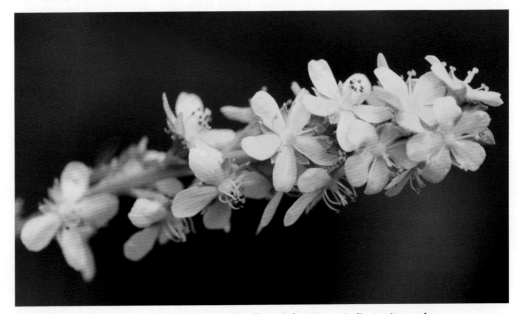

According to the doctrine of signatures, the yellow flower of agrimony indicates its use for imbalances in the solar plexus region. The color yellow is also specifically associated with the liver, gallbladder (bile), and kidneys (urine).

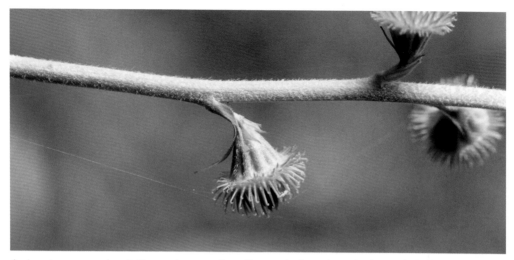

Agrimonia gryposepala gets its species name from the sepals that grip to the fur or clothing of passersby.

Where, When, and How to Wildcraft

Agrimony tends to grow in disturbed soil, alongside trails, in forest edges, and in forests proper. Collect a few leaves from a variety of plants in spring before flowering. Pick the flowers in early summer to use right away in a flower essence or dry for later use for infusions or other applications. Gather burs in late summer when they emerge.

Medicinal Uses

The aroma of agrimony, whether fresh or dried, is pleasantly sweet and makes a delicious infusion with a broad range of applications. Taking a sip, there is a slight feeling of astringency on the back of the tongue indicating its ability to tone mucous membranes while stanching discharges and bleeding.

For a blood-cleansing spring tonic, combine fresh or dried leaves of agrimony with stinging nettle, cleavers, and sassafras. Drink regularly throughout the spring to ease or diminish allergic reactions to pollen.

When the voice has become strained or hoarse, drink or gargle an infusion of agrimony to bring relief. Dilute one dropperful of a tincture of the leaves and flowers in ¼ cup of water as a mouthwash or gargle for sore throats or canker sores.

In case of diarrhea due to sluggish digestion, make an infusion of agrimony with the optional addition of peppermint and blackberry leaf or root. Agrimony also imparts its effect on the urinary system, bringing relief to cystitis and pain around the kidneys.

Apply a compress or poultice of fresh or dried leaves to new or slow-to-heal wounds, eczema, or other skin irritations.

Agrimony has a mildly relaxant effect on both physical and mental tension. The herb was once used as a treatment for insomnia aggravated by troubled emotions and intense dreams. Both the herb and the flower essence bring relief to deeply embedded anxiety or buried emotions. More specifically, the flower essence is indicated for people who are hiding their pain beneath a cheerful disposition or addiction.

Dried agrimony leaves and flowers make a sweet-smelling, cleansing incense. Sprinkle a pinch over a hot coal in a fireproof container and wash the smoke over your head, body, and home.

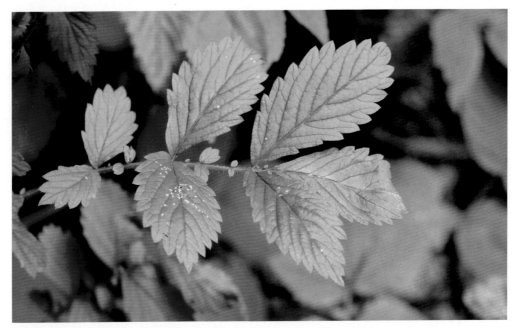

Native to Europe, Asia, Africa, and North America, agrimony has been prized for centuries for its medicinal virtues and magical uses.

⚠ Precautions

Agrimony is generally considered safe for young to elder folk. If you are taking a medication to regulate blood glucose, keep track of your levels as agrimony may lower blood sugar. Consult with your healthcare practitioner, as a dose adjustment may be warranted if you plan to continue using agrimony.

Future Harvests

Collect individual leaves, flowers, and burs from a variety of plants as opposed to harvesting the entire plant. Some species of agrimony are threatened or endangered in places throughout the Northeast. Be sure to correctly identify which species you plan to gather. Harvest mainly from the more common species, including *A. gryposepala*, *A. striata*, and introduced *A. eupatoria*. Encourage future harvests by directly sowing seeds in the spring after frost is no longer likely.

HERBAL PREPARATIONS

Tea
Standard infusion of dried leaves
Drink 4 ounces up to 3 times per day.

Tincture
1 part fresh flowers and leaves
2 parts menstruum (50% alcohol, 50% water)
or
1 part dried flowers and leaves
5 parts menstruum (50% alcohol, 50% water)
Take 20–40 drops up to 3 times per day.

Flower essence
Follow instructions for making flower essences on page 54. Take 3 drops on the tongue or in water 3 times per day or as needed.

Alnus species

European alder (*A. glutinosa*), gray or speckled alder (*A. incana*),
tag or smooth alder (*A. serrulata*), green alder (*A. viridis*)

PARTS USED bark, catkins, leaf buds, leaves, twigs

The bitter, astringent nature of alder normalizes fluid imbalance, improves lymphatic function, and stimulates digestive juices to encourage healthy gut function.

How to Identify

There are four main species of alder in the Northeast, including the introduced European alder, which is generally the largest of the species, growing as high as 60 feet. Species native to the region tend to form dense shrubby thickets near wetlands and streams. Beaver often choose alder for their dams and lodges. The bark is generally grayish and smooth. Male and female catkins or flowers are on the same plant—the male catkins are long and drooping, resembling birch catkins, and the female are shorter, cone-like, and woody. Alder imparts a sweet, spicy scent similar to birch but less potent.

The leaves are simple, ovate, and finely serrated. The appearance of the veins alternating up the leaf toward the tip give them a pleated look. European alder leaves are slightly indented at the tip while those of North American species come to a blunted point.

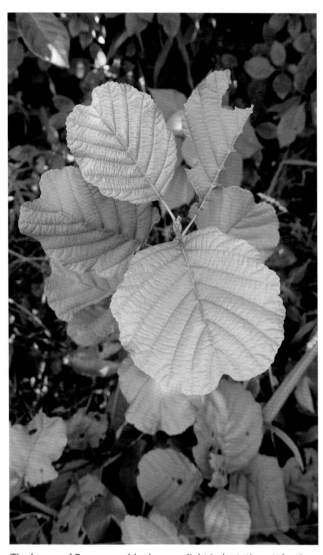

The leaves of European alder have a slight indentation at the tip.

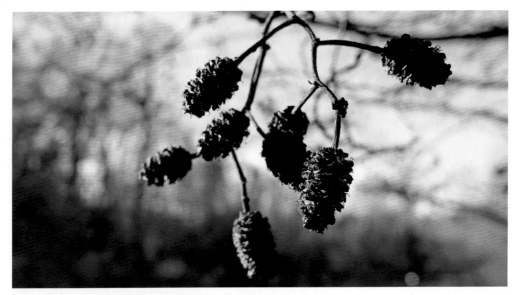
The female catkins remain on the tree through winter.

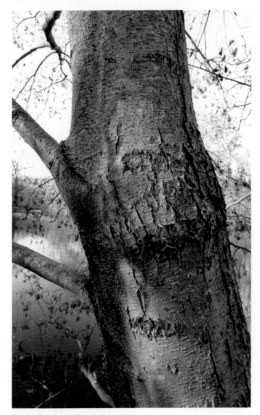
Gray or speckled alder in winter. Alder prefers having wet feet.

Where, When, and How to Wildcraft

Alders live along the shores and edges of waterways and swamps. Spring is the season for wildcrafting, when the catkins ripen. Collect the fallen twigs and branches after strong winds or storms. Cut up the twigs to tincture fresh or dry for later use. On larger branches, remove the bark by making an incision around the circumference and peeling it away. Bark is available for harvest year-round. Gather leaves as they unfold.

Medicinal Uses

Like its function in the ecosystem to restore disturbed or damaged wetland environments, alder works to normalize the fluid environments of the body, namely the lymph. Alder helps to move stuck lymphatic fluid to reduce glandular swelling in cases where the immune system is suppressed or a lingering infection is present.

Drinking a decoction of alder bark increases digestive fluids where there is gastric insufficiency, a common condition in the elder population that presents as heartburn due to low gastric secretion rather than excess. Similarly, alder stimulates digestion where there is constipation or diarrhea due to lack of tone.

Make a strong infusion of the dried or fresh leaves or a decoction of the bark and catkins to apply as a wash or compress to slow-healing or pus-filled wounds or skin eruptions, including poison ivy rash, psoriasis, or eczema.

⚠ Precautions

The yellow inner bark may induce vomiting if used in excess.

Use with caution during breastfeeding, unless there is excess milk production or if weaning is desired, as alder may dry up breastmilk.

Future Harvests

European alder is abundant and considered weedy in some locales. Tag or smooth alder, the officinal species native to the Northeast, is in good conservation status. Green alder is at risk in parts of the Northeast. Check conservation status in your area before harvesting.

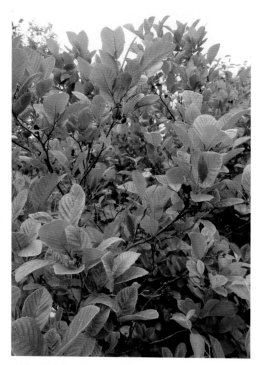

Alder thriving in a marshland.

HERBAL PREPARATIONS

Tea
Standard decoction of fresh or dried bark, catkins, leaf buds, leaves, and/or twigs
Drink 4 ounces as needed. Or use externally as a wash.

Tincture
1 part fresh bark, catkins, leaf buds, leaves, and/or twigs
2 parts menstruum (95% alcohol, 5% water)
or
1 part dried bark, catkins, leaf buds, leaves, and/or twigs
5 parts menstruum (95% alcohol, 5% water)
Take 30 drops up to 5 times per day.

American spikenard

Aralia racemosa

PARTS USED rhizomes

American spikenard is a member of the ginseng family and shares some similar characteristics with its kin, including the ability to energize the body and boost the immune system.

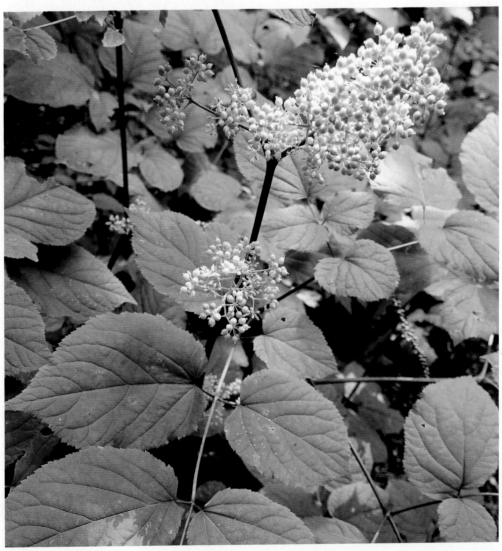

The not-yet-ripe fruit of American spikenard. Several northeastern First Peoples, including the Haudenosaunee and Algonquin (Québec), traditionally use the root as medicine.

How to Identify

American spikenard is a perennial herbaceous sometimes shrubby plant that can grow 3–6 feet in a spreading rather than upright fashion. The leaves are twice pinnately compound and are composed of large toothed, pointed leaflets that are slightly heart shaped toward the base. These grow on reddish brown to almost black stems that branch off in different directions. Green-white flowers with five triangle-shaped petals grow in clusters of small umbels emerging in early to midsummer. The edible purple-red berries ripen in autumn. The rhizomatous root is hairy at the crown and gives off an earthy, woodsy, spicy scent.

Where, When, and How to Wildcraft

Look for American spikenard in moist deciduous forests or at the edge of forest trails. Dig a small section of the rhizome in autumn, leaving or replanting the rest to continue to grow.

Medicinal Uses

A root decoction of American spikenard is warming and stimulating with blood-purifying properties lending to its broad application in cold, stuck conditions. The root itself imparts a sticky resinous trace when simmered to make a decoction. The taste is slightly sweet, acrid, and pungent, leaving a tingling warmth at the roof of the mouth. The decoction brings on sweating in case of fever and has an expectorant effect for coughs brought on by adrenal insufficiency, exhaustion, or cold, dry weather.

The reddish brown color of the stems and berries is a signature for the blood. American spikenard is used to purify the blood and was traditionally used to treat diabetes. Use the root decoction to stimulate menstruation when the uterus is cold or lacking circulation.

Make a poultice of the dried roots by simmering then mashing them or use reconstituted root powder to relieve wounds, burns, or boils. A poultice or compress is also useful for easing the pain and inflammation of sprains, broken bones, or inflamed joints.

⚠ Precautions

Do not use American spikenard during pregnancy as it can be too stimulating to the uterus.

Future Harvests

Harvest a section of the root and re-cover remaining roots in the soil after harvesting. Directly sow seeds near where you harvest in late fall to encourage the future of this valued native plant.

American spikenard is critically imperiled in Rhode Island. Check its conservation status in your area before harvesting.

HERBAL PREPARATIONS

Tea

Standard decoction of dried rhizomes
Drink 2 ounces as needed.

Tincture

1 part fresh rhizomes
2 parts menstruum (50% alcohol, 50% water)
or
1 part dried rhizomes
5 parts menstruum (50% alcohol, 50% water)
Take 5–30 drops 4 times per day.

barberry

Berberis species
Japanese barberry (*B. thunbergii*), common barberry (*B. vulgaris*)
PARTS USED bark, fruit, roots

*The medicinal virtues of barberry as a bitter liver tonic have been known
for millennia. Barberry is strongly antimicrobial and can be used in place
of endangered goldenseal for internal and topical infection.*

How to Identify

Hailing originally from Eurasia and North Africa, barberry is a deciduous shrub with arching stems. Small, ovate, alternate leaves, and sharp spines grow singly or in groups of up to three off the stem. The strongly scented yellow blooms of barberry emerge in spring in pendulous, 1- to 2-inch-long clusters donning up to twenty flowers. Small, bright red, egg-shaped berries ripen in fall.

There are two native species of barberry, though they are less common than the two introduced species. American barberry (*B. canadensis*) reaches its northern range in Pennsylvania, however it may be extirpated there. Its more prominently toothed leaves

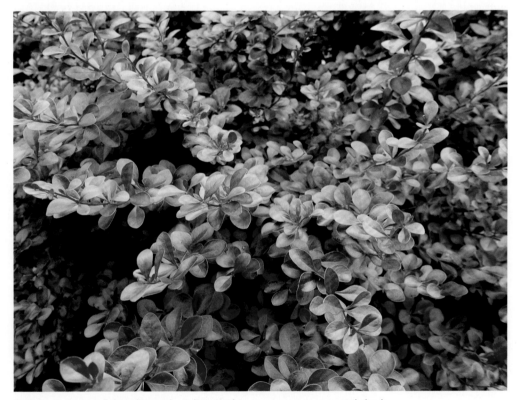

Barberry is a powerful medicine plant disguised as a common ornamental shrub.

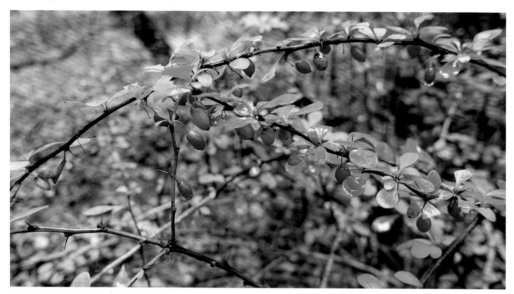
The tart red berries of barberry are antioxidant.

may help distinguish it from the introduced species. Oregon grape or hollyleaved barberry (*B. aquifolium* syn. *Mahonia aquifolium*), which has sharp-edged holly-like leaves, has sparse distribution in the Northeast. Although it is more commonly found in Western states and provinces, I mention it here because it is a fairly well-known and valued plant medicine.

Where, When, and How to Wildcraft

The first place you may notice barberry growing is in a domestic garden as a hedgerow or ornamental shrub. In the wild, barberry is abundant in disturbed habitats and nearly every other type of ecosystem, perhaps save swamps. Harvest the roots and bark of lower stems in the early winter, spring, or fall to tincture fresh or dry for later use. The roots are fairly easy to remove as they tend to be shallow, though be sure to cover well the vacant spot in the soil where you've removed the root.

Gather the red berries in late fall when they ripen. The berries are best dehydrated or kept in the freezer.

Medicinal Uses

The yellow color of barberry roots corresponds with the liver and kidneys, as well as reveals the presence of berberine, an alkaloid compound also found in goldenseal and known for its efficacy against intestinal infections such as dysentery. The roots and root bark inhibit the growth of bacteria. Use a decoction or tincture of the root to support the body in preventing or eradicating infection, especially of the intestines and blood.

Combine barberry root with goldenrod and common mallow root to ease burning and irritation associated with a urinary tract infection.

The berries are pleasantly sour, hinting at their antioxidant and cooling properties. Drink a berry infusion to reduce histaminic reactions or cold symptoms, and to reduce fever. In clinical trials, the berry extract has been found to be beneficial for regulating glucose metabolism in people with type 2 diabetes.

Use barberry instead of endangered goldenseal for systemic infections.

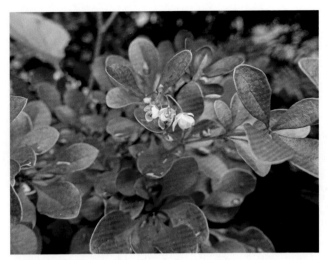
Small yellow flowers bloom in clusters in spring.

Future Harvests

The most common species of barberry in our region are introduced and considered invasive—their propagation is even discouraged in some places. In other words, harvesting barberry root could be seen as a good deed to native plant enthusiasts and those who work in forest management. On the other hand, tread lightly if you've found American barberry or Oregon grape as these native species are rare in the Northeast.

⚠ Precautions

Before using barberry, consult with a healthcare practitioner who has experience with herbal medicine. Barberry may interfere with certain medications, including antibiotics, antihistamines, blood thinners, and medications metabolized by the liver. Discontinue barberry 2 weeks prior to surgery as it may thin the blood, as well as slow heartrate, blood pressure, and respiration.

Do not use barberry during pregnancy and breastfeeding, in children younger than 2 years old, and in the elder population. The constituent berberine found in barberry may be harmful to newborns, particularly if they are premature or have jaundice.

Borrelia burgdorferi–carrying deer ticks are commonly found in these shrubs and, coincidentally, barberry is sometimes a component of formulas to treat Lyme disease. Take care when harvesting barberry from forests where ticks are plentiful. If you suspect or know you have contracted Lyme disease consult with a knowledgeable physician. You may also consider working with an experienced herbalist or naturopath who is familiar with effective herbal protocols for Lyme disease.

HERBAL PREPARATIONS

Tea
Standard decoction of dried bark and/or roots
Drink 4 ounces 3 times per day. Use topically as a wash for wounds or infections.
or
Standard infusion of berries
Drink 4 ounces 3 times per day.

Tincture
1 part fresh bark, berries, and/or roots
2 parts menstruum (50% alcohol, 50% water)
or
1 part dried bark, berries, and/or roots
5 parts menstruum (50% alcohol, 50% water)
Take 40-80 drops 3 times per day. Limit use to 2 weeks at a time unless otherwise directed by an experienced herbal practitioner.

Fagus species
American beech (*F. grandifolia*), European beech (*F. sylvatica*)
PARTS USED leaves, nuts

*The leaves of graceful, majestic beech lend a soothing
effect to burns and mucousy coughs.*

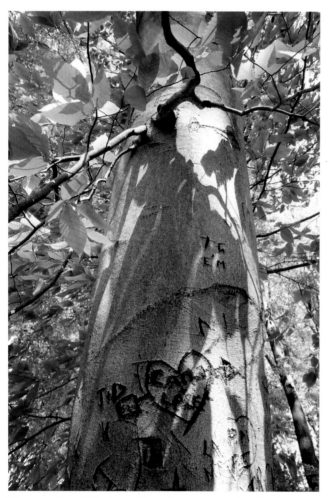

The word "beech" is derived from the same word as "book" in several Germanic languages. Before paper became commonplace, people wrote on beech wood tablets and, taking a look at beech trees in populated areas, it seems this desire is still ingrained in us today.

How to Identify

The first thing most people notice about beech is the trunk with its smooth, gray bark resembling elephant skin. In places frequented by humans, this bark is marked by stretched-out graffiti, showing the time lapse between when the markings were made and the subsequent growth of the tree. The leaves of beech are hardy, green, and toothed in the summer shifting in the fall to golden brown in American beech and reddish copper in European beech. Both species also tend to hold onto their leaves in the winter; this holding on is known as marcescence. European beech leaves have wavy, round-toothed margins as opposed to the flatter, sharper appearance of the American variety. Beech nuts are triangular and housed in bur-covered shells that drop in late summer.

Where, When, and How to Wildcraft

You'll find European beech in parks, disturbed habitats, forests, and forest edges. American

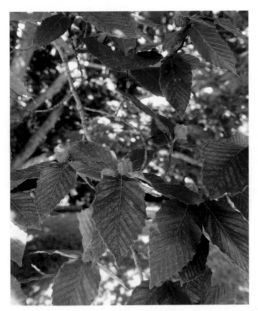

The hardy green-toothed leaves of beech interspersed with bristly bur-covered husks.

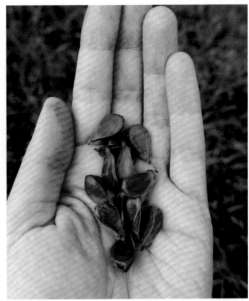

A modest harvest of the triangular nuts that you'll find at the center of the bristly husk.

beech is mostly at home in the forest. Leaves can be harvested year-round, though in some traditions the winter leaves are preferred. Collect the nuts, also known as mast, when they drop in late summer to early autumn. Remove the spiky outer husks and gently toast the nuts inside. Remove the smooth shell from the nuts before consuming or simply crush the nut in its smooth shell and simmer in a decoction.

Medicinal Uses

Beech is one of the few species of deciduous trees that sometimes holds onto its leaves in winter. The Mi'kmaq people of southeastern Canada and Maine traditionally collect these dry, brown winter leaves and the bark of beech to treat tuberculosis. Think of the rattling sound of the leaves in the wind as a signature for a rattling cough. Use an infusion of these winter leaves to bring relief to a wet cough.

Combine beech and linden leaves to make a poultice for burns. Use the winter leaves in a poultice or compress for frostbite.

Make a decoction of the nuts for a restorative tea. Gently toast the nuts for 3–5 minutes. You can grind and brew them like coffee or simply simmer in water for a nourishing drink.

Future Harvests

American beech is prone to beech bark disease—collect only prunable branches and leaves from this species.

HERBAL PREPARATIONS

Tea
Standard decoction of lightly toasted nuts
Drink 1 cup as needed.
or
Standard decoction of winter leaves
Drink ½ cup as needed. Use as a wash for frostbite, wounds, and burns.

beggarticks

Bidens species

Spanish needles (*B. bipinnata*), nodding burr-marigold (*B. cernua*), devil's-pitchfork (*B. frondosa*), three-lobe beggarticks or burr marigold (*B. tripartita*)

PARTS USED flowers, leaves, roots

This bitter, sweet, and mildly pungent herb is known for its astringency and ability to stanch bleeding both internally and externally.

How to Identify

Like its relatives in the aster family, the inflorescence of beggarticks is composed of several small flowers. In this genus, the flowers are yellow and some species have white petals surrounding the yellow inflorescence. The leaves are opposite and toothed, either entire or divided, depending on the species. The plant starts green and grows to be spindly, the stems sometimes turning reddish purple.

Where, When, and How to Wildcraft

Look for beggarticks in wet places, especially disturbed soils, meadows, fields, roadside ditches, and riparian and fresh tidal zones.

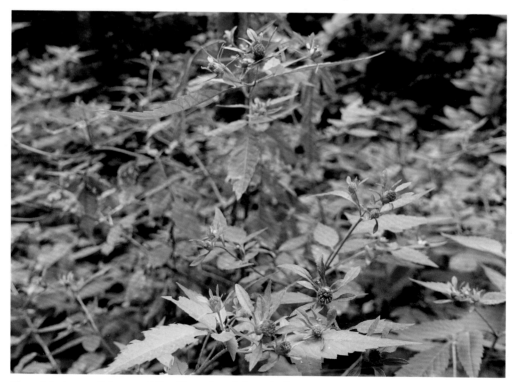

Three-lobe beggarticks, one of the 47 species of plants in this genus, likes to grow in wet habitats.

Collect the leaves in summer before flowering, the aerial parts of the plant when in bloom, and the root in fall after the flowers have gone to seed. Tincture fresh or dry for later use.

Medicinal Uses

Beggarticks is considered a tropical plant and it tends to grow in very moist habitats. This plant also happens to be effective against parasitic infections acquired in tropical or moist places, including babesia, malaria, and leishmania. Further, its antimicrobial activity and astringent nature are beneficial for a broad range of conditions affecting the moist places of the body, in other words, the mucous membranes. Use a succus or tincture of fresh herbs for systemic infections, especially of the urinary, digestive, and respiratory tracts.

The fresh or dried herb can alleviate the symptoms of benign prostatic hyperplasia.

Beggarticks, used fresh or dried, also has a strong influence on the blood and cardiovascular system. It is blood cleansing and can stop excessive bleeding, regulate blood sugar, and lower blood pressure. It is especially effective in conditions where there is or may be bleeding from the mucosa, including dysentery, ulcerative colitis, tuberculosis, uterine hemorrhaging, and cystitis.

Beggarticks also has an opening effect on the skin, making it useful in fever. An infusion of the dried herb can be used in this case.

Use a poultice or the juice of fresh leaves to treat wounds and skin ulcers.

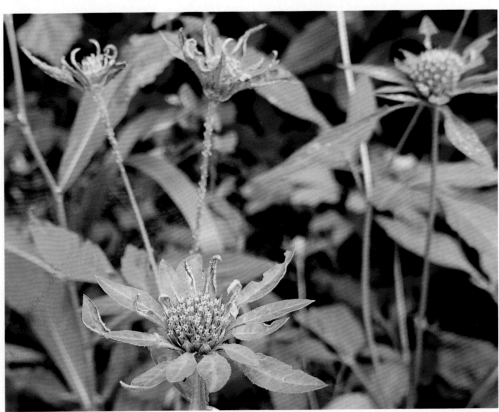

A closer look at the yellow blooms.

⚠ Precautions

Do not use beggarticks in pregnancy, especially the root and seeds as they are considered emmenagogic.

Beggarticks is safe for short-term use—using the herb for too long may lead to afflictions of the esophagus.

Be sure to consult with a knowledgeable healthcare practitioner if you are on diabetes medication, as beggarticks has an effect on blood sugar and insulin.

Beggarticks absorbs heavy metals from the soil, so take care to know the land from which you harvest. Avoid abandoned lots, waste sites, and places with a history of industrial use.

Future Harvests

The most common species of beggarticks—*B. tripartita, B. frondosa, B. bipinnata*—are considered invasive in the Northeast. However, the following are threatened or endangered in this range: *B. beckii, B. bidentoides, B. connata, B. coronata, B. discoidea, B. eatonii, B. hyperborea, B. laevis.* This is where a good dichotomous key will come in handy to determine which species you've found.

HERBAL PREPARATIONS

Tea

Standard infusion of dried flowers and leaves
Drink 4 ounces as needed. Use with the steeped leaves as a poultice on wounds.

Succus

Freeze or make a succus with the juice by adding enough alcohol to equal 25% alcohol by volume in the finished product. Take 45–90 drops up to 2 times per day. For acute conditions, take up to 1 tablespoon 6 times per day. Use externally as a wash for wounds.

Tincture

1 part fresh leaves and/or roots
2 parts menstruum (50% alcohol, 50% water)
Take 45–90 drops up to 2 times per day. For acute conditions, take up to 1 tablespoon up to 6 times per day.

Betula species

cherry, black, or sweet birch (*B. lenta*), paper birch (*B. papyrifera*), yellow birch (*B. alleghaniensis*), European or silver birch (*B. pendula*), gray birch (*B. populifolia*), downy birch (*B. pubescens*), river birch (*B. nigra*)

PARTS USED bark, catkins, leaf buds, leaves, sap, twigs

Birch has a long history of use in Eurasia and North America as a spring blood tonic and treatment for skin conditions.

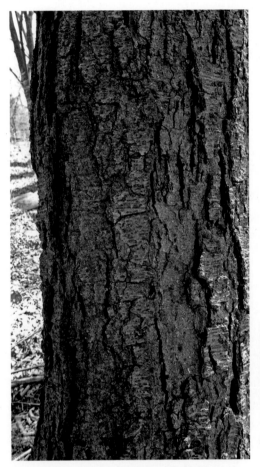

Sweet wintergreen-scented cherry birch has bark that resembles that of cherry trees.

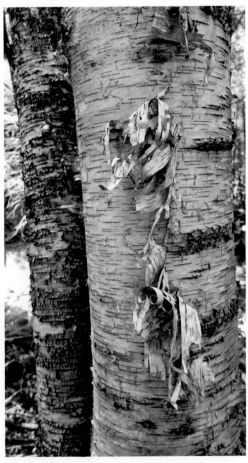

The characteristic peeling bark of paper birch is akin to peeling skin. The bark is a versatile material used for arts, crafts, and medicinal purposes. It also makes wonderful tinder for starting a campfire.

How to Identify

Birch is a lanky tree, standing out with gently fluttering leaves on thin elegant branches. The bark varies greatly between the several species of birch present in the Northeast, from brown and furrowed with prominent lenticels (cherry birch) to white and powdery with peeling bark (paper birch).

The leaves of birch are alternate and simple with finely serrated margins and range from ovate to slightly triangular in shape, depending on the species. Cherry birch and yellow birch, two common native species with bark that smells of wintergreen, have ovate leaves. Meanwhile, European birch and gray birch have leaves that are more triangular with a long, pointed tip. The leaves of paper birch, downy birch, and river birch fall somewhere between these two shapes, being slightly ovate with a broader base and narrower tip.

Like many other members of the birch (Betulaceae) family, birch is adorned with catkins, with both male and female flowers on the same tree. The male catkins hang down like long pendulums while the female ones are short and stand out straight.

Birch is an important browse for deer and is considered sacred by indigenous people of North America and Eurasia who depend on these animals for their livelihood.

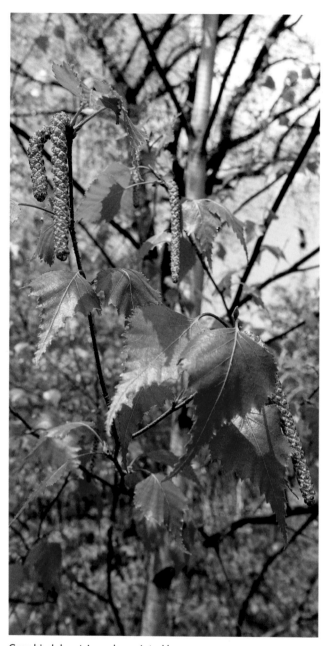

Gray birch has triangular pointed leaves.

Where, When, and How to Wildcraft

Birch is a pioneer species that favors wet places. You'll most often find birch trees at the edges of streams, in wetlands and meadows, in swamps, and in forests or forest edges.

Gather leaf buds and catkins in early spring and leaves when they emerge.

In the winter or early spring, during a full moon if possible, collect bark and twigs from pruned branches that are ½–1 inch in diameter. This is also the time to collect sap through tapping. See the maple section for details on how to tap.

Another place to look for freshly felled birch is at a sawmill or a place where firewood is processed. In both cases, it isn't the bark they are after; in exchange for the bark you can offer the landowner some birch tincture or infused oil.

Medicinal Uses

Despite their differences in appearance, all birches share similar properties for healing the skin. It is in the bark where we see the signature, the peeling away or furrowing, and the prominent lenticels. Birch is astringent and anodyne, toning the skin tissue while relieving pain and itching. Make a wash or poultice of the leaves and twigs for eczema and psoriasis. Birch leaf makes a great rinse for itchy, scaly scalp. Combine the leaves of birch with mallow root in a bath tea to alleviate itching from dry winter air. Birch also works through the skin by opening the

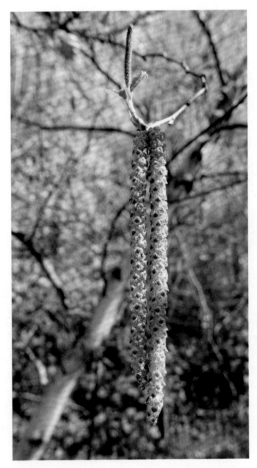

Drooping male and upright female catkins appear on birch in spring.

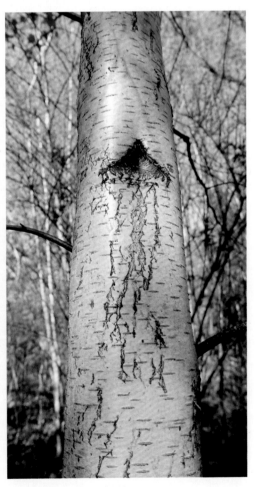

Smooth bark of gray birch.

pores and aiding the body in diaphoresis or sweating to break a fever.

Birch sap affects its action through diuresis as well, bringing relief to edema, rheumatism, arthritis, and gout. Use birch bark decoction to break up kidney stones, or to alleviate bladder irritation or infection.

Combine birch buds and twigs to make a massage oil for sore muscles and joints.

The bitterness of the bark indicates its ability to stimulate bile to tone the liver and aid elimination of waste. Birch bark decoction or birch sap make a cleansing spring tonic used alone or in combination with cleavers and sassafras.

Future Harvests

Collecting leaves and fallen twigs will not put birch at risk. However, take care when gathering directly from species that are threatened in parts of the Northeast: *B. glandulosa*, *B. minor*, *B. nigra*, and *B. pumila*. Only tap mature healthy trees of species that are not at risk and that are at least 8 inches in diameter.

HERBAL PREPARATIONS

Tea
Standard infusion of dried leaves or standard decoction of dried bark
Drink 4 ounces 3 times per day. Use externally as a hair and scalp rinse.

Infused oil
1 part fresh bark, leaf buds, leaves, and/or twigs
2 parts oil
For twigs, expose as much of the inner bark as possible by scraping away the outer bark. Chop bark, buds, and leaves before adding oil to infuse. Use topically on sore muscles or inflamed skin conditions.

Tincture
1 part fresh bark, leaf buds, leaves, and/or twigs
2 parts menstruum (70% alcohol, 30% water)
or
1 part dried bark, leaf buds, leaves, and/or twigs
5 parts menstruum (50% alcohol, 50% water)
Take 20–30 drops 3 times per day.

blackberry

Rubus allegheniensis
common blackberry, Allegheny blackberry
PARTS USED flowers, fruit, leaves, root bark

Blackberry is a rose family astringent well known for its ability to stop internal bleeding and diarrhea. The fruit and leaves fortify the blood in cases of deficiency, such as anemia.

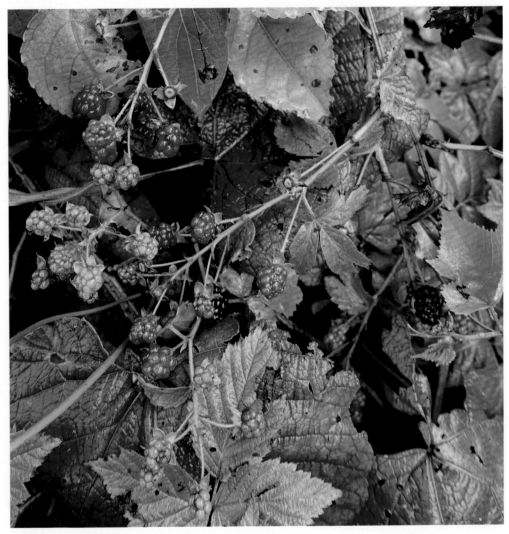

The ripening aggregate berries of blackberry are enjoyed by a variety of birds and mammals, including humans.

How to Identify

Until you take a closer look, blackberry looks quite a lot like other rose family brambles, with long arching branches in great tangles. Like some *Rubus* species, the leaves are palmately compound with three to five toothed, ovate leaflets; however, the leaves of blackberry feature prickles on their underside. On mature plants, angular stalks are covered with robust prickles. The inflorescence, a spreading raceme, is covered with stalked glands. The white (to sometimes pale pink) five-petaled flowers don numerous pistils and stamens. The edible berries start out small, firm, and green, passing through red before ripening to deep black by late summer.

Distinguish *R. allegheniensis* from Himalayan blackberry (*R. armeniacus*) by its uniform leaf color—the latter species has a downy white underside. Both can be used medicinally.

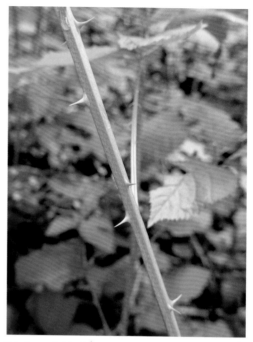

Distinguish blackberry from other *Rubus* species by its ridged green stems.

Blood-Building Syrup

Essential minerals are lacking from our modern soils and modern diets, resulting in blood deficiency, especially in women. This syrup provides vitamins A and C while helping to boost levels of iron, calcium, magnesium, manganese, and other minerals.

What you'll need:

- 3 parts dried stinging nettle leaf
- 2 parts dried blackberry leaf
- 2 parts dried yellow dock root
- 1 part dried dandelion leaf
- 1 part fresh blackberry fruit
- 1 part dried or fresh mulberry fruit

- 1 part dried hawthorn berry
- ½ part dried rosehips
- ½ part dried spearmint leaf
- Honey, maple syrup, or vegetable glycerin
- Blackstrap molasses

Combine the dried herbs and fruit in a pot. Follow instructions for making herbal syrups on page 52. Add 2 tablespoons of blackstrap molasses for every cup of syrup you make. Take 4–8 tablespoons of syrup daily. You can drink it straight up, add to sparkling water or tea, or drizzle on yogurt or pancakes.

Where, When, and How to Wildcraft

Blackberry finds itself at home in disturbed soils, forest paths, and edges as well as meadows and fields. Collect the blooms in late spring to early summer and the fruits in late summer when ripe. Ripe fruit will be purple-black, soft to the touch, and juicy. It will taste sweet instead of bitter, sour, and astringent. Gather the roots in spring or fall. Strip off the outer bark of the root and spread out to dry in a dehydrator or oven at a low setting.

Medicinal Uses

The root bark of blackberry is one of the best astringents available, a specific for treating profuse diarrhea, including dysentery or what was once known as the "bloody flux."

Blackberry is rich in vitamins and minerals and its astringent nature makes an excellent tea for someone suffering from a cold with a mucousy cough. Combine blackberry leaf with burdock root, stinging nettle leaf, and violet leaf in a decoction to clear a lingering cough.

Drink blackberry leaf infusion to tone the gastrointestinal tract and colon. To treat hemorrhoids, make a decoction of blackberry leaves, witch hazel bark, and partridgeberry leaves and stems to use in a sitz bath.

Make a blackberry infusion to use as a wash for oozing wounds. Make a compress with the infusion to apply to sore, tired eyes.

The flower essence of blackberry supports manifestation in those who procrastinate or have difficulties taking decisive action in their lives.

Future Harvests

Avoid harvesting the roots of smooth blackberry (*R. canadensis*) and showy blackberry (*R. elegantulus*), which are both at risk of becoming endangered in the Northeast.

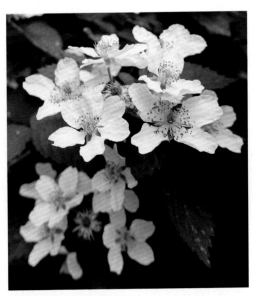

The delicate white blossoms of blackberry are beloved by pollinators and make a lovely flower essence for healing energetic imbalances in the solar plexus.

HERBAL PREPARATIONS

Tea
Standard infusion or decoction of dried leaves
Drink 1 cup 3 times per day, more frequently in cases of recurrent diarrhea. Use as a wash for wounds or a sitz bath for hemorrhoids.

Tincture
1 part fresh root bark
2 parts menstruum (50% alcohol, 50% water)
or
1 part dried root bark
5 parts menstruum (50% alcohol, 50% water)
Take 30 drops up to 4 times per day.

Flower essence
Follow instructions for making flower essences on page 54. Take 3 drops on the tongue or in water 3 times per day or as needed.

black cherry

Prunus serotina

rum cherry

PARTS USED bark, flowers, fruit

*One of three cherry trees native to the Northeast,
black cherry is a mainstay remedy for a lingering cough.*

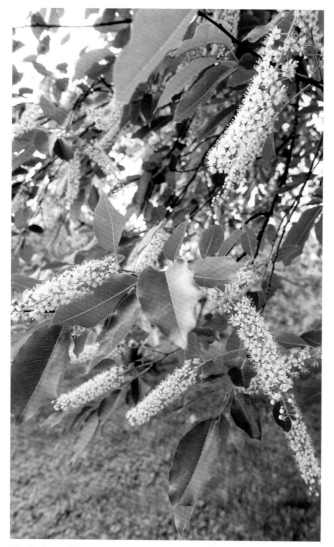

Black cherry blossoms give off the sweet scent of almonds,
hinting at the cyanogenic compounds present in the tree.

How to Identify

Black cherry is a deciduous tree with an alternate branching pattern, growing as high as 100 feet. The dark brown-gray to black bark has prominent lenticels that are more evident on the trunks of younger trees. As black cherry ages, the bark becomes thick and platy and you may have to look up to the branches to find the characteristic lenticels. Scratching the bark exposes the inner reddish bark scented of almond, revealing the presence of hydrocyanic acid.

Leaves of black cherry are simple, oblong to lanceolate, and finely serrated. The small white fragrant flowers grow on pendulous racemes, giving way to edible, dark red-black fruits with very large seeds.

Two related species, chokecherry (*P. virginiana*) and pin or fire cherry (*P. pensylvanica*), have also been historically used as medicine. Chokecherry has broader, more ovate leaves than black cherry. Pin cherry has bright red fruit and its inflorescences are

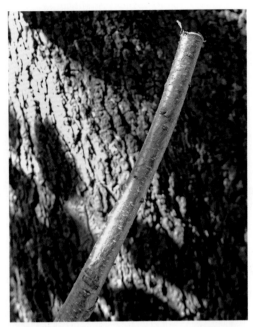

It's fairly easy to find young branches to harvest on the black cherry tree.

larger and more upright than black cherry's drooping racemes.

Where, When, and How to Wildcraft

Look for black cherry in mixed deciduous forests, disturbed soils, and on the banks of streams or rivers.

Prune young, low-growing branches for their inner bark in late summer to fall. Immediately use fresh or dry in a dehydrator or oven on a low setting for later use. Collect flowers in late spring to use in a flower essence. Gather fruit in late summer.

Medicinal Uses

Like other rose family plants, black cherry is bitter, astringent, drying, and cooling, lending itself well to conditions characterized by dampness, heat, and inflammation. Use a syrup of black cherry fruit to relieve diarrhea,

Black Cherry Bark Syrup

Got a cough that keeps you up all night? Keep some of this syrup on hand to ease the irritation and get some rest.

What you'll need:

- 1 part elderflower
- 1 part white horehound
- 1 part coltsfoot leaf
- 1 part mullein leaf
- 1 part elecampane root

- 2 parts black cherry bark
- 1 part common mallow root
- Honey
- Brandy (optional)

Combine the elderflower, white horehound, coltsfoot leaf, mullein leaf, and elecampane root in a small cooking pot. Cover with water. Simmer gently until the liquid is reduced by half, about 20–30 minutes. Take the pot off the heat and add the black cherry bark and common mallow root. Infuse for 4 hours. After infusing, strain off the liquid into a measuring cup. Compost the herbs. Note how much liquid you have and add an equal amount of honey (or use equal parts honey and brandy to add more preservative power to the syrup). Take 1–2 tablespoons as needed. Store in the refrigerator for up to 3 months.

dyspepsia, and peptic ulcers. Externally, apply a wash of black cherry bark decoction to persistent sores, skin ulcers, and burns.

The inner bark of the black cherry tree contains prunasin, a cyanogenic glycoside that may hold the key to its sedating, cough-suppressing, and heart-regulating properties. This compound is also what makes the wilting leaves and fermented bark of black cherry poisonous, so take care to use the right parts of this plant. At therapeutic doses, black cherry bark syrup, elixir, or infusion comes through for those suffering from a tight, hacking cough that keeps them up at night.

Like its relative hawthorn, black cherry bark dilates the blood vessels, lowering blood pressure. It also works to normalize a rapid or irregular heartbeat.

Black cherry flower essence helps reignite the creative spark when we are feeling stuck.

⚠ Precautions

Harvest directly from the plant or collect only freshly fallen twigs and branches, as the wilting leaves and fermenting bark of black cherry have concentrated amounts of cyanogenic glycosides and are toxic. Use the bark right away in teas or tinctures or dehydrate well in an oven or dehydrator for later use.

Future Harvests

Black cherry is a pioneer species that readily enters clear-cut land or areas affected by fire. In some places, black cherry is considered weedy or a nuisance. It is generally a prolific producer of branches suitable for harvest. That being said, a little goes a long way with black cherry and you won't need more than a small branch or two to make a decent amount of medicine.

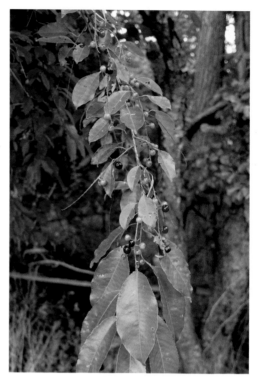

Black cherries ripen in late summer or early fall.

HERBAL PREPARATIONS

Tea
Cold infusion of dried bark
Drink 4 ounces up to 3 times per day.

Tincture
1 part fresh bark
2 parts menstruum (50% alcohol, 50% water)
or
1 part dried bark
5 parts menstruum (50% alcohol, 50% water)
Take 30–60 drops up to 4 times per day.

Flower essence
Follow instructions for making flower essences on page 54. Take 3 drops on the tongue or in water 3 times per day or as needed.

Rudbeckia hirta

PARTS USED flowers, leaves, roots

This aster family beauty has immune-boosting and blood-cleansing effects suited for clearing viral infections and healing venomous bites.

How to Identify

Black-eyed Susan is a perennial plant growing as tall as 3 feet. The stems and ovate leaves (up to 7 inches long) sport small bristly hairs. What stands out on black-eyed Susan is the bloom for which it is named. The flower features a cylindrical dark brown to black "eye" in the center surrounded by wide-open, golden-yellow petals. These bloom in summer to early fall, reaching up to 3 inches wide and presenting up to twenty-one petals.

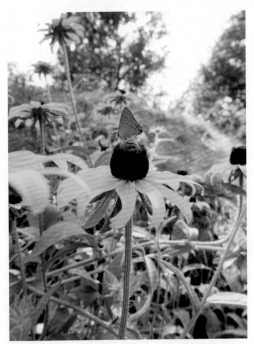

Black-eyed Susan's stems are sparsely covered in stiff hairs. The flower attracts pollinating insects, like this gray hairstreak (*Strymon melinus*).

Where, When, and How to Wildcraft

Black-eyed Susan is a popular garden plant in the Northeast, where it is also native. You'll find this aster family plant growing in disturbed soils, in meadows and fields, and at the edges of woodlands, as well as in cultivated gardens.

Gather leaves from spring to late summer. Collect the flowers in summer when they are at peak bloom. Harvest the root in fall when the flowers die back.

Medicinal Uses

The roots and flowers of black-eyed Susan stimulate the immune system, similarly to its coneflower cousin, echinacea. Use a tincture or decoction of the roots at the first signs of a cold. One of the signatures for black-eyed Susan is the concentric rings present on the cone part of the flower. "Deer eye" (*awiakata*) is a Tsalagi (Cherokee) word for this plant, again referring to the cone. Both of these are reflective of the deer tick and the concentric rings of a rash from *Borrelia burgdorferi* or Lyme disease exposure. Black-eyed Susan, a potent anti-inflammatory, is a Cherokee remedy for Lyme disease. Always consult an experienced healthcare practitioner if you have experienced a tick bite.

The cone shape is also a signature for the head and for abscess or *something that comes to a head*. The root juice is a Cherokee remedy for earache. Black-eyed Susan is antiseptic and has been traditionally used

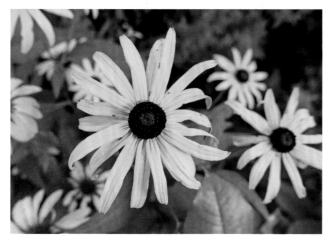

Black-eyed Susan and echinacea are related and share some medicinal uses.

gives us the strength and protection to face them with compassion. The dark center represents our shadow aspects while the golden petals represent the light of day. Black-eyed Susan allows us to sit with both parts of ourselves in balance, releasing shame and restoring love for all aspects of our being.

Future Harvests

Sow black-eyed Susan seeds directly into the soil in fall or spring to encourage future growth and harvests.

to treat snakebites. Apply a wash or poultice of the roots to venomous bites, stings, or lingering sores.

When old beliefs and hidden emotions hold us back, black-eyed Susan flower essence

Two species related to black-eyed Susan are at risk in the Northeast—orange coneflower (*R. fulgida*) in New Jersey and cutleaf coneflower (*R. laciniata*), which is threatened in Rhode Island, but abundant elsewhere.

HERBAL PREPARATIONS

Tea
Standard decoction of dried roots
Drink 4 ounces 3 times per day. Drink smaller more frequent doses, 2 ounces every hour, for acute infection.

Tincture
1 part fresh flowers and roots
2 parts menstruum (50% alcohol, 50% water)
or
1 part dried flowers and roots
5 parts menstruum (50% alcohol, 50% water)
Take 30–60 drops 3 times per day.

Flower essence
Follow instructions for making flower essences on page 54. Take 3 drops on the tongue or in water 3 times per day or as needed.

The "eye" of black-eyed Susan even boasts lush eyelashes.

black walnut

Juglans nigra
eastern black walnut
PARTS USED leaves, nut hulls, nuts

Antiparasitic, antimicrobial, and astringent black walnut has an affinity with the brain, heart, and intestinal tract. Leaf extracts have an inhibitory effect on certain kinds of tumors.

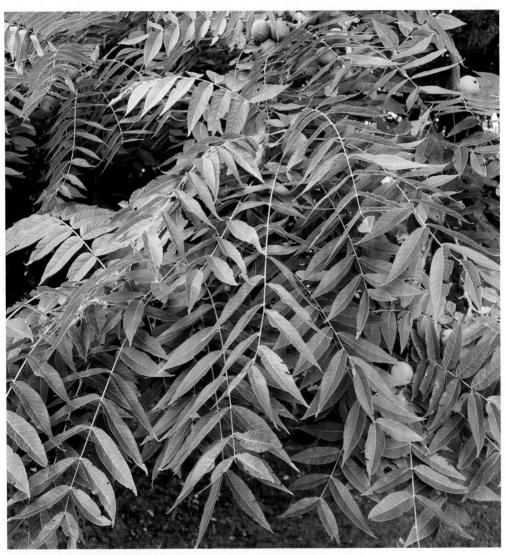

Black walnut's compound leaves give the canopy a sort of lacy look.

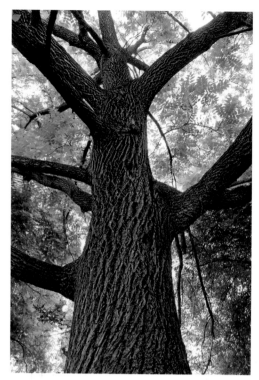
Mature bark is dark gray-brown to black and furrowed in a diamond pattern.

How to Identify

Black walnut is a deciduous tree growing as tall as 75–100 feet sporting rough, diamond-patterned, dark gray-brown to black bark. Younger trees tend to have a more draping habit while older ones have long trunks with a circular habit of high branches. The alternate compound leaves are comprised of ten to twenty-four toothed, ovate to lanceolate leaflets. There is sometimes a small terminal leaflet, but often not. In summer, green-hulled nuts form.

Where, When, and How to Wildcraft

Find black walnut in forests, meadows, fields, and disturbed areas. Collect the leaves in spring. Gather nuts in late summer to early fall when they start to fall to the ground—watch not to get conked on the head! Wear gloves when processing black walnut hulls as they stain the skin. In addition to using the green hulls in tincture, they also make a great plant dye or natural ink. For a nut harvest, remove the outer hull and dry the shelled nut for 2–3 weeks in a well-ventilated area. Alternately, place them in a large dehydrator set to 95°F for 3–4 days. Opening the shell to get to the nutmeat takes quite a lot of force. A hammer, brick, or large rock against a sidewalk should do the trick. A shop vise also works, although it may be slower going.

Medicinal Uses

The leaves and hulls of black walnut are astringent, bitter, and aromatic. The green hull and heart-shaped cross section of an unripe nut suggest an affinity with the heart center. Black walnut has a toning effect on the blood vessels and reduces hypertension.

The curling shape and structure of the nut inside correspond with the serpentine shapes of the brain. Walnuts are considered "brain food," high in mono- and polyunsaturated fats, including linoleic acid and alpha-linolenic acid, an omega-3 fatty acid. They are also high in B vitamins, antioxidants, and essential minerals. Chew on two or three per day to get your dose of these important nutrients.

Black walnut's bitter taste tells us of its action on the gallbladder and liver, ultimately aiding in digestion, assimilation, and elimination. Use black walnut leaf infusion or black walnut hull tincture to relieve constipation. An infusion of black walnut leaves or a tincture of the hulls improves the health of intestinal mucosa and eliminates parasites.

In Appalachian folk medicine, black walnut hulls are traditionally used to treat goiter or hypothyroidism. Iodine, an essential mineral for thyroid function, is found in the hulls. In cases of iodine deficiency,

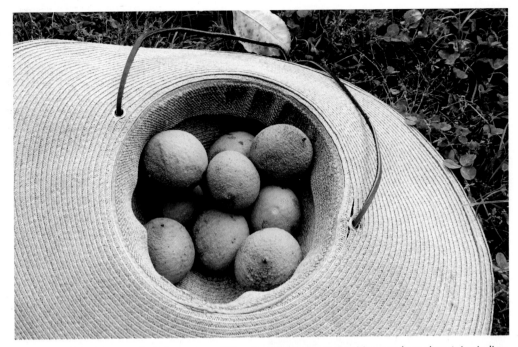

A tincture of the green nut hulls is used as a bitter digestive, an antiparasitic remedy, and contains iodine.

apply a 3-inch square of black walnut (green) hull tincture with a cotton ball or makeup brush to the inside of the arm or leg daily. Continue applying daily until the body no longer absorbs the tincture within 1 hour of application.

Externally, a leaf infusion applied as a wash or poultice eradicates ringworm. It also assuages symptoms of skin conditions such as eczema, acne, and impetigo.

⚠ Precautions

Use caution with medications for hypertension, as black walnut may lower blood pressure.

Do not use black walnut medicinally during pregnancy or breastfeeding. One of the active constituents of black walnut is juglone, which may cause deformities in the developing fetus.

Black walnut hulls stain skin and clothing, so it's best to wear gloves when handling.

Future Harvests

Collecting walnuts from the ground does not harm the tree. Picking a modest number of developing walnuts from a tree should not cause damage. To collect leaves without compromising the tree, check for fallen branches after a windstorm, or make use of ones that are available as a consequence of pruning.

HERBAL PREPARATIONS

Tea
Standard infusion of dried leaves
Drink 1 cup 3 times per day. Use as a wash for ringworm, eczema, acne, or impetigo.

Tincture
1 part fresh green hulls
2 parts menstruum (50% alcohol, 50% water)
Take 15–30 drops 3 times per day. Apply topically as an iodine supplement.

blue flag iris

Iris versicolor
harlequin blue flag
PARTS USED rhizomes

Deeply cleansing, water-loving blue flag iris is synonymous with fluid regulation.

How to Identify
Blue flag iris is a conspicuously flowering perennial herbaceous plant that forms clumping colonies in wet habitats. In spring elegant blue to purple blooms with distinct purple veins emerge. Toward the center of the three purple sepals you'll find a white background featuring prominent purple veins and a pale yellow splotch. Deep green to blue-green, narrow, lance-shaped leaves tend to overlap each other in a fanning pattern. The leaves grow up to 2 feet long with the flowers rising up another 6 inches above that. Seed capsules form after flowering. The root system is comprised of hardy rhizomes with thin, unbranching rootlets.

Where, When, and How to Wildcraft
Blue flag iris has a strong preference for water. Look for it on the edges of fresh waterways and marshes. Keep in mind where the flowers were growing in spring to early summer—harvest roots (rhizomes) from these previously noted plants in late summer to early autumn and dry for later use.

Medicinal Uses
Blue flag iris is deeply detoxifying and has a strongly stimulating action on the liver, gallbladder, and kidneys. An infusion of the dried root floods the digestive system with fluid to enhance elimination. This can go to the extreme if taken in excess, resulting in an overwhelming evacuation of fluids from the body either through vomiting, diarrhea, or diuresis. Small doses are essential to prevent undesirable effects.

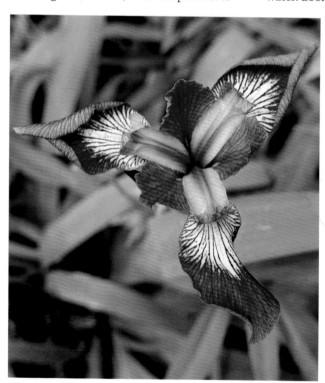

Irises are named for Iris, goddess of rainbows, who inspires beauty and artistic pursuits.

Like the excessive outcomes seen when too much of it is used, blue flag iris root treats extremes or fluctuations. Use blue flag root tincture when hormonal fluctuations of the thyroid and pituitary gland bring on extreme changes in mood and energy level.

Blue flag iris is also useful where there is dryness and burning of the digestive mucosa and the skin. Use the tincture to increase salivation in those with dry mouth and improve digestive fluid output in those with burning "dry" intestines. Make a blue flag iris poultice by mashing the reconstituted dried roots and applying to skin that is afflicted with psoriasis, acne, herpes, or festering wounds. Apply the poultice to swollen joints in case of acute or chronic injury or arthritis. Use a compress or wash to relieve sunburn.

Similarly to the herb, homeopathic *Iris versicolor* is used to treat enlarged glands, especially the thyroid, pancreas, and intestinal glands, and supports the healthy flow of hormones and digestive juices and enzymes.

Use iris flower essence to inspire artistic expression, clearing patterns of stagnation and self-limiting beliefs to make way for creativity, especially in the musical and visual realms.

⚠ Precautions

Do not use blue flag iris during pregnancy or breastfeeding.

Do not use the fresh root of blue flag iris. Use only the minimum therapeutic dose of the dried root to prevent toxic side effects that can be experienced with overdose. These include extreme inflammation and burning sensation of mucous membranes,

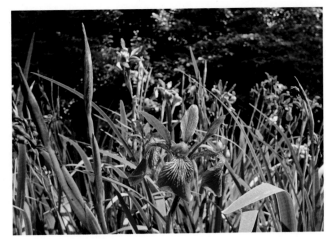

Look for blue flag iris in shallow pools of fresh water or at the edge of watery zones.

difficulty breathing, severe diarrhea, and other life-threatening symptoms, especially in people with weakened constitutions.

Wear gloves when harvesting as the fresh root can also cause skin irritation in some.

Future Harvests

Only a small amount of rhizome is needed to make an effective medicine. Take a portion of the rootstock and replant what you don't use. Blue flag iris can be propagated by dividing the roots and directly planting in the soil from which you harvested. Thinning a clump of iris encourages new growth.

HERBAL PREPARATIONS

Tincture
1 part dried rhizomes
5 parts menstruum (50% alcohol,
  50% water)
Take 1–5 drops as needed.

Flower essence
Follow instructions for making flower essences on page 54. Take 3 drops on the tongue or in water 3 times per day or as needed.

Scutellaria lateriflora
mad-dog skullcap
PARTS USED aerial parts in flower, leaves

*Antispasmodic and anxiolytic, blue skullcap is a great ally
for reducing tension as well as easing and overcoming anxiety.*

How to Identify

Blue skullcap is a perennial mint family plant native to North America. Toothed leaves up to 3 inches long and 2 inches wide grow oppositely in pairs from square stems that range from green to red-green. The leaves are darker green on the topside of the leaf than the bottom.

In summer, tubular, two-lipped, pale purple, white, or blue flowers (about ⅓ inch) bloom in pairs of up to six or seven in racemes emerging from the leaf axils. The calyx at the base of the flower is shaped like an upside-down plate, or *scutella*, and that's how *Scutellaria* got its name.

Blue skullcap spreads by seed and rhizome and can form small colonies in the right conditions.

The plant is bitter and not very aromatic.

Where, When, and How to Wildcraft

Blue skullcap likes moist soil in partially shaded areas, from marshes and the edges of waterways to meadows and fields.

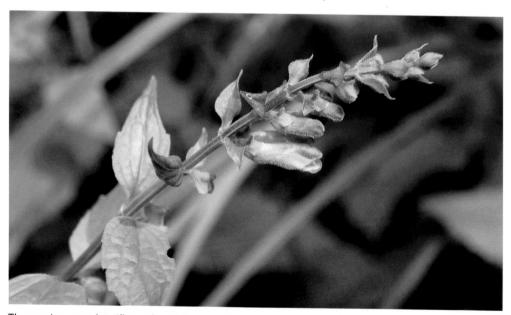

The species name *lateriflora* refers to how the flower racemes of blue skullcap grow out of the side of the leaf axils. Violet-colored flowers are a signature for the nervous system and indicate an affinity with the third eye chakra and mental processes.

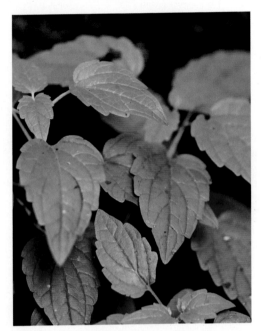

The young plant before flowering. Opposite toothed leaves grow from square stems, characteristic of mint family plants.

Collect leaves in late spring to early summer. Throughout summer, gather the aerial portions of the plant when in flower. It's best tinctured fresh and it can be dried for tea.

Medicinal Uses

Blue skullcap is a must-have nervine for any apothecary. The tincture of the aerial parts brings relief to insomnia, especially where there is stress and anxiety. With wild lettuce, mugwort, and mullein root, it helps bring on sleep where pain is involved.

It is calming to frazzled nerves; relieving to tension headaches; and settling to twitches, tics, and spasms. Combine blue skullcap and blue vervain in tincture to reduce symptoms of restless legs syndrome. Adding ginkgo leaf to this pairing may reduce tremors in Parkinson's disease.

Taken as a tonic, blue skullcap can help those who get stuck in mental processes or have a hard time letting go of heightened emotions. It brings a sense of embodiment and grounding where there is overthinking, worry, or spaciness. A few drops of blue skullcap tincture can be taken before meditation to support mental clarity and focus by helping to relax tension and dissolve discursive thoughts.

Blue skullcap, motherwort, and rose make a great team to ease premenstrual symptoms, particularly anxiety, tension, mood swings, and breast tenderness.

⚠ Precautions

Do not use blue skullcap during pregnancy as it may be too stimulating to the uterus.

Future Harvests

Blue skullcap is the most widespread and stable of this native genus, so favor this species over others that are at risk in the Northeast, including *S. incana*, *S. integrifolia*, *S. parvula*, and *S. serrata*. If these species are in good conservation status in your area, they can be used interchangeably. Propagate skullcap by seed or root division. Plant stratified seeds in moist soil.

HERBAL PREPARATIONS

Tea
Standard infusion of dried aerial parts in flower and/or leaves
Drink 4-8 ounces as needed. Use as a compress for headaches.

Tincture
1 part fresh leaves
2 parts menstruum (95% alcohol, 5% water)
Take 3-5 drops to take the edge off mild tension. Take 20-30 drops to induce sleep.

---

blue vervain

Verbena hastata
blue verbena, swamp verbena
PARTS USED flowering tops, leaves

*Blue vervain is a stunning native plant valued
for its benefits to the nervous and digestive systems.*

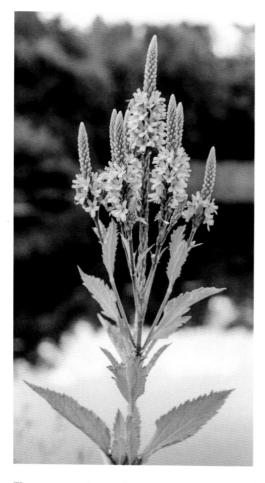

The name *vervain* or *verbena* comes from Latin,
meaning "sacred bough" or "altar plant" and refers
to European vervain (*V. officinalis*) as well as other
plants sacred to the ancient Greeks, Egyptians,
and Romans.

How to Identify
Blue vervain is a perennial herbaceous plant
growing 2–6 feet high. The lance-shaped,
coarsely toothed, short-stalked leaves grow
opposite each other up the stem. In summer,
small blue-purple flowers grow on numerous
antenna-like spikes somehow both graceful
and gangly in appearance.

Where, When, and How to Wildcraft
Blue vervain grows in open fields and meadows, as well as marshes and wetland edges.
Collect leaves and flowers from the top third
of the plant in summer to early fall when it
is in bloom. After harvesting, strip off the
leaves and flowers to tincture fresh or dry for
use in tea.

Medicinal Uses
Blue vervain suits those who are hot and
bothered, in other words chronic worriers or
perfectionists with matching chronic neck
and shoulder tension. The acrid bitterness of
this herb makes one shudder, an action that
indicates its relaxant effect on the nervous
system. Regular doses of the tincture foster
an unwinding of tight muscles, furrowed
brows, and knotted stomachs. Combine blue
vervain with chamomile and blue skullcap
in an infusion to relieve insomnia caused
by mild anxiety, nervousness, or restless
legs syndrome.

The cooling relaxant action of blue vervain is also helpful for reducing fever in people who are restless and uncomfortable, with an appearance of wanting to shake off their illness in impatience.

Like other bitter tonics, blue vervain fosters healthy liver function and stimulates bile production to aid in digestion. By helping the liver process hormones, blue vervain clears hot skin conditions, such as acne. You can also use a wash or compress of the infusion externally to treat skin inflammations.

Use the tincture of blue vervain to ease menstrual cramping and bring on delayed menstruation caused by heat and tension in the uterus.

The flower essence is akin to the medicinal uses of the plant, chiefly calming agitation, anger, and underlying bitterness.

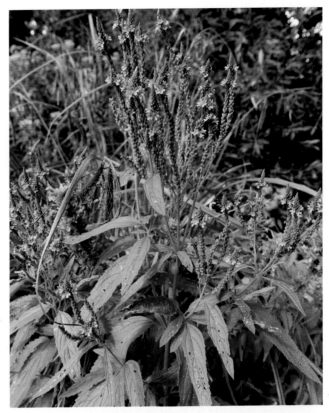

Blue vervain can sometimes have a bushy and scraggly appearance.

⚠ Precautions

Do not use blue vervain in pregnancy as it is too cooling and relaxing to the uterus.

Higher-than-needed doses can induce nausea and vomiting.

Future Harvests

Collecting select leaves and flowers from the upper parts of the plant will encourage branching. Once plants have gone to seed in fall, shake the seeds and directly plant in the soil to ensure future harvests.

HERBAL PREPARATIONS

Tea
Standard infusion of dried flowering tops and leaves
Drink 2–4 ounces as needed.

Tincture
1 part fresh flowering tops and leaves
2 parts menstruum (70% alcohol, 30% water)
Take 1–3 drops to start and up to 30 drops as needed.

Flower essence
Follow instructions for making flower essences on page 54. Take 3 drops on the tongue or in water 3 times per day or as needed.

boneset

Eupatorium perfoliatum
thoroughwort
PARTS USED flowering tops, leaves

Astringent and bitter, boneset is an antiviral, antibacterial herb that also stimulates digestion and increases appetite.

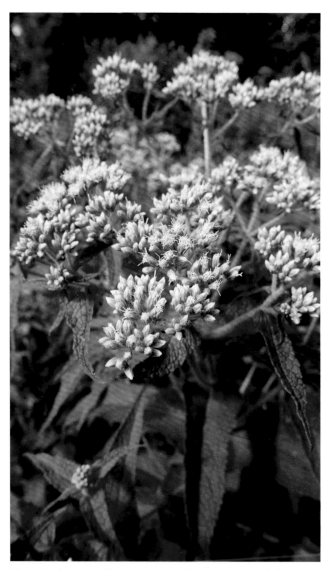

The white blooms of boneset emerge from summer to fall.

How to Identify

Boneset is a perennial herb growing up to 4 feet high with a round, upright, hair-covered stem. The dark green leaves are opposite, finely toothed, and lanceolate. Lower leaves are oppositely fused together (perfoliate) and up to 8 inches in length. Upper leaves are up to 4 inches long and fused to the stem. The foliage is rough on top and resinous and bumpy underneath. From summer to early fall, boneset blooms in a multitude of composite flowerheads with ten to twenty white florets with a shaggy appearance.

Where, When, and How to Wildcraft

Boneset is often found in wet places, from disturbed habitats to the edges of lakes, rivers, and swamps. Gather the upper third of the plant in mid- to late summer or early fall when it is in bloom.

Medicinal Uses

Boneset has been traditionally used for fever and colds, as well as for arthritis and gastrointestinal upset, applications that continue to be used in modern herbalism.

The common name *boneset* originates from its use for dengue fever or *breakbone* fever, a mosquito-borne illness once common in wet places of North America. The herb was also historically used to treat malaria.

Boneset is anti-inflammatory, antispasmodic, expectorant, and diaphoretic. Drink a warm infusion of boneset, elderflower, and spearmint to ease aching flu-like symptoms, alleviate respiratory congestion, and reduce fever.

Boneset stimulates appetite and digestion and, in some cases, eradicates parasites from the intestines. Use boneset tincture for relieving constipation, especially in those with poor appetite and weakened constitutions where the peristaltic action is compromised.

⚠ Precautions

Taking too much boneset can cause nausea, vomiting, and diarrhea. Luckily, the bitterness of this herb is usually enough to prevent those untoward effects from happening.

Future Harvests

Boneset is threatened by habitat loss. When coming across a stand of boneset be mindful of this and harvest only the aerial parts of a small portion of plants. Propagate by dividing the plants after they go to seed in fall, or in spring when young shoots appear.

HERBAL PREPARATIONS

Tea
Standard infusion of dried flowering tops and leaves
Drink 1 cup, hot, 3 times per day.

Tincture
1 part fresh flowering tops
2 parts menstruum (55% alcohol, 45% water)
or
1 part dried flowering tops
5 parts menstruum (55% alcohol, 45% water)
Take 30 drops 3 times per day.

---

borage

Borago officinalis
starflower
PARTS USED flowers, leaves

*Borage has been recognized throughout the ages
for its ability to bring joy to the heart.*

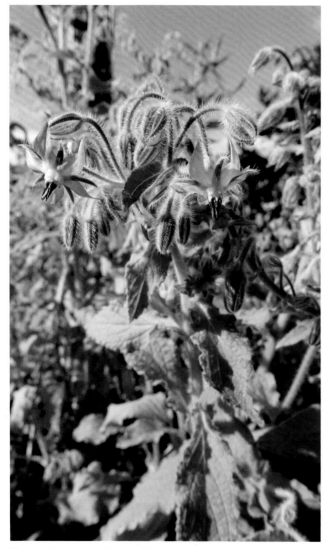

"Borage for courage" is an old adage that speaks to the herb's ability to restore the nerves and uplift the mood.

How to Identify

Borage is an herbaceous self-seeding annual plant composed of dark green, deeply veined, wrinkled leaves that are 2–6 inches long, with the lower leaves on the larger end of the spectrum. The entire plant is covered in bristly white hairs that catch the light and give it a glowing appearance. The stems are round, hollow, and branched. Bright blue, upright, five-petaled flowers with a prominent cone of black anthers adorn the top of the plant; unopened blooms droop downward sporting pink sepals covered in prickly hairs, like the rest of the plant.

Where, When, and How to Wildcraft

Borage is an introduced garden escapee found in disturbed habitats, meadows, and fields. Collect the leaves in late spring to summer or the leaves and flowers together throughout summer to use fresh or dry for later. It's best to harvest on a dry, sunny day to prevent rot or wilt.

Medicinal Uses

Soothing, cooling, demulcent borage has a restorative effect on the nervous system. Note the prominent hairs covering the entire plant and the blue flower—both features are signatures for the nerves. Take a borage infusion for nervous exhaustion or adrenal depletion, especially during hormonal fluctuations coinciding with menopause or hyperthyroidism.

Borage has an uplifting quality to the heart and mood and is traditionally used for depressive or melancholic states. Make a comforting infusion of borage with lemon balm, hawthorn, and linden blossoms to lighten a heavy, burdened, or grieving heart. Alternately, you can use the flower essence of borage to this effect.

Borage promotes diuresis and through this action conveys cooling to inflamed, feverish conditions. Borage-infused honey allays coughs, wheezing, asthma, and other lung irritations. This can be eaten off the spoon or infused in warm water as a sweet tea.

Externally, a borage poultice brings relief to damaged skin, wounds, and sores.

⚠ Precautions

Borage contains small amounts of pyrrolizidine alkaloids. Tested in animals, in isolation from the whole plant, these alkaloids have been implicated in liver disease. It is recommended that those with liver conditions avoid use of plants containing pyrrolizidine alkaloids. (Note that oil of borage and the flower essence do not contain these alkaloids.)

To keep on the safe side, limit use of borage to 6 weeks at a time.

Future Harvests

Being a prolific reproducer, the future of borage populations will not be harmed by harvesting its leaves and flowers.

HERBAL PREPARATIONS

Tea
Standard infusion of dried leaves
Drink 2–4 ounces up to 3 times per day.

Infused honey
1 part fresh flowers and leaves
2 parts honey
Take 1 teaspoon in warm water as needed.

Tincture
1 part fresh flowers and leaves
2 parts menstruum (50% alcohol,
   50% water)
Take 3–5 drops 3 times per day.

Flower essence
Follow instructions for making flower essences on page 54. Take 3 drops on the tongue or in water 3 times per day or as needed.

bull thistle

Cirsium vulgare
spear thistle
PARTS USED flowers, leaves, roots

Standing tall and prickly, bull thistle is useful where there is stabbing pain or in joint pain caused by arthritic conditions.

How to Identify

Bull thistle is a robust biennial herbaceous plant starting its first year as a basal rosette of dark green, deeply lobed, downy, prickle-covered leaves. The lobes and leaf tips end in tan spikes. In the second year, thorny wings adorn the upright stem. Magenta flowers, 1½–2 inches wide, emerge in mid- to late summer. The petals of the flower appear as one big tuft on top of a spiky head. Bull thistle can grow up to 6 feet tall.

Where, When, and How to Wildcraft

It's hard to miss bull thistle in open fields, meadows, and in the edge. Collect the taproot in fall of the first year through early spring of the second. From summer to fall, gather the leaves of the first-year basal rosette, which will yield more plant material than the small second-year leaves. Collect flowers from late summer to early fall when in bloom.

Protect your skin while harvesting this bristly plant. Wear sturdy gloves and

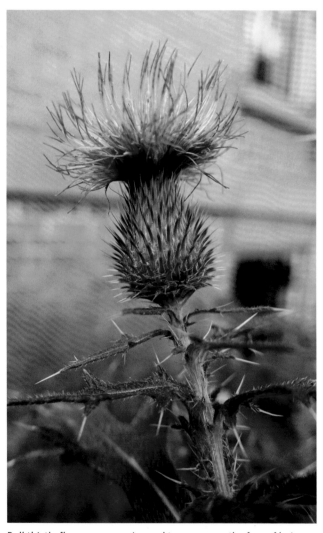

Bull thistle flower essence is used to overcome the fear of being bullied or trapped, and it imparts the confidence to communicate—especially with authority figures—from a grounded place.

thick long-sleeves to prevent
scratches or irritation.

Medicinal Uses

Take a look at this formidable
plant covered in spikes. Looks
like it might hurt, right? This
suggests its efficacy in relieving
stabbing pain. The Haudenosaunee discovered bull thistle's
usefulness in treating bleeding
hemorrhoids—also known
as "piles"—and the first-year
growth of leaves is like a pile
of something that would make
one's behind bleed if they sat
upon it. Make a bull thistle leaf infusion to
use as a sitz bath to treat hemorrhoids.

Use the tincture to relieve joint pain
from conditions such as rheumatoid or
psoriatic arthritis.

If you are having a difficult relationship
with someone in a place of authority, bull
thistle flower essence gives you confidence
to stand your ground and speak your
truth confidently.

 Precautions

Pay close attention when harvesting, so
as not to poke yourself with the spines.

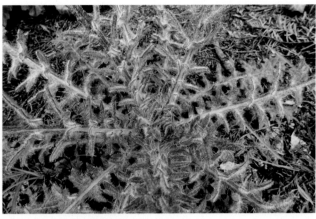

First-year leaves of bull thistle form a basal rosette covered in
down and thorns.

Future Harvests

Bull thistle is considered a difficult to eradicate
or noxious weed, so you'd be doing a service to
harvest and utilize this plant for medicine.

HERBAL PREPARATIONS

Tea

Standard decoction of dried roots
*Drink 1 cup 3 times per day. Use as a sitz bath
for hemorrhoids.*

Tincture

1 part fresh basal leaves
2 parts menstruum (50% alcohol,
   50% water)
Take 40–60 drops 3 times per day.

Flower essence

*Follow instructions for making flower essences
on page 54. Take 3 drops 4 times per day or as
needed.*

burdock

Arctium species

PARTS USED leaves, roots, seeds

While some may regard burdock as a highly invasive, noxious weed, those in the know have come to love this hardy, tenacious plant with great value as a restorative tonic that balances intestinal flora.

How to Identify

Burdock is an introduced plant that begins as a basal rosette of stemmed leaves growing from a central taproot. The young leaves are spade or heart shaped. As they get larger, the soft, green leaves resemble a long, frilly-edged tongue with a prominent central vein. The leaves are downy white on the underside, distinguishing burdock from other "dock" plants. Depending on environmental conditions, burdock can act like a biennial or a perennial that takes 4 or more years to develop into its "biennial" form. When it does reach this next phase of growth, burdock sends up a branching stalk from its center, adorned with alternate leaves similar in appearance to the young basal leaves. In summer, globe-shaped flowers topped with purple and silver tufts bloom, covered in green hooked barbs. These become the burs that famously stick to clothing and animal fur.

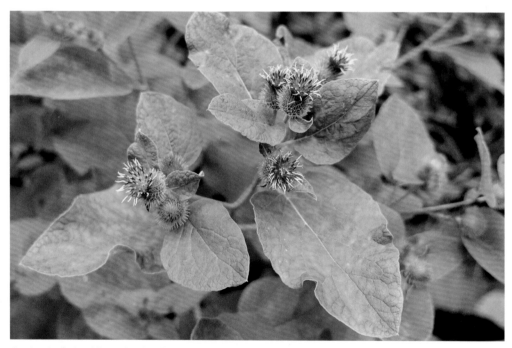

Arctium is derived from the Greek *arctos* or "bear," and burdock is considered bear medicine, or a nourishing herb that brings about great healing, in the lands where it grows.

Where, When, and How to Wildcraft

Burdock loves the edge. You'll find the first- and second-year plants growing in disturbed soils, at the dripline of trees, and at the margins of forested areas.

Harvest the roots in fall of the first year through spring of the second year while most of the plant's energy is down in the earth. To find burdock roots at the right stage, look for the previous year's dead stalks covered in brown burs. The younger plants growing nearby are the ones from which to harvest. Burdock isn't picky about soil conditions and is often growing in compacted earth. Digging roots after rain or choosing plants growing in sandier soils will ease the process. It takes quite a bit of digging and you may not get all the root. Clean the roots well, chop them and dry them for use in infusions. I like to julienne and sauté fresh roots in oil, soy sauce, and mirin to make a Japanese appetizer called kinpira gobo. The fresh or dried roots also make a nutrient-dense addition to broths.

Collect leaves in peak season, from late spring to early fall. Gather seeds (if they don't find you first!) after the flower dies back.

Place seedheads in a paper or burlap bag. Roll over the bag firmly several times with a rolling pin or take the bag outside and smash it with a rubber mallet. For this next part, put on rubber gloves, a mask, and work clothes that you don't mind getting covered in burdock fluff. Pour the crushed seedheads into a relatively flat bowl or basket and take outside. Standing with your back to the wind (or a fan) winnow the seeds from the chaff by flipping the bowl away and toward your body while allowing the wind to take the outer hairs of the seed. The seeds should collect in the bottom. Alternately you can separate the pieces with a utensil like a fork or spoon. Crush or powder the seeds and tincture promptly.

Medicinal Uses

Burdock draws nutrients up to nourish the soil and in turn the root does the same for

---

Release Ritual

This ritual has the power to help you release anything which isn't serving you.

Find a large burdock leaf. Take a comfortable seat, outside if you can. Bring your attention to your body. Where do you feel tension and gripping? What sensations or emotions are you holding in these areas of your body? Listen within. We hold memories, ideas, and emotions in our bodies that we aren't even aware of, sometimes for years. When you become aware of what you are holding, think about whether it serves you. When you realize what you'd like to release, write it down on the leaf. For example, "I am releasing my feelings of anger toward my brother," "I am releasing my feelings of unworthiness," or "I am releasing my relationship with an estranged friend." Get as specific as you can.

Once you've finished writing as much or as little as you'd like, fold up your leaf and secure it closed with something compostable, such as twine or another plant's stems. Hold the bundle to your heart and state out loud, "I am ready to release what isn't serving me." Find a place outside to release your bundle. You could bury it or throw it off a cliff or into a river. Or you could just toss it into the woods or into a big patch of burdock. Release it in a place that calls to you.

us by facilitating healthy digestion, assimilation, and elimination. Burdock root makes a rich, nourishing, mineral-full decoction that serves as a deeply restorative tonic after illness or depletion. Taken regularly over weeks or months the root decoction brings health and detoxification to the whole body, especially the liver and intestines. Burdock root contains inulin, a prebiotic fiber that feeds beneficial gut bacteria, altering the terrain of the body toward balance.

In restoring function to the liver and cleansing the blood of toxins, burdock clears inflammatory conditions, such as acne, eczema, psoriasis, and arthritis.

As deep as the roots go in the soil, burdock moves stagnant anger stored deep in our bodies. (The liver is the seat of anger.) Work with burdock root or flower essence to heal ancestral wounds and deep-seated emotional patterns. Partnered with meditation and the adjacent "Release Ritual," burdock brings emotional, physical, and psychic relief to old hurts.

Take burdock seed tincture as a diuretic to reduce swelling in the joints. Add burdock seed and echinacea root tinctures to a bit of water to use as a mouthwash for toothache relief.

Use burdock leaf poultice to treat acne and infected boils.

⚠ Precautions
Do not use burdock seed during pregnancy.

Future Harvests
Burdock is considered highly invasive, grows in a variety of soil conditions, and is a prolific seed setter. At this time there is no concern over its future in the Northeast.

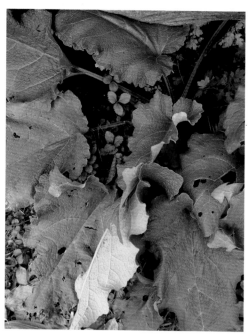

Burdock leaves feature downy white undersides, distinguishing this plant from other unrelated yet similar-looking dock plants.

HERBAL PREPARATIONS

Tea
Standard decoction of fresh or dried roots
Drink 4–6 ounces 3 times per day.

Tincture
1 part fresh roots
2 parts menstruum (40% alcohol, 60% water)
Take 30–90 drops 3 times per day.
or
1 part dried seeds, crushed or powdered
5 parts menstruum (60% alcohol, 40% water)
Take 10–25 drops up to 3 times per day.

Flower essence
Follow instructions for making flower essences on page 54 . Take 3 drops on the tongue or in water 3 times per day or as needed.

catnip

Nepeta cataria
PARTS USED flowering tops, leaves

Catnip is a mildly sedating mint family herb that helps soften the edges of anxiety and calm tension held in the stomach. Catnip has a cooling effect with a pleasantly acrid, pungent, aromatic taste.

How to Identify

Catnip is a perennial herb with a square stem from which emerge opposite, heart-shaped, scallop-toothed leaves. The entire plant, which can grow 2–3 feet tall, is covered with soft, downy hairs giving it a pale gray-green hue. The leaves and blossoms have a distinctive aroma, slightly skunky and minty. Small white to pale pink-purple flowers grow densely packed on stout spikes in summer.

Where, When, and How to Wildcraft

Catnip is a garden escapee and mainly grows in edges and disturbed habitats. Collect the upper leaves from late spring to early summer and flowering tops of the plant in summer. Tincture catnip fresh or dry for later use.

Medicinal Uses

Catnip is well known by feline lovers as a stimulating herb that instigates a state

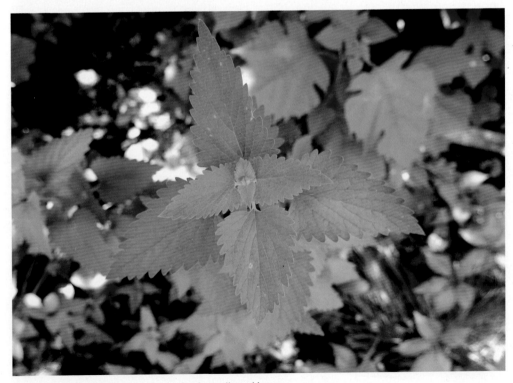

Catnip features a lovely symmetry of soft, scalloped leaves.

of euphoria in cats. While it doesn't quite induce the same feeling in humans, catnip does offer great benefits to the nervous system with its anti-spasmodic, mildly sedative effects. Drink catnip infusion to calm feelings of "edginess" and soothe stomach upset caused by nervousness. Take the infusion to alleviate mild bouts of insomnia and to support lucid dreaming.

Catnip is gentle enough for babies and small children and works well to ease colic, tense tummies, and teething symptoms. Combine catnip with chamomile and lemon balm for a belly-soothing tea. Craft a calming massage oil infused with these three herbs for infants with gassiness and bloating.

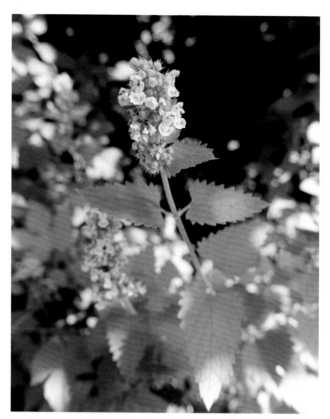

Catnip is a softening, opening, and cooling herb, assisting digestion and aiding release of heat through the pores of the skin.

This uniquely scented mint is also a well know remedy for menstrual cramps. It is a mild emmenagogue, so it can be helpful for bringing on delayed menstruation.

The cooling effect of catnip works on fever by opening the pores to encourage sweating.

Having many overlapping properties with chamomile, catnip makes a good substitute for those allergic to aster family plants.

Catnip also has insect-repelling properties and combines well in tinctures with other aromatic mint family plants to create an "aromatic pest confuser," aka, bug spray.

⚠ Precautions

Do not use with sedative drugs as catnip may increase their effects.

Future Harvests

Catnip is a popular garden herb and introduced plant that is not currently at risk in the Northeast.

HERBAL PREPARATIONS

Tea
Standard infusion of dried flowering tops and/or leaves
Drink 4–8 ounces as needed.

Tincture
1 part fresh flowering tops
2 parts menstruum (50% alcohol, 50% water)
Take 20–40 drops as needed.

---

chickweed

Stellaria media
common starwort, common stitchwort
PARTS USED aerial parts

Diminutive chickweed packs a surprising amount of medicinal power for its size. It aids in the assimilation of nutrients, soothes irritated mucous membranes, heals external wounds, and so much more.

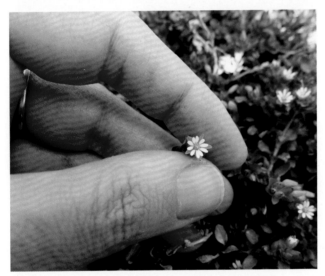

Stellaria is named for its star-shaped sepals and earned the common name chickweed for its use as nourishing fodder for chickens.

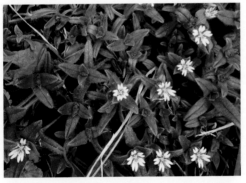

Edible mouse-eared chickweed (*C. fontanum*) looks a lot like *Stellaria* chickweed but isn't known for the same healing properties.

How to Identify

Chickweed is a delicate, succulent, low-growing perennial herb that tends to form tangled mats. The ovate leaves are arranged oppositely and in pairs up the stem. Running up the side of the stem is a single line of fine hairs that changes direction with each leaf node. Splitting the stem in half reveals a fine inner thread-like core. At first glance, the petite, white flowers of chickweed appear to have ten petals, but upon closer inspection you'll find five deeply divided petals. Cradling the petals are five hairy green sepals forming a star. Unopened flower buds nod downward like tassels on drooping stalks.

There are several species of *Cerastium*— or mouse-eared chickweed—which could be mistaken as *Stellaria* chickweed. The leaves of mouse-eared chickweed tend to be narrower, more lance-like, and fuzzier in their appearance. *Cerastium fontanum* is likely to be most easily mistaken for *S. media*. Both are edible and nutritious, but *Stellaria* is better known for its medicinal value.

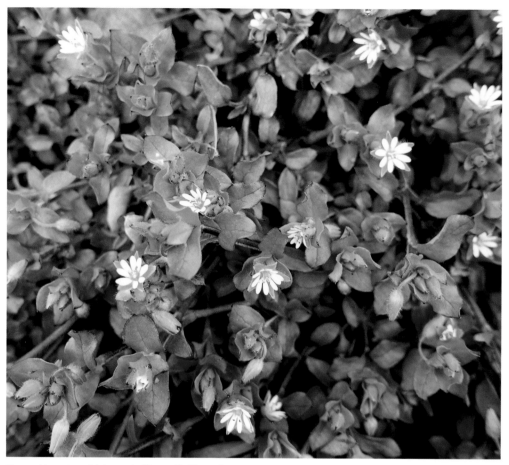

Ground-hugging chickweed offers relief for inflammation and injury, and makes a tasty, nutritious salad ingredient to boot.

Where, When, and How to Wildcraft

Chickweed might be easy to miss if you weren't looking closely at the ground. This humble plant likes cooler, slightly shady spots in the edges—hugging logs, fences, and erratic stones in disturbed habitats, meadows, and fields.

Chickweed is at its peak in spring though you may be able to find some in summer in shaded areas. Gather the entire aerial portion of the plant by hand or with small scissors. Chickweed can be dried, though it's preferable to use fresh, as a juice or succus, or in tincture.

Medicinal Uses

Despite its miniature stature, chickweed is a dynamic herb with a cooling, moistening, anti-inflammatory action for hot, dry conditions.

The deeply divided flower petals are a signature for cuts or bleeding, while the tiny hairs along the stem allude to chickweed's usefulness for the skin and nervous system. A chickweed poultice halts bleeding of fresh wounds while providing pain relief and protection against potential infection.

Chickweed takes the burning and itching out of insect bites and rashes. Make

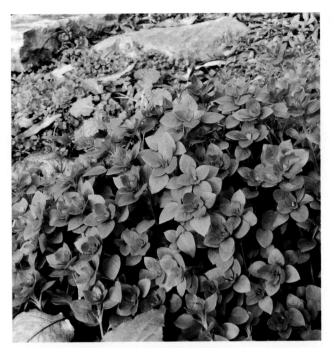
A particularly lush patch of chickweed.

Drink an infusion or take the tincture of chickweed to loosen thick, mucus-heavy coughs and ease intestinal inflammation. An infusion or tincture is also beneficial in cases of cystitis or other urinary tract inflammation, especially when combined with other demulcent, vulnerary, antimicrobial herbs such as common mallow and violet, or cleansing diuretics such as horsetail.

Future Harvests
Chickweed is a widespread, introduced plant that is not under threat of overharvesting.

chickweed ice cubes by juicing or blending the herb with water to have on hand for scrapes, burns, and bites. A salve made with chickweed-infused oil brings relief to dry, itchy winter-chapped skin. Use a chickweed compress or bath to bring relief to inflamed sore, aching joints and menstrual cramps.

A daily dose of vinegar infused with chickweed serves as a nourishing tonic to help the body assimilate nutrients while also breaking down excess fat.

Chickweed has a dissolving action on respiratory and digestive congestion, as well as on cysts and benign tumors. Massage chickweed-infused oil into breasts, lymphatic tissue, and the abdomen to break up congestion in these areas of the body.

chicory

Cichorium intybus

PARTS USED flowers, leaves, roots

Chicory is a classic bitter digestive herb that supports liver health, improves skin conditions, and relieves constipation.

How to Identify

Chicory is a perennial herb that starts as a basal rosette of deeply lobed, toothed leaves. At first glance one might mistake them for dandelion leaves; however, unlike dandelion, which has downward-pointing symmetrically opposed lobes, the lobes of chicory are at more of a right angle and tend to be alternate. Turning over the leaf of chicory reveals a hairy central rib (dandelion is smooth, sometimes with sparse, wooly hairs that lie flat).

In summer, chicory sends up stiff branching stalks covered in small, clinging stemless leaves and flower buds. One chicory plant on its own appears very spindly, while a colony of chicory plants looks like a low sprawling shrub reaching 2–3 feet high. The numerous pale blue (rarely pink) ray flowers open in the morning when the sun has not reached its apex. The flowers usually close as the day heats up. Chicory has a bitter-tasting tan-white taproot.

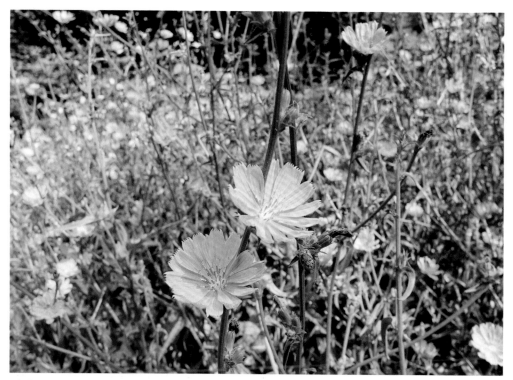

Glimpse the ethereal blue flowers in the morning before they close up with the afternoon sun.

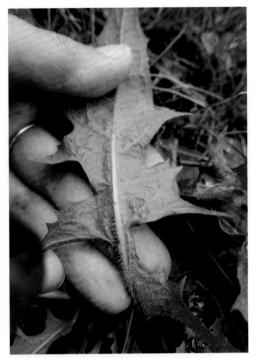

The midrib of chicory has an erect row of hairs along it, distinguishing it from its related lookalike dandelion.

Where, When, and How to Wildcraft

Chicory often graces roadsides, the edges of paths, meadows, and fields. Collect leaves in early to midspring before extreme bitterness sets in. Harvest the root in fall or early spring before the plant flowers. Gather summer-blooming flowers in the morning just as they open and before the sun becomes too intense.

Medicinal Uses

Chicory root makes a pleasantly bitter decoction that stimulates the appetite and digestion. The root is most often roasted, giving it a flavor reminiscent of coffee, for which it is often used as a substitute. Chicory has an energizing quality without being overstimulating and is diuretic without depleting the body of minerals.

Drinking the root decoction as a tonic restores intestinal balance and energy, especially useful while recovering from illness. It encourages elimination with a mild laxative

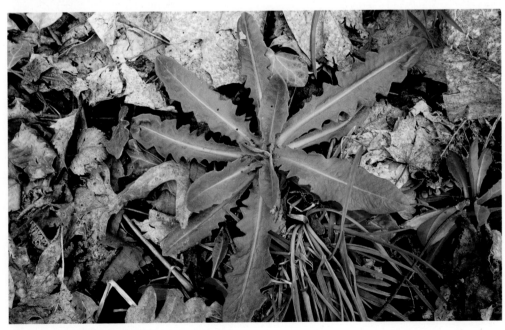

A basal rosette of young chicory leaves in spring.

effect and supports the liver through gentle detoxification. In working through the liver to improve processing of hormones and cleansing the blood of toxins, chicory clears up skin conditions such as acne and eczema. When taken over a course of weeks or months, this clearing action also benefits the joints, alleviating the pain and swelling associated with arthritis.

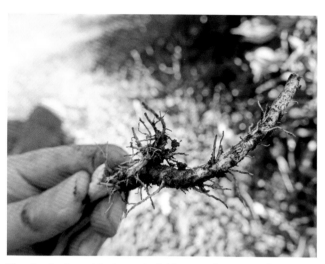

The slender tan-white taproot of chicory makes an excellent detoxifying and nourishing tonic.

The leaves and flowers are bitter as well and can be eaten in salads as an appetizer to enhance assimilation of nutrients from a meal.

Use the fresh milky latex from the stem to treat common warts.

Chicory flower essence benefits those who are controlling and overbearing in relationships, often seeking attention and praise for their deeds. The essence moves one to love more unconditionally without grasping.

⚠ Precautions

You're likely to see chicory growing abundantly at roadsides or other highly impacted areas that aren't healthy places to harvest roots for medicine. Knowing the soil conditions where you harvest from is especially important in this case.

While chicory is generally considered safe, consuming too much too frequently may lead to untoward digestive effects, including bloating and flatulence.

Future Harvests

Chicory is an abundant, introduced plant that is often considered invasive. There is currently no concern over its future in the Northeast.

HERBAL PREPARATIONS

Tea
Standard decoction of roasted roots
Add milk of your choice for a delicious, healthful coffee substitute. Drink 1 cup as desired.

Tincture
1 part fresh roots
2 parts menstruum (50% alcohol, 50% water)
or
1 part dried roots
5 parts menstruum (40% alcohol, 60% water)
Take 30–60 drops up to 3 times per day.

Flower essence
Follow instructions for making flower essences on page 54. Take 3 drops on the tongue or in water 3 times per day or as needed.

cinquefoil

Potentilla species
five finger grass
PARTS USED flowers, leaves, roots

Several species of cinquefoil, both native and introduced, grow in the Northeast. Like other members of the rose family, the astringent and cooling nature of cinquefoil is beneficial for a range of afflictions of the mucous membranes.

How to Identify
Cinquefoils, or plants in the *Potentilla* genus, are generally low-creeping—sometimes upright—perennial plants with palmately compound leaves of five toothed leaflets. They spread by runners, from which the flowers and leaves grow on individual stalks. The blossoms consist of five yellow heart-shaped petals and five green sepals.

Where, When, and How to Wildcraft
Look for cinquefoil in disturbed areas, along paths, in fields and meadows, and along streams. Collect leaves from spring through

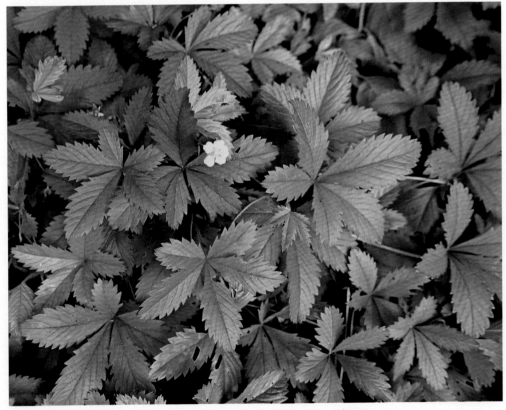

Cinquefoil translates as "five leaf," from Old French, Middle English, and Latin.

fall. Roots are ready for harvest in late summer to fall. Gather flowers to make flower essence in summer.

Medicinal Uses

Cinquefoil is a cooling, astringent herb with a toning effect. A mouthwash made from cinquefoil root decoction relieves mouth sores and tightens gum tissue to reduce looseness of teeth.

Like its fellow rose family astringent agrimony, cinquefoil has an antispasmodic quality that eases gripping pains that cause one to clench and hold their breath. Make an infusion of cinquefoil leaves or roots to alleviate stomach upset, bloating, gas, and diarrhea.

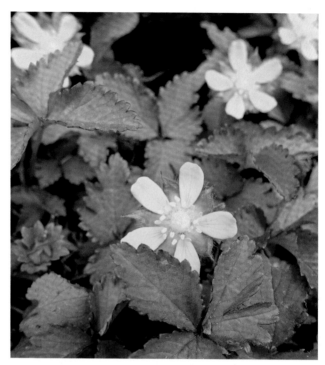

The five-petaled bright yellow flowers bloom from midspring through September.

Apply a wash or compress of cinquefoil leaf infusion to soothe topical burns.

Drink an infusion of cinquefoil, goldenrod, and strawberry leaf to bring balance to delicate tissues where candida is present.

Cinquefoil flower essence instills greater self-appreciation and self-love to those who are critical of or disconnected from themselves.

The hand-shaped leaf of cinquefoil is a sign to "keep your hands off," and the plant, both physically and metaphysically imparts a sense of unbinding. Cinquefoil is utilized in folk magic rituals to establish healthy boundaries, especially with those who overstep their bounds in your personal, work, or home life.

Future Harvests

Cinquefoil is generally considered weedy in many places where it grows. However, bushy or paradox cinquefoil (*P. paradoxa*) is threatened or endangered in parts of the Northeast. Check local conservation status and be certain of species identification before harvesting.

HERBAL PREPARATIONS

Tea

Standard decoction of dried roots
Drink 6–8 ounces as needed.

or

Standard infusion of leaves
Drink 6–8 ounces as needed. Or use as a wash for burns.

Flower essence

Follow instructions for making flower essences on page 54. Take 3 drops on the tongue or in water 3 times per day or as needed.

cleavers

Galium aparine
bedstraw, goosegrass, sticky Willy
PARTS USED aerial parts

Cleavers is a common introduced plant with cooling, detoxifying properties making it a go-to for inflamed conditions, especially of the lymphatic and urinary systems.

How to Identify

Cleavers is an herbaceous perennial that begins as a small, upright, weak-stemmed plant and grows to a gangly, flopping stature, clinging to itself and neighboring plants for dear life. The entire plant is covered in bristles which give it its characteristic stickiness. Whorls of six to eight leaves grow up the length of the square stem. Tiny white flowers grow individually or in small clusters up to three in number, followed by a small, globe-shaped, bur-like fruit.

Where, When, and How to Wildcraft

You'll find cleavers growing in semi-shaded areas with damp soil, at the edges of gardens

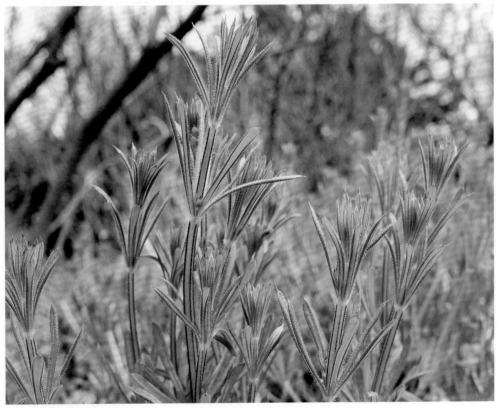

The sticky hairs of this plant inspired the common names of cleavers and sticky Willy.

and paths, overtaking ground cover in thick clusters. Collect the aerial parts all together in early spring to use as a fresh tonic and in late spring when in flower as the coumarin content increases, indicated by a sweet vanilla-like scent.

Medicinal Uses

Salty, sweet, astringent, and cool, cleavers is a useful anti-inflammatory and blood-cleansing herb that benefits nearly every system of the body. Cleavers aids the body in detoxifying from conventional cancer therapies and can be used during and after treatment.

Drink an infusion of cleavers to soothe inflammation in the urinary tract, especially in conditions such as cystitis, urethritis, and prostatitis. Sip the juice of cleavers or a cool infusion to relieve hot, inflamed conditions, including tonsillitis and glandular fever or mononucleosis infection.

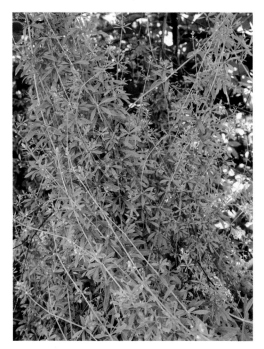

Cleavers forms tangled mats of sticky stems and whorled leaves that envelop the plants in its path.

Combine cleavers with stinging nettle and chickweed in apple cider vinegar for an antioxidant spring tonic or when recovering from illness to move stagnant lymphatic fluids. Take by the spoonful daily, either alone, in water, or as a medicinal salad dressing.

Use cleavers internally as an infusion or tincture and externally as a wash to ease inflamed skin conditions—including acne, eczema, psoriasis—and to treat wounds.

⚠ Precautions

Avoid use of cleavers in those taking blood-thinning agents and blood pressure medication, as it could increase the effects of these treatments.

Future Harvests

Cleavers is a prolific, persistent—albeit short-lived—introduced plant that can sustain a good harvest. In other words, in the Northeast, there is no harm in putting generous amounts of cleavers to good medicinal use.

HERBAL PREPARATIONS

Tea
Standard or cold infusion of fresh or dried aerial parts
Drink 1 cup as needed, up to 4 times per day.

Infused vinegar
1 part fresh aerial parts
2 parts apple cider vinegar
Take 1–2 tablespoons in water. Or use with oil as a salad dressing.

Tincture
1 part fresh aerial parts
2 parts menstruum (50% alcohol, 50% water)
Take 60 drops up to 4 times per day.

coltsfoot

Tussilago farfara
filius ante patrem (the son before the father)
PARTS USED flowers, leaves, stalks

Demulcent, expectorant coltsfoot is an effective remedy for respiratory congestion and, applied topically, provides relief from itchy, red rashes.

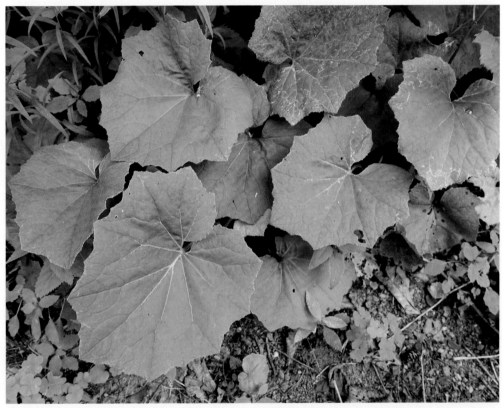

The genus name *Tussilago* hails from Latin, where *tussis* means cough, and *ago,* means to cast aside or depart.

How to Identify

Coltsfoot is a perennial herbaceous plant that prefers acidic soil and can often be found in ditches and gutters along roadsides. Coltsfoot is unique in that it blooms before its leaves form—this is where the name *filius ante patrem* (the son before the father) is derived. In early spring bunches of golden ray flowers bloom on scaly erect stems. When the flower begins to go to seed, the simple, barely lobed, heart-shaped leaves begin to emerge. The leaf has a downy white underside and its shape is somewhat reminiscent of a horse's foot, hence the name "coltsfoot."

Where, When, and How to Wildcraft

Coltsfoot is found in disturbed soils and is common along places where water gathers, such as ditches, riversides, and lakesides. Harvest flowers, including the stalks, in spring when they emerge. Collect leaves in summer.

Medicinal Uses

Moistening and expectorant, coltsfoot leaves make an excellent infusion to alleviate persistent, dry cough from bronchitis or asthma. The root has also been used historically to ease respiratory complaints, including tuberculosis. Drink an infusion of coltsfoot leaf, agrimony, and violet to soothe a scratchy sore throat and restore the voice in cases of laryngitis.

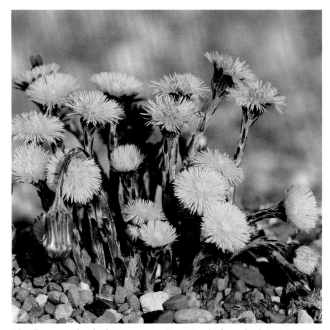

The flowers of coltsfoot emerge in spring before the leaves. Flowers and stalks are used topically for inflamed and irritated skin conditions.

Make an infusion of the leaves, flowers, and stalks to soothe the itching and redness of insect bites and to relieve symptoms of eczema.

⚠ Precautions

Coltsfoot is not recommended during pregnancy, breastfeeding, or in children. Do not use coltsfoot in those with liver disease.

There has been much debate over the use of coltsfoot and other herbs containing pyrrolizidine alkaloids (PAs). In isolation and in large doses, PAs are toxic to the liver. Use your own discretion when using PA-containing plants such as coltsfoot, comfrey, and borage, but avoid drinking tea from them if you are pregnant. If you do use coltsfoot, take the lowest effective dose and do so for short-term treatment—no more than 6 weeks at a time. When in doubt, choose another herb to suit your needs or consult with a professional herbalist or other health-care practitioner with herbal knowledge.

Future Harvests

Coltsfoot spreads fairly easily through its root system and by seed and is often considered a weed. Be sure to correctly identify coltsfoot as lookalike plants, particularly native *Petasites*, are at risk in some parts of the Northeast.

HERBAL PREPARATIONS

Tea
Standard infusion of dried flowers, leaves, and/or stalks
Drink 2–6 ounces as needed. Use topically with or without flowers and stalks.

---

comfrey

Symphytum officinale
knitbone
PARTS USED flowers, leaves, roots

*Commonly used as a fertilizer, comfrey is a fast-spreading garden herb
that is highly effective at healing wounds, both internal and external.*

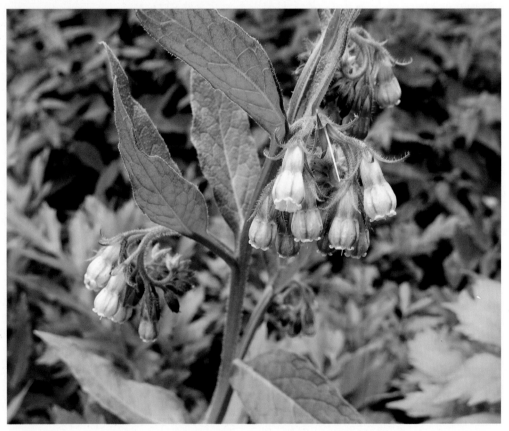

Comfrey flowers present in a range of colors, from white to pink to purple. Comfrey flower essence is used for healing deep-seated or trapped emotions.

How to Identify

Comfrey is an herbaceous perennial plant that grows in abundant colonies, each plant reaching 1–3 feet in height. The dark green, entire, bristly haired leaves are lance shaped. Basal leaves are prone to an arching habit and extend to about 8 inches in length. Upper leaves are shorter and point fairly straight out from a hairy, winged angular stem. Drooping clusters of bell-like flowers range in color from white to pink to purple. Roots are stout and dark brown.

Where, When, and How to Wildcraft

Comfrey is a common, introduced garden plant that jumped the fence. You'll find it growing in disturbed soils, meadows, and fields. Collect the leaves on a dry morning, from late spring through summer. Harvest flowers in late spring. Infuse flower buds and flowers in honey, use them in a poultice, or craft a flower essence with them. Gather roots in fall to infuse in oil or dry for later use.

Medicinal Uses

Comfrey is an unparalleled wound healer. Externally, a comfrey root salve or leaf infusion is so effective on cuts that it has been known to knit the skin back together over infected tissue, trapping it inside. Take care to clean wounds well before applying comfrey and save it for superficial cuts, as well as areas that are clear of pus and debris.

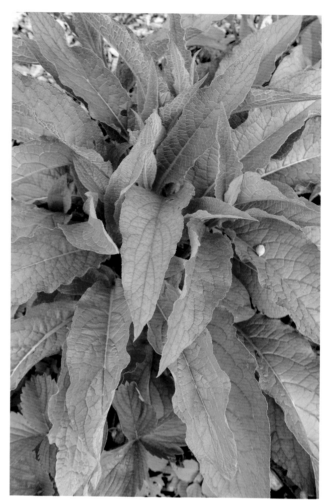

Comfrey leaves are used internally and externally to heal injured tissue, from skin and bone to stomach lining.

This seemingly magical ability to heal skin tissue also extends to the internal connective and structural tissue. Apply a poultice of comfrey leaves and mashed roots or reconstituted root powder externally to areas affected by bruises, sprained ligaments, strained tendons, and even fractured bone. Another caveat here—be sure the bones are set properly as comfrey can heal connective tissue and bone so rapidly and thoroughly that if it is out of place it may have to be rebroken.

Internally a comfrey leaf infusion heals ulcers, internal hemorrhaging, and diarrhea.

Drink comfrey leaf infusion or take honey infused with comfrey leaf to alleviate irritated bronchioles due to a dry, hacking cough. Although comfrey has been used internally for millennia, discretion must be taken due to the presence of potentially liver-damaging alkaloids. This is especially true for those with liver conditions, children, and in pregnancy and breastfeeding.

Comfrey flower essence is used to heal deep emotional wounds.

⚠ Precautions

Comfrey is not recommended during pregnancy, breast-feeding, or in children. Do not use comfrey in those with liver disease.

It is advisable to only use comfrey root externally. Do not use comfrey leaf or root on deep or open wounds or infected cuts or ulcerations. Cleanse the wound thoroughly and allow infections to clear before applying comfrey.

As with coltsfoot and borage, use your own discretion when using comfrey internally as it contains potentially liver-damaging pyrrolizidine alkaloids (PAs). If you do use comfrey, do so only in the short-term or in short cycles. When in doubt, choose another herb to suit your needs or consult with a professional herbalist or other healthcare practitioner with herbal knowledge.

Future Harvests

Comfrey is an introduced plant that easily spreads itself. Its future is not currently at risk.

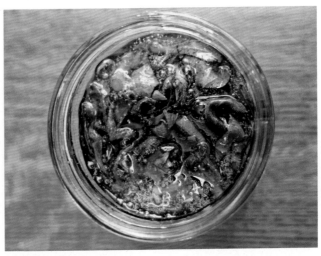

Comfrey-infused honey combines the antimicrobial action of honey with the tissue-growing abilities of the herb.

HERBAL PREPARATIONS

Tea
Standard infusion of dried leaves
Drink 4 ounces up to 3 times per day.
or
Standard decoction of roots
Use externally as a wash or compress for wounds and inflammation.

Infused oil or salve
1 part fresh roots
2 parts oil
or
1 part dried roots
4 parts oil
Use as a massage oil for strengthening connective tissue, or as a salve for wound care.

Infused honey
1 part flowers and leaves
2 parts honey
Take by the teaspoonful as needed.

Flower essence
Follow instructions for making flower essences on page 54. Take 3 drops on the tongue or in water 3 times per day or as needed.

common mallow

Malva neglecta
cheese mallow, cheeseweed
PARTS USED flowers, fruit, leaves, roots

Cooling and moistening common mallow conveys a soothing effect to irritated tissues of the respiratory, digestive, and urinary tracts.

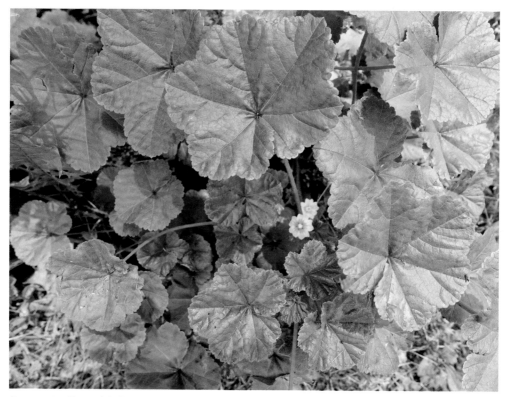

Common mallow, while being one of the more unassuming members of the mallow family, is a useful demulcent herb like its relatives.

How to Identify

Common mallow is a self-sowing annual with a spreading habit of roundly palmate, roughly scalloped leaves growing on fuzzy vining stems. Leaves grow to about 3 inches across and impart a slimy quality when chewed. Flowers—from one to three in number—present in summer on a short stalk below the leaves, fairly hidden from view. The white, pink, or pale violet flowers are just under an inch across and feature five notched petals. The fruit of common mallow is wheel-shaped, like a cheese wheel, from which derives the common names "cheese mallow" and "cheeseweed." Common mallow has a tannish white taproot.

Where, When, and How to Wildcraft

Common mallow is at home in the edges of disrupted areas, along roadsides, in parks, fields, and meadows. Collect a few leaves from each plant you find throughout the growing season, from late spring to fall. Dig the roots in late summer to fall. If you find a particularly prolific patch, take the whole plant, as every part has medicinal value.

Medicinal Uses

Reach for common mallow where there is heat, redness, and irritation, either internally or externally. Make a spit poultice for insect bites, poison ivy rashes, or minor abrasions. Brew a common mallow infusion to use in a compress for tired inflamed eyes.

Common mallow imparts mucilage when infused in cold water. This makes a soothing tea for digestive upset and constipation, especially for children. Common mallow cold infusion also relieves irritation in the urinary tract, making it useful for conditions like cystitis or urethritis. Combine common mallow with meadowsweet to ease the pain of stomach ulcers.

Future Harvests

Just as the name suggests, common mallow is a fairly ubiquitous plant that is not currently at risk of overharvesting.

HERBAL PREPARATIONS

Tea
Cold infusion of fresh or dried leaves, fruit, and/or roots
Drink 2-6 ounces as needed.

Tincture
1 part fresh roots
2 parts menstruum (40% alcohol, 60% water)
Take 30-60 drops as needed.

Viburnum opulus

European highbush cranberry, cranberry bush,
or guelder-rose (*V. opulus* var. *opulus*), American highbush
cranberry or American cranberry bush (*V. opulus* var. *americanum*)

PARTS USED bark, fruit, twigs

*Antispasmodic and sedative, crampbark brings relaxation to tight,
aching muscles and has an affinity with the uterus and kidneys.*

How to Identify

Crampbark is a tall deciduous shrub with opposite, simple, three-lobed, toothed leaves that are 2½–5 inches long. The leaves are similar in shape to maple leaves.

Dish-like clusters of white flowers (2–3 inches across) bloom in late spring to early summer. The outer ring of the inflorescence features larger five-petaled flowers while the center is comprised of smaller creamier yellow-white flowers. A cluster of egg-shaped, fleshy fruits reminiscent of cranberries (*Vaccinium* spp.) in appearance, but not taste, ripen to bright red in late summer to fall. European highbush cranberries are terrible tasting and extremely bitter, whereas the native highbush cranberry tastes much like a cranberry. When both species are available to birds, forager Sam Thayer says that the birds refuse to eat the European highbush cranberries until late winter, while the native highbush

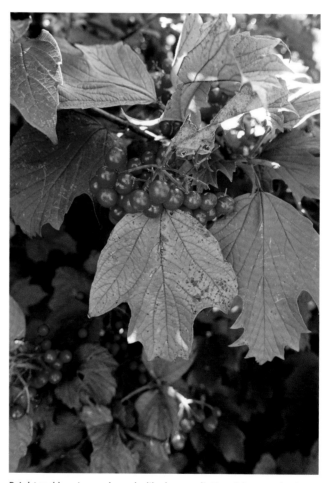

Bright red berries and maple-like leaves distinguish crampbark from other wild deciduous, fruit-bearing shrubs in the Northeast except for the native *V. edule* that shares the common name highbush cranberry.

cranberries are picked clean by the end of November.

Where, When, and How to Wildcraft

Crampbark prefers moist soil and tends to grow at the edges of forests and riparian zones or near lakes, marshes, and swamps. Prune the outer twigs and branches in spring before leafing or in late summer to fall before the leaves change color. Peel off the outer bark to process fresh in tincture or oil or dry for later use. Harvest berries when bright red and ripe in fall.

Medicinal Uses

Crampbark is as the name suggests useful for cramping conditions, from menstrual cramps to spasmodic cough. Crampbark has an affinity with the uterus and the bark has been traditionally used for preventing miscarriage. Take crampbark tincture to alleviate asthmatic symptoms, gripping pains in the abdomen, or nervous tension.

Crampbark also works well for renal colic, or pain in the kidneys from stones. Make a decoction of crampbark, spotted Joe Pye weed root, burdock seed, common mallow root, and uva-ursi leaf to ease the passage of kidney stones.

Rich in vitamin C, the berries of crampbark are anti-inflammatory and antioxidant, and can be tinctured fresh or dry to tone the heart and lower blood pressure.

Future Harvests

Carefully pruning crampbark for twigs will not harm the plant and may actually be helpful for its future growth. Do not harvest root bark from American highbush cranberry, which is rare or endangered in parts of the Northeast. It is challenging to distinguish from European highbush cranberry—one clue lies in the glands on the petiole (the leaf stalk). American highbush cranberry has more bulbous, rounded, or convex glands while the European species has flat to concave glands. Easier to see, the middle lobe of the leaves of the American highbush cranberry is long and pointed, while the middle lobe of European highbush cranberry is blunt and serrated.

Both species are susceptible to viburnum leaf beetles, which could decimate populations of *Viburnum* plants. For more information on how to identify viburnum leaf beetles and prevent their impact, visit the Cornell University's Department of Horticulture website.

HERBAL PREPARATIONS

Tea
Standard decoction of fresh or dried bark or twigs
Drink 4 ounces up to 4 times per day.

Tincture
1 part fresh bark or twigs
2 parts menstruum (50% alcohol, 50% water)
or
1 part dried bark
5 parts menstruum (50% alcohol, 50% water)
Take 30–90 drops up to 4 times per day.

Tincture
1 part fresh berries
2 parts menstruum (50% alcohol, 50% water)
or
1 part dried berries
5 parts menstruum (50% alcohol, 50% water)
Take 30–90 drops up to 4 times per day.

cranberry

Vaccinium species
large cranberry (*V. macrocarpon*), small cranberry (*V. oxycoccos*)
PARTS USED fruit

*Cranberry is an antiseptic, diuretic herb well known
for its cooling and drying actions on the urinary tract.*

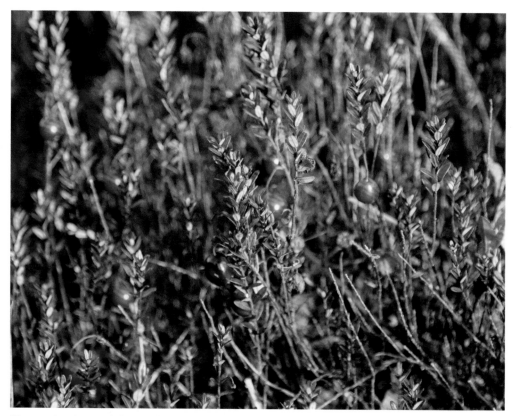

Ripe cranberries amid the matching fall foliage.

How to Identify

Cranberry is a low, spreading shrub with long, horizontal stems that reach up to 6 feet long. From the stems grow short, upright branches covered in small glossy, alternate, ovate leaves that curl under a bit at the edges, especially in small cranberry. Nodding flowers with upturned pink petals and prominent red-orange anthers bloom in late spring. Hardy, bright red, egg-shaped fruit ripen in fall and can be found through the winter.

Where, When, and How to Wildcraft

Cranberry naturally grows in wetland areas, near marshes, lakesides, or riparian zones. Cranberry harvest is in fall and even into

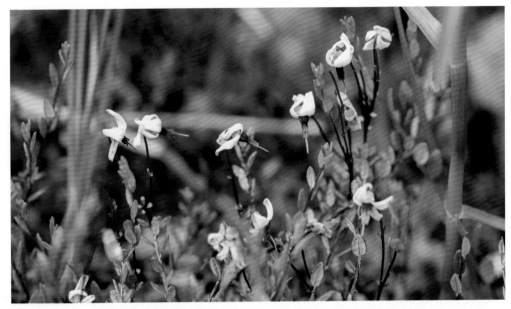

Cranberry was once called "craneberry" for its flower's resemblance to a crane's head.

winter. You're likely to find bushes on slightly drier terrain, but if you'd like to venture out into a bog or fen be well equipped with the appropriate waterproof gear. It will help to have a small bucket to tie to your waist for collecting berries.

Medicinal Uses

In precolonial times, people native to the Northeast relied on cranberry as a food, adding it to pemmican, a nutrient-dense mixture of fat, meat, and (often) fruit. The tart flavor of cranberry reveals its high levels of vitamin C, an essential nutrient for immune function and tissue repair. Our bodies need vitamin C to absorb iron, so this combination created by Algonquian people was a genius pairing—the addition of cranberry to the mixture provides not only balanced nutrition, it acts as a preservative as well.

Cranberry has a reputation for preventing and treating urinary tract infections due to its astringent, anti-inflammatory, and antimicrobial actions. Fresh-pressed cranberry juice, tea, or tincture taken frequently throughout the day can thwart an oncoming infection when early signs and symptoms appear.

Future Harvests

Carefully collecting berries from large stands of cranberries will not harm the future of the plant. As always, take only what you need and leave plenty for our animal kin.

HERBAL PREPARATIONS

Tea
Standard decoction of fresh or dried berries
Drink 1 cup 3 times per day.

Tincture
1 part fresh berries, crushed
2 parts menstruum (60% alcohol,
    40% water)
or
1 part dried berries
4 parts menstruum (60% alcohol,
    40% water)
Take 40–60 drops 4 times per day.

dandelion

Taraxacum officinale

PARTS USED flowers, leaves, roots

This extremely common and often-maligned herb holds a treasure trove of medicine, particularly for liver, skin, and joint health.

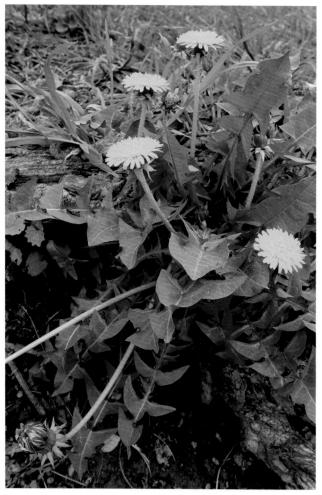

The genus name for dandelion, *Taraxacum*, may come from the Greek *taraxos*, meaning disorder, and *akos*, meaning remedy. Or it may be that Al-Razi, tenth-century Persian physician and polymath, called the plant "tarashaquq" or "tarkhashqun," the same word for chicory and endive. *Officinale* indicates the long history of use as a medicine.

How to Identify

Dandelion is a perennial, low-growing herb with a basal rosette of deeply toothed leaves. One yellow composite flowerhead grows on each green to reddish round hollow stem. The flowerhead is separated from the stem by a ring of reflexed green bracts. The stems emit a milky latex-like substance when broken. Dandelion's taproot is fleshy, whitish tan, gangly, and tenacious.

When dandelion goes to seed it looks like a ball of fluff sitting atop the stem.

Distinguish dandelion leaves from those of chicory by noting the downward-pointing direction of the teeth and the lack of erect hairs underneath the midrib; dandelion's hairs lay flat.

Where, When, and How to Wildcraft

Dandelion is hard to miss in lawns, parks, and fields. My favorite spring ritual is collecting the golden blossoms, a sign that spring is in full swing. Use the blossoms right away—leaving them to dry will only result in closed-up packages of seed fluff. Eat them fresh in salads or as fritters. Some like to remove the bitter bracts before frying, but I quite like the bitterness and leave them attached. Another way to capture their medicine is in a pain-relieving oil.

Leaves are best in spring or fall as they can be very bitter in summer. It's okay to harvest them in summer, though, especially if you are looking for bitter medicine. Collect the roots in fall by loosening the soil around the crown and gently digging with a stick or trowel. You might not get it all and that's okay, next year's growth will come back even stronger.

Medicinal Uses

Dandelion is a highly versatile bitter, cooling herb with medicine in every part. It's full of minerals and vitamins, making it a nutritive tonic. A root decoction has a healing effect on the liver, which in turn helps cleanse the blood and clear up skin conditions such as acne, eczema, and psoriasis. Dandelion root contains inulin, a prebiotic fiber that helps feed beneficial bacteria in the gut. It also acts as a gentle laxative, normalizing digestion and elimination.

Roast the root and combine with roasted chicory root for a healthy coffee substitute.

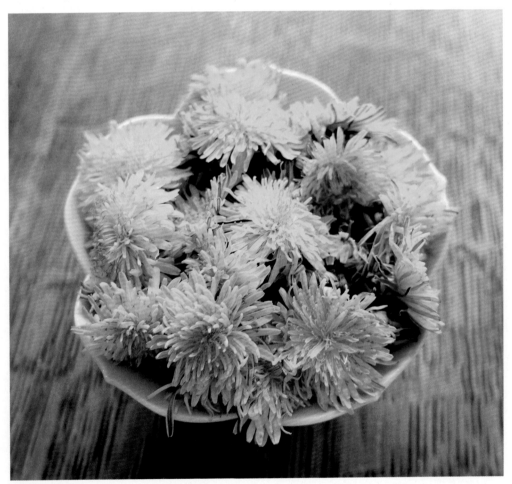

Craft a dandelion blossom oil for sunshine in a jar all year long.

They can be ground and brewed like coffee or simmered as a decoction. Both ways are delicious.

Dandelion root is effective for clearing inflammation in the joints. Drink a daily decoction for arthritis until symptoms clear.

Dandelion leaf is a gentle diuretic that doesn't deplete essential minerals, such as potassium. Use an infusion of the leaves to alleviate swelling in the kidneys or the urinary tract. Dandelion can be especially helpful to relieve edema-induced hypertension.

Make an infused oil with dandelion blossoms to use as a mild pain-relieving balm. Dandelion has a special affinity with the solar plexus and massaging the abdomen with the oil brings circulation and relief to congestion in this region.

The flower essence helps release patterns of rigidity and stubbornness, both a sign of imbalance in the solar plexus energy center.

Use the fresh sap of dandelion stems to treat topical warts.

Future Harvests

This humble plant is tenacious—if you try to rip out dandelion it will only grow back stronger. It's easy to spread the seeds. Pick one, blow the seedhead, and make a wish! Now you've just helped ensure the future of dandelions (not that they need our help).

HERBAL PREPARATIONS

Tea
Standard decoction of dried roots
Drink 4 ounces up to 3 times per day.
or
Standard infusion of dried leaves
Drink 4–8 ounces up to 3 times per day.

Tincture
1 part fresh leaves and/or roots
2 parts menstruum (50% alcohol,
  50% water)
Take 30–60 drops 3 times per day.

Infused oil
1 part fresh blossoms
2 parts oil
Use as a pain-relieving massage oil.

Flower essence
Follow instructions for making flower essences on page 54. Take 3 drops on the tongue or in water 3 times per day or as needed.

---

eastern cottonwood

Populus deltoides

PARTS USED leaf buds, twigs

Water-loving eastern cottonwood serves as a balm to painful conditions, from menstrual cramps to arthritis.

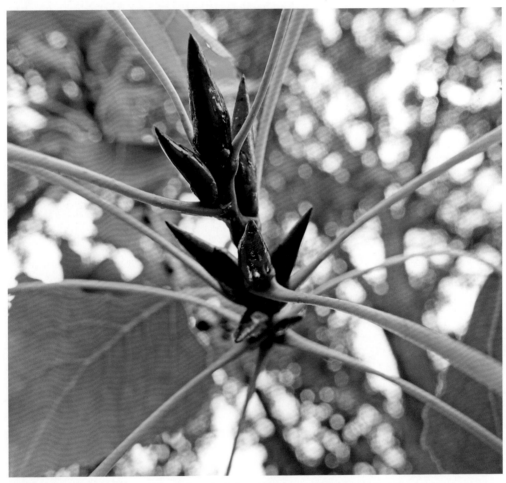

The sticky buds of eastern cottonwood can be infused in oil or made into a tincture to use as a massage oil or liniment for muscle aches.

How to Identify

Eastern cottonwood is a rapidly growing deciduous tree of the willow family that can reach up to 100 feet in height. The bark is ridged and grayish. Leaves are shiny, dark green, coarsely toothed, and roughly triangular in shape with a prominent point at the tip. In early spring, male and female catkins form on the same tree. Male catkins are red to yellow and emerge in clusters while female catkins are drooping and greenish. Once pollinated, the female flowers develop into a dangling cluster of green fruits. In late spring, the fruits burst open releasing puffs of cottony seed fluff to blanket the earth and disperse to the wind and nearby waterways.

Where, When, and How to Wildcraft

You'll find eastern cottonwood's roots holding the soil together at the edges of waterways or nearby in floodplains. Collect the sticky buds—which should have a sweet, resinous scent—in mid- to late winter. Gather twigs that have fallen after a late winter or early spring storm.

Medicinal Uses

Like its willow brethren, eastern cottonwood contains salicin, the pain-relieving and anti-inflammatory precursor to aspirin. Use the tincture internally to relieve headache, menstrual cramps, and fever in adults.

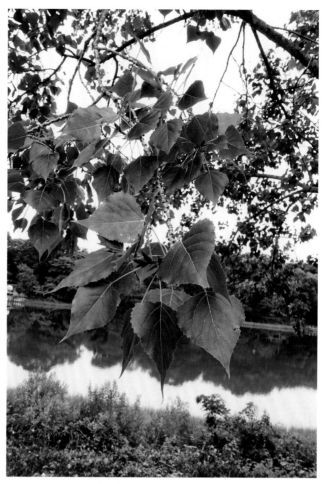

Eastern cottonwood makes its home at riversides and near streams and lakes.

Externally, eastern cottonwood bud–infused oil offers relief from muscular and joint pain. Combine with oils infused with Saint John's wort flowers, dandelion blossoms, and mugwort to ease muscle tenderness from overwork or arthritic conditions. You can also massage this oil over the womb to relieve menstrual cramps or after-birth pains.

For relief from cough, craft a chest rub oil containing cottonwood buds, eastern white pine pitch, prickly ash, and mint. Drink a cottonwood bark or twig decoction or take the tincture to clear up chest congestion.

⚠ Precautions

Although rare, aspirin- and salicylate-producing plants may lead to the development of Reye's syndrome in children. For this reason, it is advised to avoid using eastern cottonwood internally as a fever-reducer in children.

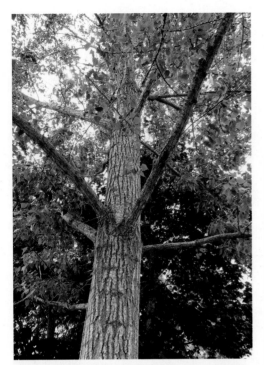

A fast-growing pioneer tree, eastern cottonwood brings balance to wetland ecosystems and provides shelter for birds like bald eagles and vital forage for bees.

Future Harvests

A sustainable way to collect twigs and branches (which might even have buds on them) from eastern cottonwood is after an early spring storm or a day of strong winds. Mindfully gathering a select amount of buds directly from the tree does not put it at risk.

HERBAL PREPARATIONS

Tea
Standard decoction of fresh or dried twigs
Drink 4 ounces as needed.

Tincture
1 part fresh leaf buds and twigs
2 parts menstruum (75% alcohol,
  25% water)
Take 15–30 drops as needed.

Infused oil
1 part fresh leaf buds
4 parts oil
Use as a massage oil for sore muscles or in a chest rub formula for cough.

Juniperus virginiana
pencil cedar, eastern juniper
PARTS USED cones, leaves, twigs

*Eastern redcedar, like fellow junipers, is valued for
its stimulating, blood-purifying, and diuretic properties.*

How to Identify

Eastern redcedar—not technically a
cedar, but in the cypress family—is
a conical to spreading evergreen tree
with reddish brown bark that peels
away in finely shredded strips. The
wood is enjoyably fragrant. Two types
of leaves are present on the tree. One
is more needle-like and prickly and
grows on new shoots and seedlings
and the other, on older branches, is
scaly and a bit less prickly. What the
majority of us call berries are actually
the female cones. Most varieties of
eastern redcedar have either male or
female cones on individual trees—
in rare cases both are present. Cones
are an important food source for
birds, especially the cedar waxwing.

Common juniper (*J. communis*) can be
used analogously to this species.

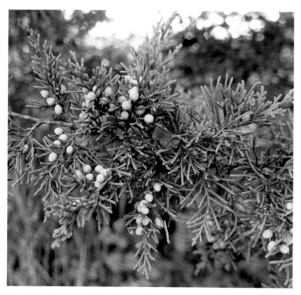

Look for the waxy blue, berry-like cones of eastern redcedar
to harvest and infuse in tea, tincture, or oil.

Where, When, and How to Wildcraft

Look for eastern redcedar in forests, at the
edges of forests, and in abandoned farmland
or fields where they are a pioneer species.
To prevent the spread of cedar-apple rust, ten-
ders of apple orchards are likely to fell whole,
young, healthy eastern redcedar trees. If you
know any apple farmers with volunteer eastern redcedar trees, this may be a good chance
for you to get an abundant harvest of leaves
and branches for a variety of applications.

Collect female cones when they are mature
and blue in color, from late fall through
early winter. Use fresh, freeze, or let dry in
a well-ventilated area and store in an airtight
container for later use. Gather twigs and leaves
throughout the year to use fresh or dried.

Medicinal Uses

Eastern redcedar's twigs, leaves, and berry-
like cones are stimulating and warming with
specific action in the respiratory tract,
kidneys, and uterus.

For an unproductive or slow-to-resolve
cough, eastern redcedar "berry" tea strengthens

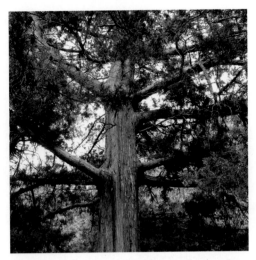

The color red is indicative of blood in the doctrine of signatures and eastern redcedar stimulates the uterus to encourage menstrual flow.

the cough reflex to help expectorate mucus. The warming quality of the herb also relieves dryness and irritation in the throat and lungs. In addition to drinking the tea, make a steam by gently simmering the crushed cones in water in a small pot for 5 minutes. Turn off the heat and let the infusion steep for another 5 minutes, covered. Place the pot on a sturdy table, then bring your face as close to the pot as is comfortable with a towel over your head—being careful not to scald yourself. Inhale the pleasantly spicy fragrance until the heat dissipates.

Eastern redcedar encourages the kidneys to quicken the flow of urine. When there is a feeling of fullness or pressure on the bladder without a satisfying release of urine, combine eastern redcedar berries with soothing anti-inflammatory herbs such as common mallow root and barberry fruit. Drink an eastern redcedar leaf or berry infusion to move fluid built up in the tissues of the limbs that cause swelling, pain, and discomfort.

Use oil infused with eastern redcedar cones, leaves, and twigs to massage into stiff joints and sore muscles. You can also massage this oil topically on the abdomen to relieve congestion in the uterus.

Bundle and dry eastern redcedar twigs and leaves and then burn them as incense to release their pleasant, cleansing scent. Alternately you can burn the crushed berries or bits of the leaves on charcoal in a fireproof container.

⚠ Precautions

Do not use eastern redcedar internally if your kidneys are compromised by injury or infection. Eastern redcedar is stimulating to the uterus and therefore should not be used in pregnancy.

Future Harvests

Gathering modest amounts of eastern redcedar twigs, leaves, and berries should not damage the tree. While the conservation status of eastern redcedar is secure in most of the Northeast and the tree is sometimes perceived as weedy, it is considered vulnerable in Québec.

HERBAL PREPARATIONS

Tea
Standard infusion of fresh or dried cones and/or leaves
Drink 2–4 ounces as needed or use as a steam.

Tincture
1 part dried cones and leaves
5 parts menstruum (75% alcohol, 25% water)
Take 20–40 drops up to 3 times per day.

Infused oil
1 part fresh cones, leaves, and/or twigs
2 parts oil
Use for massage or in a chest rub formula.

Echinacea species
coneflower, purple coneflower, snakeroot
PARTS USED flowers, leaves, roots

Most often thought of as a cold and flu herb, echinacea is no one-trick pony.
This immune-stimulating herb offers a host of benefits for the nervous,
lymphatic, respiratory, and digestive systems as well.

How to Identify

Echinacea is a perennial
herbaceous plant with an
upright growth pattern, growing 2–4 feet tall and usually
unbranched. Leaves arranged
mostly alternately on the stem
are lance-shaped, toothed, and
very bristly and rough like a
cat's tongue. There is no softness about echinacea, except
maybe the pink to purple petals
surrounding the stiff spiky
cone or seedhead. Echinacea
is frequented by bees, butterflies, and when it goes to seed,
birds. Moving slowing over the
Velcro-like seedheads, it almost
seems as though bees adhere to
the bristly surface when they
visit to collect nectar.

E. purpurea roots are pale,
thin, and scraggly, while other
Echinacea species have dark
brown taproots.

Where, When,
and How to Wildcraft

Echinacea is typically a prairie
plant and not technically
native to the Northeast. It can
be found in scattered locales

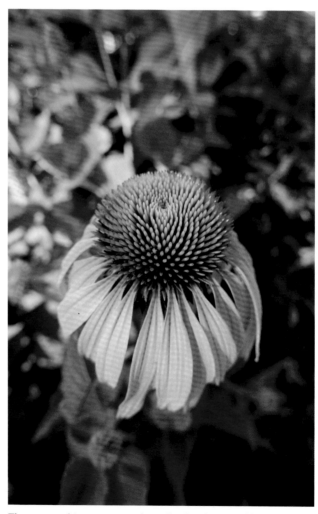

The name echinacea comes from the Greek root *echino-*, meaning
spiny or prickly. *Echinos* also means hedgehog or sea urchin and
it's easy to see this flower's resemblance to both.

around the region with a mostly southerly existence—though it is sometimes seen as far north as Maine and Ontario. If you find a patch, most likely they are garden escapees that have found a new home in open woodland areas, fields, or meadows. The species you'll encounter in the wild, if you do, will be *E. purpurea* or *E. pallida*. The aerial parts, that is the leaves, stems, and flowers, of all species are used medicinally and can be harvested when in flower. The roots vary from species to species, but the time to dig them is in the fall after at least the third year of growth. Unearth the roots and divide the plants by the crown, replanting portions to continue growing for future harvests. Alternately, you can cut pieces from the root ball and replant the remaining roots attached to the crown.

Medicinal Uses

All parts of echinacea, but especially the root and flowers, are sweet, pungent, cooling, and stimulating. Take a nibble of the root or a drop of the tincture and you'll find one of the great benefits of echinacea—that tingling sensation that brings your attention only to that sensation. This numbing quality is brought on by the alkamides present in the plant and is a reason that echinacea is sometimes called "toothache plant." It also makes echinacea a great partner for relieving sore throat caused by infection such as *Streptococcus pneumoniae*. Gargle at least 30 drops of the tincture every hour for 30 seconds at a time to heal sore throats, do the same but swish for mouth sores and toothache.

At the onset of cold or flu, take frequent, copious doses of echinacea root or whole plant tincture, up to 1 fluid ounce straight up every hour until symptoms cease. If the first dose instigates nausea, add the next dose to 2 ounces of water and continue with the protocol. The addition of red root tincture

or infusion can speed the recovery process. A distinction needs to be noted with the use of echinacea for acute infections. Echinacea tincture can help prevent a full-blown manifestation of cold or flu at the *onset* of illness to stimulate the immune system to fight infection, and it's recommended to limit use to cycles of 7–14 days. Echinacea is not generally used as a tonic herb to prevent infection over the long-term. For those cases, using immune-supportive tonic herbs such as elderberry or burdock may be more appropriate.

Echinacea root decoction is not as effective as the tincture for kicking a cold, rather, the tea conveys benefits for digestive health. Like burdock and other root herbs, echinacea contains inulin, a prebiotic fiber that normalizes gut flora. Drinking a decoction of echinacea stimulates digestion and assimilation, supports the liver, and brings balance to the intestines. The result of this can also lead to improved skin in cases of acne or eczema. For acne caused by bacterial infection, apply equal parts water and tincture externally to the affected area. Taking a course of the tincture or decoction internally will aid in healing.

Snakeroot is another common name for echinacea, for its efficacy in treating venomous bites or stings. However, this is where scientific names are essential to be sure you have *Echinacea* and not *Ageratina altissima*, a poisonous perennial herb known as white snakeroot. For snakebites, use the tincture internally in a short course of teaspoonful doses every hour and apply externally directly to the affected site. Plantain tincture or poultice could prove a useful addition to this treatment. This same protocol can be used for external wounds as well.

Echinacea flower essence is used for grounding and maintaining a strong sense of self through the healing of trauma or

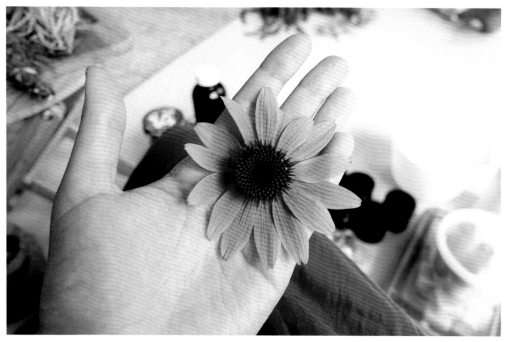

Echinacea blossoms are equally prized as, and more sustainable than, the roots.

through big transitions. Like the shedding of a snake, echinacea ushers us into feeling comfortable in our own skin on the other side of change.

⚠ Precautions

There is no substitute for rest and recovery when our bodies are worn down and prone to infection. Taking repeated courses of echinacea tincture for recurring illness can lead the body into a detrimental cycle of exhaustion and depletion. It's best to save echinacea for short-term use, no longer than 14 days at a time.

Future Harvests

Echinacea is endangered in many parts of the continent. Favor the aerial parts of the plant over the roots, which take several years to develop. When harvesting roots, divide mature plants by the crown and replant what you don't plan to use.

HERBAL PREPARATIONS

Tea
Standard decoction of fresh or dried roots
Drink 1 cup up to 4 times per day. Use externally as a wash for wounds and bites.

Tincture
1 part fresh flowers, leaves, and roots
2 parts menstruum (60% alcohol,
  40% water)
For acute use: Take 60–90 drops or up to 1 fluid ounce hourly until symptoms resolve. Back off to a lower dose if nausea is induced. Use diluted in equal parts water externally for acne, wounds, and bites.

Flower essence
Follow instructions for making flower essences on page 54. Take 3 drops on the tongue or in water 3 times per day or as needed.

elder

Sambucus nigra
PARTS USED flowers, fruit, leaves, twigs

*Cooling, bitter, and acrid, elder is a veritable medicine chest with
purifying, protective, and immune-, blood-, and bone-building qualities.*

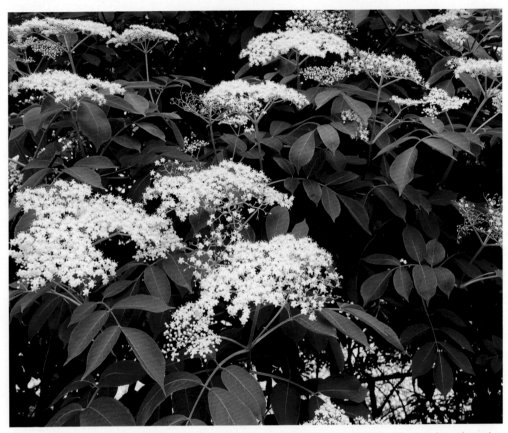

In some accounts, the name "elder" is derived from the Anglo-Saxon word *aeld* for "fire" and in others the
name comes from Holda, goddess of wisdom, winter, and protector of the housewife and mother. The
genus name *Sambucus* comes from the sambuca flute that was carved from the branches (or vice versa).

How to Identify

Elder is a spindly shrub growing 5–30 feet
tall. Its opposite branches sport lenticels
(braille-like bumps) that easily break off
from the light, hollow-feeling branch. Leaves
are compound in odd numbers, five to seven,
with toothed margins. Creamy white,
musty-sweet flowers grow in umbels or
"dishes" in late spring to early summer.
Small, dark purple berries replace the
flowers, appearing in drooping clusters
in midsummer.

180]

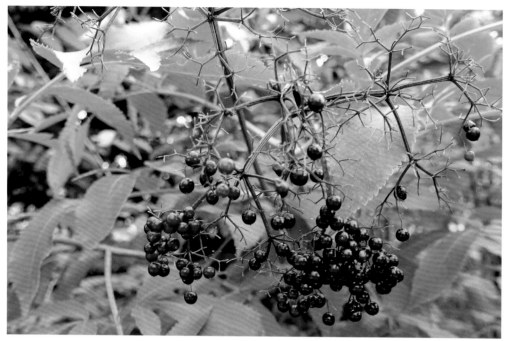

Elderberries are antiviral, immune stimulating, blood cleansing, laxative, and diuretic, just to name a few of their beneficial actions.

Where, When, and How to Wildcraft

Find elder in forests or at the forest's edge. Mindfully collect the blossoms in late spring, by gently rocking the inflorescence stalk at the node or using a small knife to carefully pop off the stalk. Leave plenty of flowers behind for berry development, and for our animal friends. Harvest clusters of berries in summer when all berries in the cluster have ripened to black, again, leaving plenty for birds and other animals. Collect leaves and twigs from spring through fall to use fresh or dry.

Medicinal Uses

From flower to stem, elder is a generous plant with a broad range of medicinal applications. The berries and flowers are useful for supporting the immune system during cold and flu season. A classic tea recipe to treat the acute symptoms of cold and flu

includes elderflower, yarrow, and mint—adding boneset would increase the pain- and fever-relieving potency. Drink this infusion and consider adding elderflower-infused honey for its mild calming effect and sweet taste to balance the bitterness.

Another time-honored recipe is elderberry syrup which can be taken throughout cold and flu season for prevention of illness. There are several ways to make it, all beneficial for boosting the body's defenses against infection and for building the blood. One way is to gently simmer dried elderberries in fruit juice for 20 minutes—adding herbs like burdock root, lemon balm, and monarda will enhance the immune-boosting effects of the blend. After simmering, let steep for 20 more minutes before processing through a food mill or tincture press to squeeze all of the goodness from the herbs. Add equal parts honey or vegetable glycerin and store in the refrigerator. See page 52 for detailed instructions on making herbal syrups. By adding yellow dock, rosehips, and stinging nettle, you can transform this versatile syrup into a blood-building blend for those suffering from mild anemia or as a postpartum strengthener.

Make a decoction of elder leaves and stems to use internally and externally for repairing injured or brittle bones. Add horsetail, stinging nettle, red clover, and comfrey leaf for added bone-building effect.

Elderflowers and leaves are applied externally to improve the health of skin. Craft an infused oil for making skin-protective lotions or salves. Apply elderflower-infused vinegar or leaf poultice to sunburns, rashes, and wounds.

⚠ Precautions

Consuming raw leaves, stems, or berries— especially reddish, unripe berries—in large amounts can lead to a build-up of toxic cyanogenic glycosides in the body.

Future Harvests

Harvesting a modest share of blossoms, berries, leaves, and stems will not harm elder shrubs. When harvesting blossoms leave enough behind for berries to grow. When harvesting berries leave enough for the birds and other creatures.

HERBAL PREPARATIONS

Tea
Standard infusion of dried flowers
Drink 4–6 ounces 3 times per day. Drink hot in cases of fever.

Infused honey
1 part fresh flowers
2 parts honey
Take by the teaspoonful as needed.

Tincture
1 part fresh flowers or berries
2 parts menstruum (50% alcohol,
   50% water)
Take 20–40 drops 3 times per day.

Syrup
Using the flowers or berries, follow instructions for making herbal syrups on page 52. Take 1–2 tablespoons daily by the spoonful, in sparkling water, or drizzled on yogurt, breakfast porridge, or pancakes.

Inula helenium
elf dock, horse-heal
PARTS USED flowers, roots

Elecampane has long been valued as medicine, having great effect on the respiratory, immune, and digestive systems.

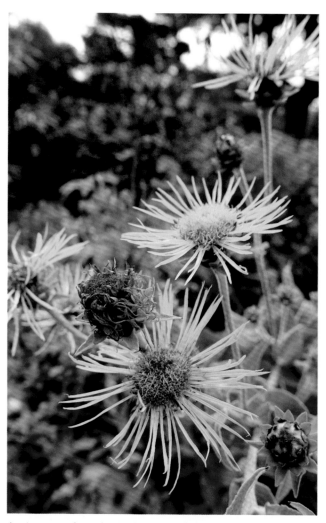

Ancient texts from the Anglo-Saxons describe a condition known as "elf-shot" where folks would be afflicted by sudden pains, purportedly from the prick of an elf's arrowhead. Elecampane treats this condition and that's where the name "elf dock" comes from.

How to Identify

Elecampane is a perennial herb with a stiff, upright habit growing 4–5 feet tall. The hardy, thick, green stem has deep creases down its length. The lower part of the plant boasts a rosette of large, stalked, toothed, egg- to lance-shaped leaves that are pointed at the tip and 1–1½ feet long and 4½ inches wide. Smaller upper leaves clasp the stem. The entire plant is covered in a soft down. Sunny yellow composite flowerheads (up to 2 inches in diameter) bloom in summer. The branching taproot is mucilaginous, resinous, tan-brown, and has a woodsy, spicy, earthy scent.

Where, When, and How to Wildcraft

Elecampane is endemic to Europe and Asia and was introduced to the Northeast by European colonists. Look for elecampane in fields, meadows, and disturbed habitats. Collect flowers in summer when they are in peak bloom. Fall is the time to harvest roots, and it's best to choose a larger, older plant for greater yield. You may have to work hard to dig up the tenacious roots, but it's worth the effort.

Medicinal Uses

Warming, stimulating, and drying, elecampane root lends itself to cold, stuck conditions, such as mucousy coughs that are slow to go. Combine the root with a balance of moistening, cooling herbs like violet leaf and red clover in a decoction or syrup to encourage recovery and soothe irritation from coughs. Another way to take the root for respiratory complaints is infused in honey. Flowers can be taken this way as well.

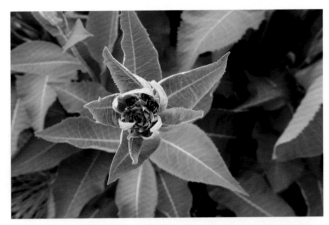

This young elecampane plant will grow a couple more feet before blooming about 2 months later, in summer.

As a gentle blood-cleansing and antimicrobial tonic, elecampane aids the body in elimination of toxins through the liver and kidneys. A tincture or decoction made of elecampane root contains high amounts of inulin (*inula* is right there in the scientific name), which encourages the proliferation of healthy gut bacteria. Elecampane root tones lax tissues and makes a nice addition to bitters blends to stimulate elimination in those with sluggish digestion. The root is also antiparasitic and can help eradicate intestinal parasites, such as roundworms.

Elecampane flower essence instills confidence when we are feeling guarded or isolated, helping us shine our unique light in the world.

⚠ Precautions

Do not use elecampane in pregnancy as it may be too stimulating to the uterus.

Future Harvests

Elecampane is an introduced plant; however, know that when you dig up the roots, you are ending the life of the plant in this form.

HERBAL PREPARATIONS

Tea
Standard decoction of fresh or dried roots
Drink 4–8 ounces up to 3 times per day.

Infused honey
1 part fresh roots
2 parts honey
Take by the teaspoonful or in tea as needed.

Tincture
1 part fresh roots
2 parts menstruum (60% alcohol, 40% water)
or
1 part dried roots
5 parts menstruum (60% alcohol, 40% water)
Take 10–30 drops up to 4 times per day.

Flower essence
Follow instructions for making flower essences on page 54. Take 3 drops on the tongue or in water 3 times per day or as needed.

English ivy

Hedera helix
PARTS USED **leaves**

Though little used in North America, English ivy is a valuable remedy for spasmodic coughs and constricted airways.

How to Identify

Originally hailing from Europe and Britain, English ivy is a commonly introduced ground cover and climbing vine in the Araliaceae—it's a cousin to native ginseng, American spikenard, and wild sarsaparilla. The rootlets of English ivy become tenacious suckers to attach the vine to trees and buildings. You'll often see it climbing the sides of buildings and up trees—it becomes invasive in forests and parks where there is minimal land management and plenty of room for it to roam.

The evergreen leaves appear in three shapes: elongated cordate, and three- and five-lobed palmate. Their color can be uniformly green or a blend of red and green with prominently contrasting lighter-colored veins. In late summer, small, green-yellow flowers bloom in 1½–2½ inch umbels. In winter, fertilized flowers ripen to small black berries hanging from the umbel on green stems.

Where, When, and How to Wildcraft

Look for English ivy in areas disturbed by human activity, in parks and forests, and growing up buildings and trees in your neighborhood. Spring is the traditional time to gather leaves, though you can collect them any time of year to tincture fresh.

The evergreen leaves of English ivy range in color and shape, from dark green to red-green and from palmate with three or five lobes to an elongated heart shape.

Medicinal Uses

English ivy leaves are primarily used as a remedy for respiratory congestion and relief of chronic lung inflammation. Take the tincture to help expel mucus from wet coughs and reduce airway constriction.

The binding nature of the plant, its ability to climb and strangle out trees, hints at its use for pain that stems from a sense of binding or pressure at the site. Anti-inflammatory and antispasmodic, it's been used traditionally as a treatment for arthritis, rheumatism, and gout. Try a compress of ivy leaf infusion with the optional addition of comfrey, mugwort, or periwinkle to relieve joint pain and pressure.

The ancient Greeks bound wreaths of ivy around their heads to prevent drunkenness—look at images of Dionysus and Bacchus and you'll see what I'm talking about. While wearing an ivy crown may not have such a direct effect, English ivy is used homeopathically for relieving intracranial pressure, so maybe the ancient Greeks and Romans were onto something.

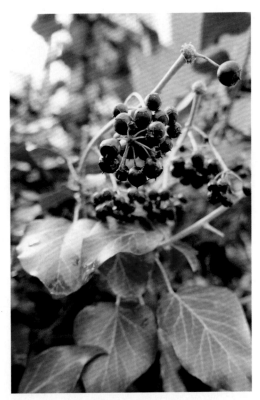

Seeming to never die, evergreen plants were associated with longevity and immortality by ancient Europeans.

⚠ Precautions

English ivy is generally regarded as safe, even for children as young as 2. There are rare reports of allergic reactions to English ivy, so as with any plant, try a small dose before proceeding with a therapeutic one.

Future Harvests

Good luck overharvesting English ivy. While perhaps not as widespread as some introduced species, it is a hardy evergreen that people either love or loathe for its tenacity.

HERBAL PREPARATIONS

Tincture
1 part fresh leaves
2 parts menstruum (50% alcohol, 50% water)
Take 30–40 drops 3 times per day.

Syrup
Make a standard infusion of the leaves then reduce by half over low heat. Add equal amounts of honey or vegetable glycerin. Take 1 tablespoon 3 times per day.

evening primrose

Oenothera biennis
PARTS USED flowers, leaves, roots, seeds

Evening primrose is a nourishing, restorative herb that brings balance to the nervous system.

How to Identify

Evening primrose is a biennial herbaceous plant that starts its first year as a basal rosette of lance-shaped, wavy-edged leaves with distinctive light-colored midveins. In the second year, a woody stalk emerges covered with tightly packed, shallowly toothed leaves growing in an alternate pattern. Fragrant, pale to bright yellow, four-petaled flowers (1–2 inches wide) bloom throughout summer. As the common name suggests, the flowers open in the evening to give moths easier access to their nectar and for pollination. The flowers bloom from the bottom up, leaving in their wake conspicuous green seed capsules that are edible to humans and other animals. Foragers enjoy the pleasantly spicy taste of the flower buds, fresh and withered flowers, and reddish brown seeds.

Where, When, and How to Wildcraft

You'll find evening primrose in areas disturbed by human activities, dry open fields, and in clearings near woodlands. Dig the roots in fall of the first year while the energy is still down in the earth. Gather leaves in spring, flowers in summer, and seed capsules in late summer through the fall.

Medicinal Uses

Just as evening primrose flowers are open and receptive in the evening, our bodies— though resting at night—are busy recovering from the stresses of the day and repairing damaged tissue. Evening primrose aids the body in these

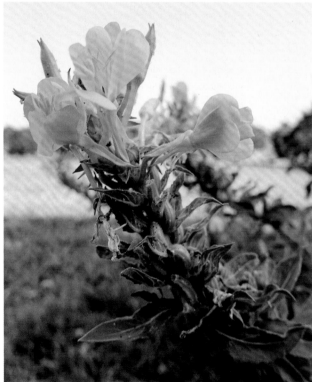

Evening primrose brings moisture and lubrication to skin and organs, in contrast to the sandy, dry soil that it grows in.

restorative processes that occur during the evening hours, helping to bring balance where there is fluctuation due to stress. Evening primrose nourishes the nervous system, restoring healthy patterns of energy, hormones, heartrate, and digestion.

For a soothing evening tea to gently bring on sleepiness and improve digestion, combine evening primrose with catnip and chamomile. Drink evening primrose infusion, or take the tincture combined with antispasmodic herbs such as motherwort and crampbark, to ease painful menstruation and abdominal cramping from conditions like irritable bowel syndrome.

Evening primrose has a moistening, cooling effect on dry coughs and works well in syrup form with valerian, mullein, and wild cherry to alleviate coughing and bring on restful sleep.

Topically, roots and leaves can be made into a poultice to treat bruises and connective tissue inflammation. Massaging with evening primrose–infused oil (not to be confused with the commercially produced seed oil) brings relief to tender breast tissue, abdominal and menstrual cramping, and sore muscles. You can also use the oil to help heal scaly, dry skin conditions and to make a protective skin lotion or salve.

Evening primrose flower essence sheds light on and helps heal early emotional pain and rejection, enabling the establishment of healthy commitments and relationships.

Future Harvests

In some places, evening primrose is a prolific producer and considered invasive. Look for these large patches to collect from and regenerate your harvest by spreading the seeds when they burst from their capsules in fall.

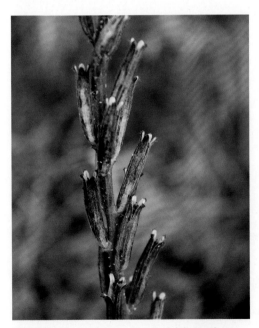

Evening primrose "shakers" full of deliciously spicy seeds. The seeds of evening primrose are extracted commercially for their oil, which is rich in gamma-linoleic acid (GLA).

HERBAL PREPARATIONS

Tea
Standard infusion of dried flowers
Drink 2–4 ounces as needed.

Tincture
1 part fresh flowers, leaves, roots, and seeds
2 parts menstruum (50% alcohol, 50% water)
Take 15–30 drops as needed.

Infused oil
1 part fresh flowers
2 parts oil
Use as a massage oil for the abdomen, breasts, or inflamed joints.

Flower essence
Follow instructions for making flower essences on page 54. Take 3 drops on the tongue or in water 3 times per day or as needed.

feverfew

Tanacetum parthenium
PARTS USED flowers, leaves

Feverfew is known as a remedy for migraines, especially when they occur at the onset of menstruation. The herb in tincture and tea form provides relief from pain as well as being a bitter digestive.

How to Identify

Feverfew is a perennial herb in the aster family that is similar in appearance to chamomile in its spreading habit of abundant little daisylike flowers. What differs in feverfew, mainly, are the leaves which are alternate, deeply divided, toothed, and pinnately lobed—somewhat resembling parsley leaves. The stem is furrowed and covered in very short, fine hairs. The plant has a strong, bitter smell.

Where, When, and How to Wildcraft

Feverfew is an introduced garden herb that jumped the fence. In the wild, you're most likely to find it in disturbed habitats, meadows, and fields. Collect leaves and flowers from late spring through early summer.

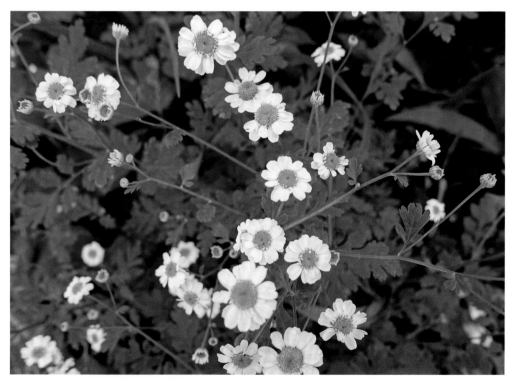

Feverfew derives from the Latin word *febrifuge*, which means "to drive away fever." (Feverfew, feverfew—phew, there goes my fever.)

Medicinal Uses

Feverfew stimulates circulation to the periphery of the body, providing warmth and pain relief to the head, neck, and extremities. This action can be useful for those suffering from migraines, peripheral arterial disease, or Raynaud's syndrome. Combine with Saint John's wort for additional nervous system support—both can be used internally as tincture and externally as oil.

Drinking feverfew tea before or after a meal stimulates the flow of saliva and other digestive fluids, supporting the body in digestion and elimination. Combine with rose and lemon balm to soothe nervous tension that presents as a headache or stomachache.

Apply feverfew-infused oil topically to the abdomen to relieve gas and bloating. The infusion is also useful as a wash to alleviate the pain and itching of insect bites.

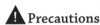 Precautions

Do not use feverfew during pregnancy as it is too stimulating to the uterus.

Caution is advised in those taking blood-thinning medications as feverfew may inhibit blood clotting.

Stop taking feverfew 2 weeks prior to surgery to prevent bleeding.

Future Harvests

Mindfully gathering the leaves and flowers of feverfew will not put this introduced plant at risk.

HERBAL PREPARATIONS

Tea
Standard or cold infusion of dried flowers and leaves
Drink 2-4 ounces as needed.

Tincture
1 part fresh flowers and leaves
2 parts menstruum (70% alcohol, 30% water)
or
1 part dried flowers and leaves
5 parts menstruum (70% alcohol, 30% water)
Take 15-20 drops up to 4 times per day.

Infused oil
1 part fresh flowers and leaves
2 parts oil
Use as a massage oil for pain relief.

---

field garlic

Allium vineale

crow garlic

PARTS USED bulbs, leaves

Milder than the cultivated species, field garlic is a useful, palatable remedy for cold symptoms when taken as a tea or in broths.

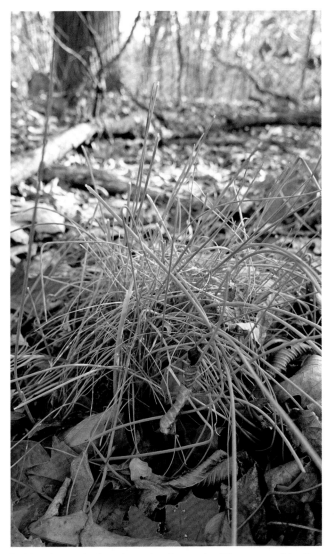

Field garlic can be found growing for much of the year, making it a readily available medicine.

How to Identify

Field garlic is a perennial plant that may look like a tangled clump of grass from a distance. Upon closer inspection, you'll notice the long tubular leaves and upon sniffing you'll catch the aroma of garlic or onion. Apparently this plant blooms little purple pompom flowers in spring, but often it doesn't. Best to go by smell as this is the most identifiable characteristic and it would be hard to miss. The garlic leaves or chives grow out of a small system of little bulbs surrounded by a tan papery sheath.

Where, When, and How to Wildcraft

You'll notice field garlic growing in the cooler months emerging from a blanket of leaf litter in shaded, forested areas. Collect just the leaves or unearth the whole plant to use fresh in teas or broths.

Medicinal Uses

Like its cultivated relative, field garlic has a strong affinity with the heart and lungs. It helps

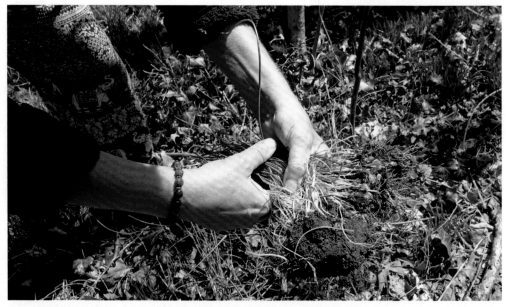

Harvesting field garlic bulbs is as easy as using a knife to cut a circle at an inward angle around the base of the plant, loosening up the soil, and lifting out a whole mess of bulbs. Oh, and you get the chives this way, too.

open the airways and gets blood flowing, lending itself well to asthmatic conditions and coughs. Infuse honey with the bulbs and leaves to take for nasal and chest congestion. Add this honey to violet, mullein, and elder-flower infusion to relieve cold symptoms.

Field garlic supports the circulatory and digestive systems and tends to grow in the colder months when our bodies need it most. Add field garlic, burdock, dande-lion root, red clover, stinging nettle, and chickweed to the pot when making bone or vegetable broth to boost the nutrient con-tent. Sipping this vitamin- and mineral-rich brew daily can be a boon to health, especially during cold and flu season or when recover-ing from illness.

Future Harvests

Field garlic may be considered a bit weedy; however, know that when you harvest the roots you are taking the life of the plant.

Meadow garlic (*A. canadense*), a related spe-cies with larger shoots and bulbs covered in a mesh of fibers, is endangered or threatened in some parts of the Northeast. Harvesting the leaves of this species and field garlic is a more sustainable way to use the medicine of these plants.

HERBAL PREPARATIONS

Tea
Standard infusion of fresh or dried bulbs and leaves
Drink 2–4 ounces as needed. Alternately, add-ing the bulbs and leaves to a broth would be a tasty way to take in the medicine of this plant.

Tincture
1 part fresh bulbs and leaves
2 parts menstruum (50% alcohol,
  50% water)
Take 20 drops as needed.

forsythia

Forsythia species
weeping forsythia (*F. suspensa*), green-stemmed forsythia (*F. viridissima*)
PARTS USED flowers, fruit

One of the first flowering plants of spring, forsythia lends a cooling action to burning hot conditions such as tonsillitis and fever.

How to Identify

Forsythia is an introduced ornamental deciduous shrub with a large spreading habit of arching branches. It is most recognizable when in bloom—its four-lobed yellow flowers blanketing the entire shrub before the leaves emerge. The bark is yellowish brown and covered in lenticels. Opposite, toothed, ovate green leaves appear after flowering and can appear simple or compound in groups of three. The fruit is a green to yellow capsule that is shaped like an inverted teardrop—as

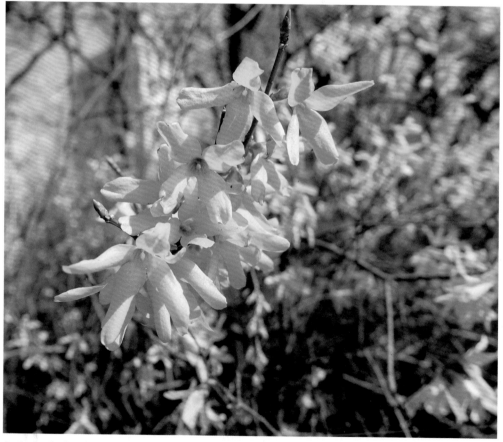

Antimicrobial and anti-inflammatory forsythia brings relief to allergies and respiratory infections.

it dries the capsule turns brown and splits in half, looking sometimes like a baby bird's beak reaching up for food.

Where, When, and How to Wildcraft

You'll find forsythia planted in parks and common areas, along forest trails and as ornamental hedgerows. Collect flowers in early spring as they bloom. Gather the unripe green fruits in summer to tincture fresh. Harvest the yellow ripe fruit in fall if you want to dry it for later use. If you plan to gather from a person's yard, be sure to ask permission and whether they use any chemical treatments on the land.

Medicinal Uses

Forsythia is native to China and its fruit is a fundamental herb of Chinese medicine. Used alone or in combination with other herbs forsythia dispels heat, dissolves swelling, and clears infection. Take a decoction or tincture to overcome fever, shrink swollen glands, or ease the burning of a urinary tract infection. A combination of forsythia fruit and burdock seed tincture can resolve tonsillitis. Drink a decoction of forsythia fruit and honeysuckle flower at the early signs of cold or flu to stave off full-blown illness.

Forsythia is taken internally and applied externally to clear up acne, and especially painful, hot boils or carbuncles. Work with forsythia fruit and burdock seed tinctures externally and internally to encourage clear skin in those with persistent skin eruptions.

Pair forsythia fruit–infused honey with honeysuckle flowers to reduce burning, itching, reactive symptoms during allergy season.

⚠ Precautions

Forsythia is recommended for treating acute conditions in those with an otherwise robust constitution. It is best avoided in those with chronic digestive issues or weakened immune systems, or those who are generally depleted.

Forsythia is not recommended for use during pregnancy or early postpartum as it may be too cooling.

Future Harvests

Mindfully harvesting the fruits of forsythia does not compromise the health of this hardy, introduced plant.

HERBAL PREPARATIONS

Tea
Standard decoction of dried fruit
Drink 2–4 ounces as needed.
or
Infusion of fresh flowers
Gather ¼ cup of flowers and infuse in 1 cup of boiling water. Steep for 10–15 minutes. Drink as needed.

Tincture
1 part fresh green fruit, crushed
2 parts menstruum (50% alcohol, 50% water)
or
1 part dried yellow fruit, powdered
5 parts menstruum (50% alcohol, 50% water)
Take 20–30 drops as needed.

---

garlic mustard

Alliaria petiolata

PARTS USED flowers, leaves, roots, seeds

Let's make use of what many consider a nuisance plant for its tasty bitter leaves and spicy roots and seeds that stimulate perspiration and respiration to clear tightness and congestion in the lungs.

How to Identify

An introduced biennial, garlic mustard starts out as a clumped rosette of heart-shaped leaves with deep veins and conspicuously scalloped edges. In its second year it shoots up a stalk with alternating leaves that are more triangular in shape, sporting sharper teeth and a pointed tip. Topping off the stalk, white four-petaled flowers in a cross pattern give away this plant as a member of the mustard (Brassicaceae) family. In midspring, long, thin seedpods called siliques begin to emerge, alternating at an upward angle from the stem. Inside are tiny black spicy-tasting seeds.

Leaves, flowers, and siliques have a distinctly garlic-like taste and smell. The slender white taproots have been likened to mini horseradish roots.

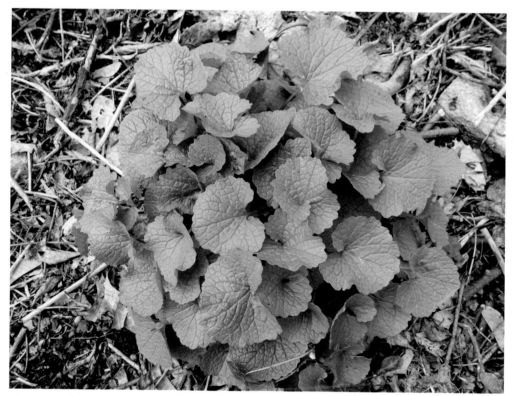

First-year garlic mustard emerges in early spring, often growing in bushy clumps.

Where, When, and How to Wildcraft

Garlic mustard is common in moist soils in forested areas and edges, particularly areas where there is human activity. You might also find it in floodplains near rivers or streams.

The leaves are tastiest and tenderest in early spring before it gets too hot. They have a nice balance of garlicky bitterness. The flowers and flower buds before they open and are still green are also quite delicious and tender. As the temperature warms, garlic mustard becomes extremely bitter. If this is what you are looking for, have at it. If you are sad you missed out on the good stuff in spring, not to worry. A second, less-bitter harvest comes again in fall when things cool down.

You can also nibble the green seedpods (siliques) as a trail snack. In summer, once the siliques dry on the plant, this is a good time to collect them for the spicy seeds inside. To separate out the seeds, place the silique in between your two palms and rub it back and forth. Catch the falling seeds in a bowl or jar. Be sure to do this indoors to avoid inadvertently spreading the seeds of this highly prolific plant.

Dig the roots in spring or fall to use as a horseradish substitute.

Medicinal Uses

Garlic mustard is a powerhouse of nutrients, rich in vitamin C and with more vitamin A than spinach. Incorporate garlic mustard into nourishing spring tonic tea blends, add it to green juice for a boost of nutrients, or blend it into pesto with stinging nettle, field garlic, sunflower or olive oil, and pumpkin seeds.

In a hot infusion, the leaves, roots, and seeds stimulate sweating to help break a fever. Drink this brew or take the tincture to alleviate constriction in the lungs from asthma or bronchitis.

Make a spit poultice of the leaves to relieve itching, particularly of insect bites.

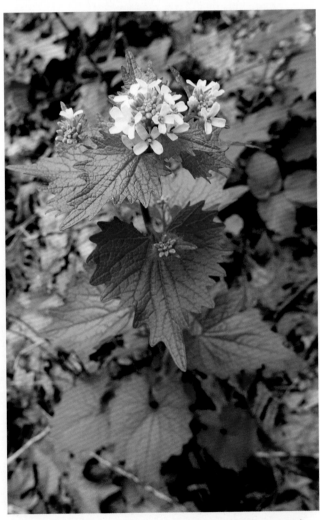

Second-year garlic mustard in flower. In spring, the flowers make a delightful addition to salads.

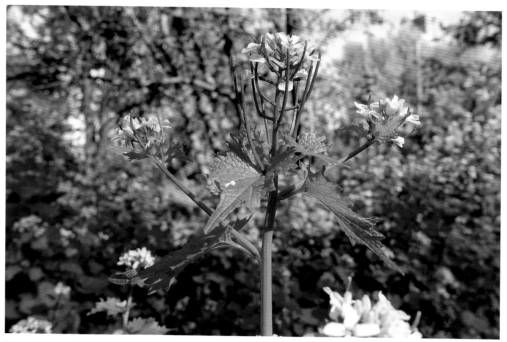

The siliques of garlic mustard just starting to emerge beneath the flowers in midspring.

Future Harvests

Garlic mustard is plentiful in the Northeast.

Contrary to popular belief, and according to a Boston University study, garlic mustard does not exude harmful chemicals in the soil to prevent other plants from growing near it. It encourages leaf litter decomposition and nutrient cycling, improving soil conditions of forests. Perhaps it's time to shift perceptions around this plant's status as a noxious, invasive species.

HERBAL PREPARATIONS

Tea
Standard infusion of fresh or dried leaves and/or roots
Drink 4 ounces as needed. Add to soups or broths.

Tincture
1 part fresh leaves, roots, and seeds
2 parts menstruum (50% alcohol, 50% water)
Take 15–20 drops as needed.

Succus
Blend garlic mustard with a splash of water and strain it or juice it in a juicer. Add enough alcohol so the finished product is 25% alcohol by volume. Take at the first sign of a cold or when you are feeling rundown.

German chamomile

Matricaria recutita

German mayweed

PARTS USED flowers

German chamomile is well known and loved for its ability to calm frazzled nerves and upset stomachs. But there's even more to chamomile than these common uses, including its fever-reducing properties.

How to Identify

German chamomile is a self-seeding annual that can grow up to 2 feet tall. The deeply divided leaves have a delicate, fringy, frayed look. The small, sweetly scented flowers have white petals that fold down from yellow cones.

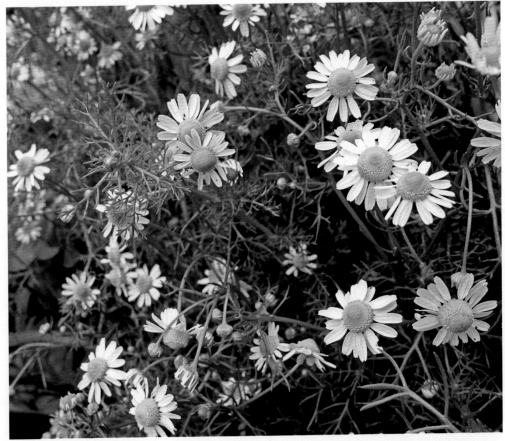

The name chamomile comes from both Latin and Greek meaning "earth apple," referring to its scent and growing habit. *Matricaria* refers to either the uterus (Latin, *matrix*) or mother (Latin, *mater*) reflecting the historical use of German chamomile for women's health issues.

Pineapple weed (*M. discoidea*) is a related species that is more widespread and can be used almost analogously to German chamomile. Roman chamomile (*Chamaemelum nobile*), also known as "true chamomile," is less widespread and has similar properties to German chamomile.

Where, When, and How to Wildcraft

German chamomile is a much-beloved garden plant that jumped the fence. You'll find it growing in disturbed habitats, meadows, and fields. Gather blossoms in late spring through summer to use fresh or dry for later.

Medicinal Uses

While German chamomile is recognized as a gentle, child-friendly herb, there is great strength in its medicine. German chamomile has an affinity with the nervous system, reflected in the signature of fine, frayed-looking leaves. Drink a warm German chamomile infusion to relieve mild anxiety, acute insomnia, and menstrual cramps.

The anxiety-reducing and antispasmodic capacities of German chamomile also extend to the digestive system, bringing calm to stress-induced stomach upset. In infants and toddlers, digestive distress often coincides with the pain and discomfort of emerging teeth. A small dose of chamomile infusion or glycerite alleviates both, reducing tears and headache for both child and caregiver.

German chamomile is bitter, particularly when steeped longer than 5 minutes. This taste hints at its action in the liver and gallbladder—German chamomile stimulates bile production to facilitate absorption of fats and fat-soluble vitamins. Drinking a cup of warm German chamomile infusion with meals enhances digestion and assimilation of nutrients. Taking German chamomile regularly benefits those with irritable

bowel syndrome, Crohn's disease, and peptic ulcers.

German chamomile is a calming agent for eruptive, irritated, or burning skin conditions. A cool infusion can be used as a wash or compress for sunburn. Infuse oil with chamomile to craft a salve or use it straight up on diaper rash, chafing, and other uncomfortable skin conditions. German chamomile is also an effective fever reducer; drink the warm infusion every 2 hours until symptoms abate.

⚠ Precautions

People who are allergic to plants in the aster family should avoid this herb. Chamomile can cause dizziness in some, and nausea if taken to excess.

Future Harvests

Chamomile is an introduced plant that is fairly easy to grow. If you'd like to ensure its future, directly sow seeds in mid- to late spring, after the frost date has passed for your growing zone.

HERBAL PREPARATIONS

Tea
Infuse 1 tablespoon of dried flowers per cup for 5–10 minutes. Drink 1 cup as needed.

Tincture
1 part fresh flowers
2 parts menstruum (50% alcohol, 50% water)
or
1 part dried flowers
5 parts menstruum (50% alcohol, 50% water)
Take 20–60 drops as needed.

Ginkgo biloba
maidenhair tree
PARTS USED leaves, seeds

A hardy, ancient tree species most often seen as a street tree or in parks,
ginkgo is a circulatory stimulant, and brain and lung tonic.

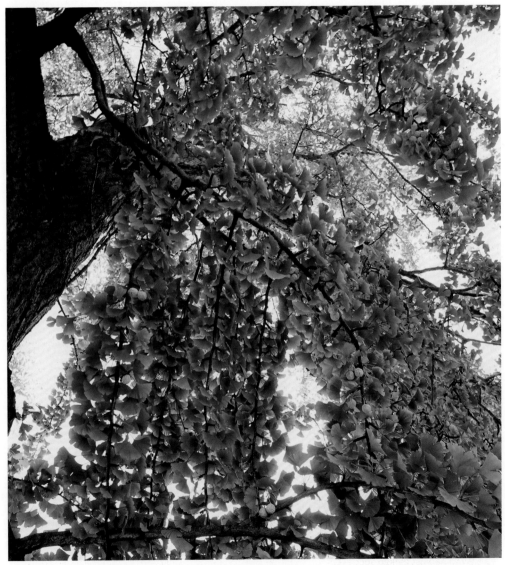

Ginkgo branches cascade from the tree, full of ripening fruit in fall.

How to Identify

Ginkgo is a tall (upward of 100 feet) deciduous conifer tree classified as a gymnosperm, or plant that does not produce flowers nor fruit to encase the seed. It's sometimes called a shadeless shade-tree for, despite its height, its upright branches give it a slender habit. Fan-shaped leaves with nearly parallel veins often feature an indentation at the center that forms two lobes—hence the specific name "bi-loba." Ginkgo trees are dioecious, meaning there are male and female plants. Male trees don pale green pollen cones in spring. Wind-pollinated female trees form fleshy, extremely stinky, orange-yellow "fruit" in fall—the seeds inside are edible when properly cooked.

Where, When, and How to Wildcraft

You'll most likely see ginkgo planted as a street tree or in parks in the lower range of the Northeast, specifically New Jersey, New York, and Pennsylvania. Collect the green leaves from fallen branches or low branches in summer to tincture fresh or dry for use in tea. Gather yellow leaves and fruit in fall—it is perfectly acceptable and convenient to pick these from the ground. Wearing gloves to remove the outer flesh of the fruit while harvesting will help leave the stink outside.

Medicinal Uses

Ginkgo is an ancient tree that almost went extinct. Thankfully humans who revered ginkgo for its beauty and medicine brought it back from the brink.

Looking at the (usually) two-lobed leaf, one is reminded of the anatomy of both the brain and lungs. And in these areas of the body, ginkgo proffers benefits. In recent years, ginkgo leaf has become popular as a treatment for cognitive function, namely improving memory and mental clarity. Brew a tea of the green or yellow leaves for an energizing, brain-stimulating tonic.

Ginkgo stimulates circulation to the periphery, making it beneficial for conditions such as peripheral neuropathy, peripheral arterial disease, and Raynaud's syndrome. Ginkgo also aids in reducing tinnitus due to poor circulation and helps mitigate altitude sickness.

The yellow leaves are utilized for assuaging respiratory ailments, including asthma, allergic wheezing, and coughs. The roasted or boiled seeds are used for a similar purpose.

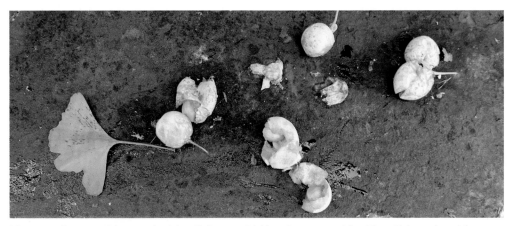

It's easy to harvest ginkgo seeds right off the ground. Use gloves to avoid getting stinky and peel the outer flesh in situ before bringing your harvest home.

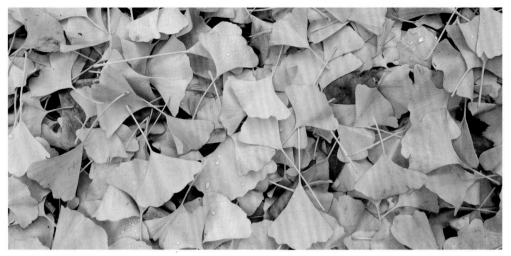

Autumn's yellow ginkgo leaves and seeds are useful for treating asthma, wheezing, and coughs.

Preparing and Eating Ginkgo Nuts

Raw ginkgo nuts are toxic, so cooking them is essential. They make a delicious food-as-medicine complement to rice dishes or are just as satisfying on their own. Here are two methods for preparing and eating freshly gathered ginkgo seeds.

Boiling method: Place unshelled (but hulled of the outer yellow flesh) and washed ginkgo seeds in a small saucepan along with 1 tablespoon of sea salt. Add enough water to cover the seeds. Gently boil for 10 minutes. Strain and rinse in cold water. Remove the shells with a nutcracker and peel away the skin. Enjoy as is or chopped up in rice.

Roasting method: Preheat the oven to 300°F. Clean off any pulp or dirt from the exterior of the shells. Spread the ginkgo seeds on a baking sheet and roast for 30 minutes. Crack and peel the shell and skin and enjoy.

⚠ Precautions

Use caution if taking blood-thinning medications, or if you have a blood clotting disorder.

Do not use ginkgo in pregnancy.

The seeds are purportedly toxic in large quantities, so it is advised not to exceed 10–15 seeds per day for adults and 5 for children. Wear gloves when collecting the seeds to reduce the risk of skin irritation, and to keep your hands stink-free.

Future Harvests

Respectfully collecting the leaves and fruit of ginkgo does not endanger this hardy tree.

HERBAL PREPARATIONS

Tea
Standard infusion of dried leaves
Drink 2–4 ounces up to 3 times per day.

Tincture
1 part fresh leaves
2 parts menstruum (60% alcohol, 40% water)
Take 30–60 drops up to 3 times per day.

Solidago species
Canada goldenrod (*S. canadensis*), tall goldenrod (*S. altissima*),
early goldenrod (*S. juncea*), giant goldenrod (*S. gigantea*)
PARTS USED flowering tops

*Partner with sunny goldenrod for its effectiveness in urinary
tract infections, seasonal allergies, and sore joints and muscles.*

How to Identify

There are at least 100–120 species of goldenrod worldwide, with a great concentration in
North America and especially the Northeast.
In general, these perennial plants share
the following characteristics: small, golden,
composite flowers that bloom from top to
bottom, commonly in pyramidal panicles or

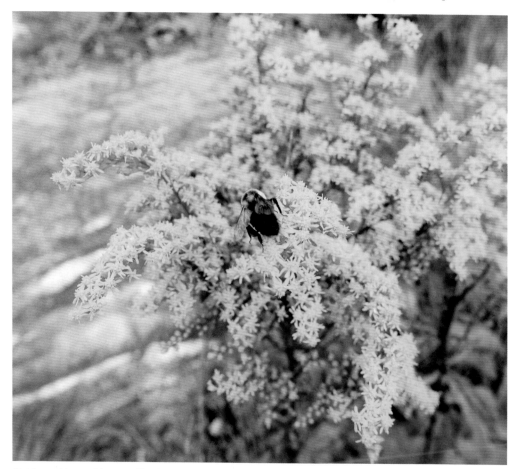

Goldenrod is a golden candle shining in summer to fall as the sunlight wanes.

in some species in a raceme or flower spike; simple, toothed, lanceolate leaves with small rough hairs growing uniformly alternate up a stiff, upright stem.

Canada goldenrod and tall goldenrod are two of the most common species and in good conservation status—some even call them weeds. They grow 2–6 feet tall with sharply toothed lanceolate leaves 4–6 inches long with a central vein and two prominent veins parallel to it. The stem is smooth at the base and hairy near the top. The yellow flowers are very small, under ⅛ inch long, and grow in a pyramidal panicle.

Where, When, and How to Wildcraft

Depending on the species, goldenrod blooms from late summer to fall in places as varied as sandy coastal areas, open fields, in and at the edge of forests, and at the edge of lakes and rivers. Harvest the top third of the flowering plant carefully by hand or with clippers. Leave plenty of the flowers for the bees, who busily collect the pollen and nectar through the fall when other flowers have died back. All parts—leaves, stems, flowers—can be used fresh or air dried. Because the flowers go to seed fairly soon after picking, dry the flowering tops in a paper bag, either lying on a flat surface in a single layer or hanging with the bag loosely tied around it.

Medicinal Uses

Glowing golden yellow in the waning light of summer, goldenrod brings relief to afflictions of the solar plexus region of the body. Goldenrod has an affinity with the urinary tract, reducing pain and inflammation of

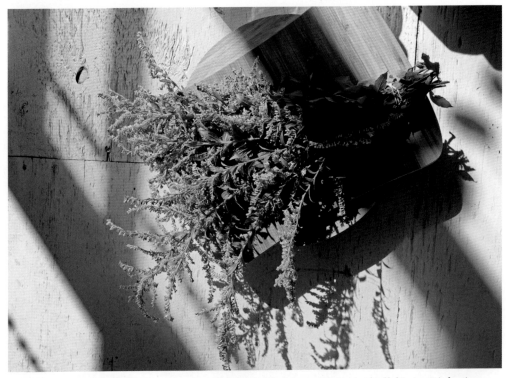

Versatile medicine, goldenrod can be infused in water, oil, vinegar, honey, or alcohol to treat infection, allergies, and pain.

the kidneys and urethra when infection is present. Combine goldenrod, spotted Joe Pye weed, crampbark, and common mallow to ease the passage of kidney stones. Infuse oil with goldenrod to use as a solar plexus massage oil to ease abdominal pain and bloating.

The infused oil can also be used to relieve sore muscles and joints in conditions such as arthritis and carpal tunnel syndrome. Add oils infused with Saint John's wort, dandelion blossom, and mugwort to craft a pain-relieving balm.

Goldenrod infusion reduces allergic symptoms, particularly runny nose and watery eyes. The infusion is rather bitter and astringent, and adding spearmint, elderflower, rosehips, and nettle will improve the taste as well as add to its antihistaminic and anti-inflammatory properties.

The astringent nature of goldenrod helps to tone tissues of the digestive tract, putting diarrhea in check. Topically, goldenrod can stanch bleeding of wounds.

Goldenrod is antifungal and adding monarda and cinquefoil in tincture or infusion form along with an anti-candida protocol can eradicate yeast infections.

Future Harvests

Several species of goldenrod are endangered, threatened, or extirpated in parts of the Northeast. Check local conservation status to be sure you are not harvesting a plant that is endangered in your area. Collect from more abundant species, such as Canada goldenrod, tall goldenrod, early goldenrod, and giant goldenrod to ensure the diversity of this valuable native plant.

HERBAL PREPARATIONS

Tea

Standard infusion of dried flowering tops
Double strain the infusion to filter out fine hairs that could cause irritation. Drink 1 cup up to 4 times per day.

Tincture

1 part fresh flowering tops
2 parts menstruum (50% alcohol, 50% water)
Take 30–60 drops 3 times per day.

Infused oil

1 part fresh flowering tops
2 parts oil
Use for massage. Add to a salve with other pain-relieving or wound-healing herbs.

Aegopodium podagraria
ground elder, bishop's elder, bishopswort, goatweed
PARTS USED leaves, roots

A tasty potherb akin to celery, goutweed is a diuretic,
sedative plant that provides relief for gout and rheumatism.

How to Identify

Goutweed is an introduced perennial herb that easily overtakes the understory of forests and disturbed soils in shaded areas. It is fairly low-growing, except for its flowers which grow on slender smooth erect stems. The tiny white flowers appear in an umbel or dish, resembling elderflowers and

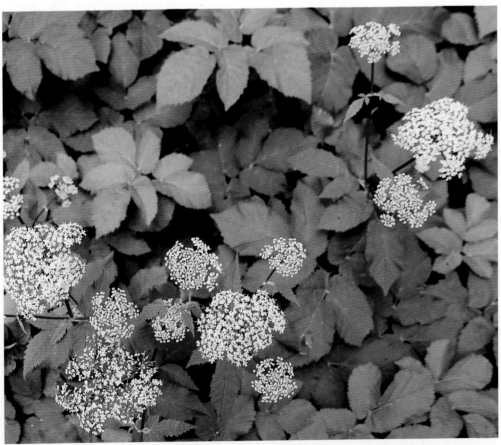

The genus name *Aegopodium* derives from the Greek words for "goat" (*aix, aigos*) and "foot" (*pous, podos*), as the leaves kind of resemble a goat's foot. The species name hails from the Latin word for "gout," *podagra*, telling us of its traditional use for this condition.

blooming around the same time, hence the common name ground elder. The flowers are also reminiscent of wild carrot or Queen Anne's lace, to which it is related. You'll often find bees buzzing about the blooms collecting pollen.

Tender, toothed leaves are inconsistently divided into two or three leaflets, some of which are similar in appearance to a goat's footprint—goatweed is an older and lesser-used common name. Stems have a triangular shape. Crushing any part of the plant reveals a celery-like scent. Goutweed extends itself readily by a network of thin tan-white rhizomes.

Where, When, and How to Wildcraft

Goutweed spreads out in the shady edge, blanketing forest floors, garden borders, and park paths, much to the chagrin of native plant enthusiasts. Pluck the leaves, stem and all, from spring through early summer—they are more tender before flowering, so this is the time to harvest if you plan to eat them. Better yet, dig up the entire plant, aiming to get as much of the root as possible. Every part is medicinal and this extremely widespread invasive plant will reproduce rampantly if given the chance. Be sure not to inadvertently introduce the plant into a garden by way of compost, as it will readily take over wherever it can get a roothold.

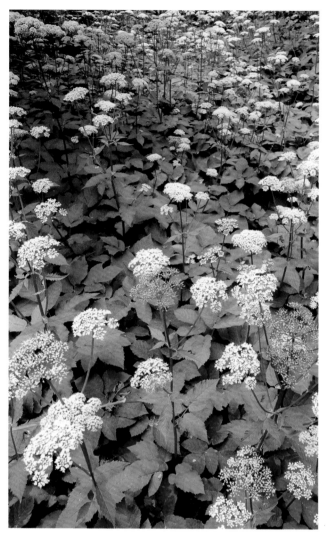

Sometimes called bishop's elder or bishopswort, goutweed was planted in medieval monastic gardens as an edible and medicinal herb to treat what was once called the "disease of kings." Those of means had access to rich food and drink that would contribute to elevated uric acid in the blood, leading to gout.

Medicinal Uses

Goutweed has been used since ancient Roman times for its diuretic, sedative, and pain-relieving effects. A tea or tincture of the leaves brings relief to gout. Eating the leaves is another way to take in the medicine.

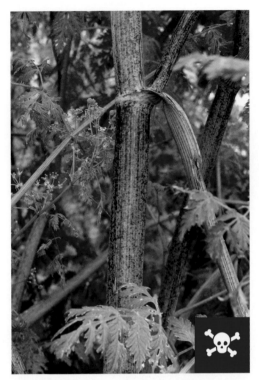

Sip a decoction of goutweed, dandelion root, and Japanese knotweed root to reduce the pain and swelling of arthritic conditions. Externally, make a poultice of goutweed leaf or root, with the optional addition of comfrey leaf or root, to further alleviate rheumatic and arthritic symptoms.

Future Harvests

Goutweed is a very difficult to eradicate introduced plant. Harvesting the entire plant for food or medicine will make the jobs of people working in forest management a bit easier and will make room for other understory plants.

Although goutweed is not terribly similar looking to its toxic relative, poison hemlock (*Conium maculatum*), it's still prudent to be able to distinguish the two from one another. The opposite compound leaves of poison hemlock are lacy and very symmetrical. In its second year, poison hemlock has feathery leaves growing oppositely up a smooth, hollow stem dotted with purple splotches at its base. Also, the scent would be a giveaway—goutweed smells of celery and poison hemlock has an unpleasant musty scent.

HERBAL PREPARATIONS

Tea
Standard infusion of dried leaves
Drink 1 cup up to 3 times per day.

Tincture
1 part fresh leaves
2 parts menstruum (50% alcohol, 50% water)
Take 20–40 drops up to 3 times per day.

Poultice
Simmer chopped root for 20 minutes. Place boiled root along with some of the cooking liquid into a piece of cloth. Place on affected area for 25–30 minutes and repeat as needed.

ground ivy

Glechoma hederacea
creeping Charlie, gill-over-the-ground
PARTS USED aerial parts in flower, leaves

A common, introduced, weedy plant, ground ivy has a long history of use as a remedy for headaches, congestion, kidney complaints, and digestion.

How to Identify

Ground ivy is a low-growing perennial herb in the mint family. Colonies of ground ivy often form a dense mat of scalloped, overlapping, kidney-shaped leaves. Closer inspection reveals the leaves growing opposite each other in pairs. In midspring when small blue-purple flowers emerge, the leaves appear more heart shaped with a slight point at the tip. Stems are square, typical of many other mints. Crushing the plant reveals a warm, sharp, minty aroma.

Where, When, and How to Wildcraft

Ground ivy grows in full to partial sun at the base of trees or at edges of paths in areas disturbed by human activity. Gather the aerial parts of the plant by hand in spring when in flower or the leaves from spring through fall.

With its low-growing habit, ground ivy is likely to be covered in dirt, especially after a hard rain. Since the herb contains valuable volatile oils that washing would remove, collect clean-looking ground ivy on a dry morning, if possible.

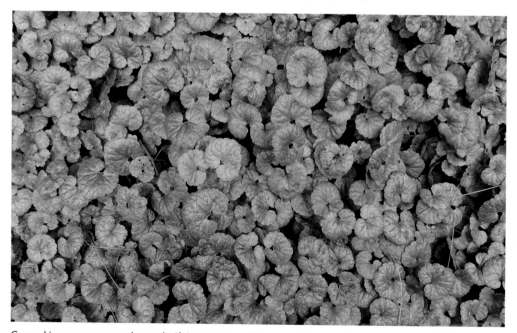

Ground ivy was once used as a clarifying agent and flavoring in beers—the common name "gill" (as in gill-over-the-ground) comes from the French word *guiller*, or "to ferment."

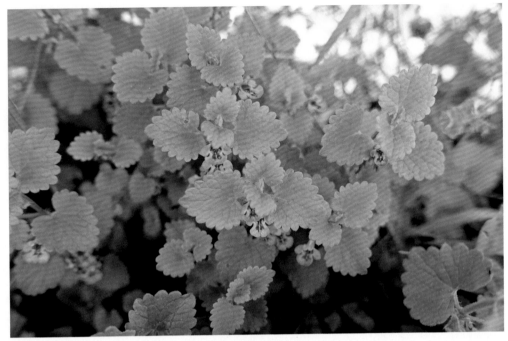

As ground ivy flowers, the leaves tend to become more heart-shaped.

Medicinal Uses

Bitter, aromatic, and astringent, ground ivy has long been used for its toning effect on the mucous membranes.

Pairs of kidney-shaped leaves grow opposite one another on the plant, like a pair of kidneys. You could also liken this to a pair of ears or a pair of lungs. Ground ivy is balancing for all of these organs. The infusion or tincture is an effective remedy for afflictions of the ears including tinnitus, earache, and fluid trapped in the middle ear (glue ear).

As a mild expectorant, ground ivy breaks up congestion in the lungs and sinuses. Drink warm ground ivy infusion to relieve headache due to sinus congestion and alleviate cough due to stuck mucus in the lungs. Make a steam treatment of ground ivy, mint, and elderflowers to aid the process.

Ground ivy has a stimulating effect on the kidneys and digestive tract, encouraging elimination of toxins from the body. Use the tincture or tea for inflammation of the kidneys and to alleviate constipation.

Externally, a poultice of the fresh leaves soothes stings, bruises, and minor scrapes. Combine with yarrow and chickweed for added effect.

Future Harvests

Ground ivy is a common introduced herb that readily reproduces.

HERBAL PREPARATIONS

Tea
Standard infusion of dried aerial parts
Drink 4 ounces as needed.

Tincture
1 part fresh aerial parts
2 parts menstruum (50% alcohol, 50% water)
Take 15–20 drops as needed.

hawthorn

Crataegus species

PARTS USED flowers, fruit, leaves, thorns

Hawthorn is a magical, protective ally for physical and energetic ailments of the heart.

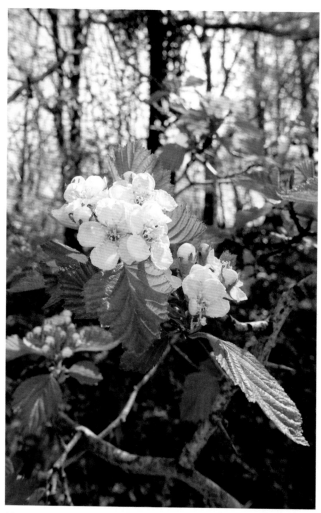

The genus name *Crataegus* derives partially from *krátaios*, the name that Greek physician Dioscorides gave this tree in the first century CE. The Greek root of *Crataegus* is *krátys*, meaning "strong" or "hard," and "akis" meaning sharp. Hawthorn allays sharp stabbing pains of the heart, a symptom of angina.

How to Identify

Native to Europe, Asia, and North America, hawthorn comprises 100–200 species in deciduous tree or shrub form. There is great variation within the *Crataegus* genus in habit, flower size, fruit size, and leaf shape.

In general, hawthorn has a crooked, worn shape similar to its crabapple relative. As you get closer to the tree or shrub, you'll notice the thorns. Hawthorn has true thorns, which unlike the prickles of roses, have the potential to become branches. Look up into the branches in winter and you're likely to see a bird's nest tucked in safely. This speaks to the protective nature of hawthorn.

Leaves are fairly leathery and range from sharply toothed to deeply lobed. Creamy white to pink, five-petaled flowers emerge in midspring, aligning with May Day celebrations where the hawthorn tree stands as a maypole and the old tradition is to wear hawthorn flower crowns. The flowers have a sweet scent with a hint of fruity sharpness. Some liken the scent to a rotting fish odor—thanks to trimethylamine, a fragrance that attracts carrion insects.

Tart, edible berries (more accurately, pomes or thornapples) ripen to a bright red in late summer to autumn, in time for harvest festivals. Depending on the species, the number of seeds in the fruit ranges from one to five.

Where, When, and How to Wildcraft

Being a boundary tree, hawthorn frequents edges and understories of forests, and is often planted in parks. Historically, hawthorn was used as hedgerow and the two words are nearly synonymous when you get to the root of them—"haw" is derived from an old English word for hedge.

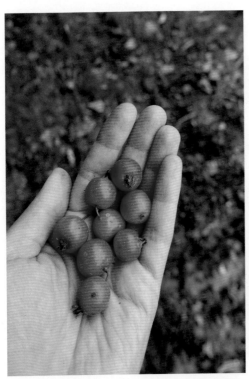

It is perfectly okay to collect freshly fallen hawthorn fruit from the ground. Check to be sure no critters have nibbled the berries or taken up residence inside before taking home your harvest.

Gently pick the flowers when they bloom in midspring. Be mindful to leave plenty of flowers behind as, once pollinated, they lead to fruit. Pluck leaves from spring through fall. Gather only healthy, green leaves—hawthorn, like other rose-family plants, is prone to rust from redcedar trees. Carefully remove thorns by hand, being cautious not to damage the branch.

Berries will let you know when they are ready for harvesting. If you spy a few already on the ground, it's likely time to harvest from the tree. Gather the fallen fruit as well as any berries that easily come off the branch. If you tug on them and they don't come loose, leave those to ripen more. Also leave plenty for the birds to sustain them through the colder months.

Medicinal Uses

Hawthorn thorns, leaves, flowers, and berries are all used medicinally to strengthen the heart. Thorns, or plant parts that can prick you and make you bleed, are a signature for applications in the blood and heart. The red berries are another signature for the blood. Their tartness hints at vitamin C content, indicating antioxidant and anti-inflammatory effects and a protective quality to the cardiovascular system. Hawthorn improves blood flow to the heart, helping to normalize or balance blood pressure, blood lipids, and heart rhythm. Take the tincture or berry infusion daily to correct arrhythmia, improve blood cholesterol, reduce atherosclerosis, and regulate hypertension.

In Chinese medicine, hawthorn fruit is taken to aid digestion. The sweet/sour berries, in the form of a syrup, jelly, infusion, or decoction help remove stagnation from the intestinal tract, breaking down blockages and undigested food (especially meat) in the small intestines.

Working on an energetic level and coupled with its mild sedative effect, hawthorn can help heal a broken heart. Taking an elixir or tea in times of grief can help one process their feelings with an open heart. Use the flower essence alone or with the herb to heal emotional wounds related to loss or death.

⚠ Precautions

If you are using cardioactive pharmaceuticals like digoxin, consult with a physician who has herbal knowledge. The cardiotonic effect of hawthorn may necessitate a lower dose of medication.

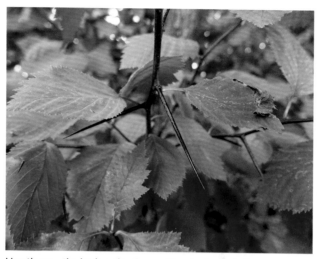

Hawthorn—the hedge, the thorned border tree—helps us navigate liminal spaces, establish healthy boundaries, and process pain and loss, especially in matters of the heart.

Avoid ingesting the seeds as they contain cyanogenic compounds (as does any plant part that smells strongly of almonds when crushed).

Future Harvests

Collecting flowers, fruit, leaves, and thorns with good attention and intention will not put hawthorn at risk. Being that hawthorn is linked with fairies, it wouldn't hurt to leave a gift of honey or sweetened milk in exchange for your harvest.

HERBAL PREPARATIONS

Tea

1 hour infusion of dried berries
Drink 1 cup 3 times per day.
or
Standard infusion of flowers and leaves
Drink 4 ounces up to 4 times per day or as needed.

Tincture

1 part fresh flowers, fruit, leaves, and thorns
2 parts menstruum (50% alcohol, 50% water)
Take 60–90 drops up to 4 times per day.

Flower essence

Follow instructions for making flower essences on page 54. Take 3 drops on the tongue or in water 3 times per day or as needed.

hops

Humulus lupulus
PARTS USED strobiles

Hops is more than just a bittering agent for beer. The fruit of this hemp family plant calms the nerves, aids digestion, and helps nursing mothers with healthy milk production.

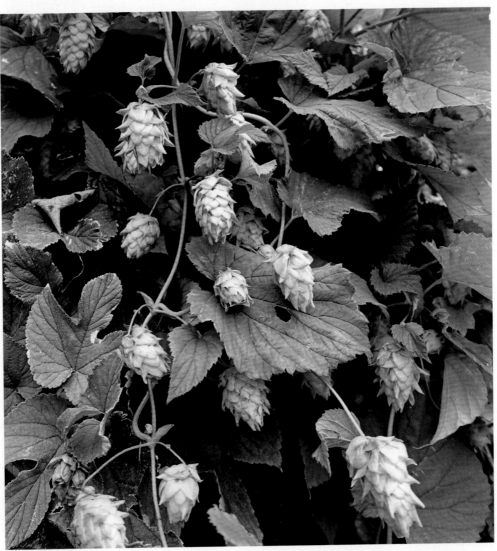

In all the places they are native to, *Humulus* species have long been utilized as a remedy for pain and nervous tension.

How to Identify

Native to Europe, Asia, and North America, hops is a perennial climbing, twining vine (bine) in the hemp family that grows up to 30 feet. Toothed, rough leaves range from heart shaped to three-lobed to palmately lobed (roughly hand shaped). Hops is dioecious, meaning there are separate male and female plants, and in early summer their flowers emerge. On male plants, five-petaled yellow-green flowers grow in drooping panicles. Inconspicuous yellow-green pistillate flowers emerge on females. Once pollinated the female flowers become strobiles (fruit) that are harvested for medicinal use. The strobiles are resinous with a pine-like scent.

Where, When, and How to Wildcraft

Look for hops at the edges of forested areas, often near rivers or lakes, where it will be growing thickly up trees and shrubs. Harvest strobiles in late summer to early or mid-fall. The outer layer will feel papery with light browning at the edges of some of the petals. The inner layers should contain a yellow, sticky substance called lupulin—pressing the strobile together will release its resin and pine scent. Wear gloves and long sleeves while picking strobiles as the rough leaves can irritate skin.

Medicinal Uses

Known primarily as a bittering and preservative agent for beer, hops in tea or tincture form provides a relaxing tonic to the nervous system. The bitter taste of hops exposes its ability to aid digestion and works especially well in those who suffer from indigestion due to nervousness. Drink a warm cup of hops tea before or after meals to reduce bloating, gassiness, and abdominal pain while enhancing the body's ability to assimilate nutrients. Add catnip and chamomile for added effect.

Sedative and hypnotic, hops are conducive to relaxation and sleep. Drink hops tea in times of stress to help induce restful slumber. Skullcap and blue vervain make good companions to hops where there is anxiety-induced head and neck tension.

Hops is a great herb for new mothers, improving breastmilk production while simultaneously soothing frayed nerves.

Hops has an antimicrobial effect, particularly against gram-positive bacterial infections such as those caused by *Streptococcus* and *Clostridium*. Combining hops with barberry root, echinacea, blackberry, and mallow root could help eradicate colitis caused by *C. difficile* bacteria.

⚠ Precautions

Hops may have an anaphrodisiac effect (reducing sex drive) on some people which, depending on circumstances, may be seen as a benefit or side effect.

Future Harvests

Picking the strobiles of hops will not endanger the future of this plant.

HERBAL PREPARATIONS

Tea
Standard infusion of dried strobiles
Drink 4–8 ounces as needed.

Tincture
1 part fresh strobiles
2 parts menstruum (65% alcohol, 35% water)
or
1 part dried strobiles
5 parts menstruum (65% alcohol, 35% water)
Take 30–90 drops up to 3 times per day. Lower doses induce calm while larger doses assist in falling and staying asleep.

Dream Sachet Ritual

Herbal medicine isn't restricted to what we ingest or put on our skin. There is great healing power in employing all the senses, and in performing rituals. Another potent opportunity for healing is in our dreams. Dreams hold threads of meaning for our daily lives and provide us with beneficial guidance, if we practice asking and listening.

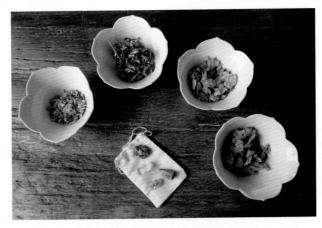

Plants are our allies in awakening to the potential of our dreams.

The following herb-crafting ritual can help you tap into the healing messages of your dreams.

What you'll need:

- Small pouch or sachet
- Herbs for dreaming (see list below)
- Small crystal or stone that holds significance for you

Start with your intention. Do you have a question about an aspect of your life? Is there a goal you'd like to achieve or something you'd like to shed light on? If you wish, you can write this on a small piece of paper to include in the sachet. Now feel into which herbs you'd like to work with. We all have personal associations with certain plants and this could guide you. Or look to the following list to assist you in choosing, based on your intentions.

- hops—to induce restful, healing sleep
- catnip—to face fears with curiosity and a playful attitude
- rose—to open your heart; for questions of love and the future
- yarrow—for divination and protection
- mullein—to enhance connection with spirit guides
- blue vervain—to balance emotions and communication
- mugwort—to stimulate lucid dreams, to cross thresholds

You can work with one or several of these herbs. Place a pinch of each herb you are working with into your sachet, thinking about your intention or question. Call on the plant spirits for guidance and healing. Take your stone or crystal and speak your question into it, then place it into the sachet. Seal the sachet and place it inside your pillowcase. When you get into bed, call on the plant spirits again. As you drift off to sleep, keep your intention or question in mind. Record your dreams as soon as you wake. You can work on the same question for several nights or longer, depending on what you derive from the dream messages.

Equisetum species
field horsetail (*E. arvense*), scouring-rush (*E. hyemale*)
PARTS USED aerial parts

Ancient, mineral-rich horsetail strengthens the structural elements of the body—bones, connective tissue, skin, hair, and nails. It's also a diuretic and lends itself well to herbal blends for healing urinary tract imbalance.

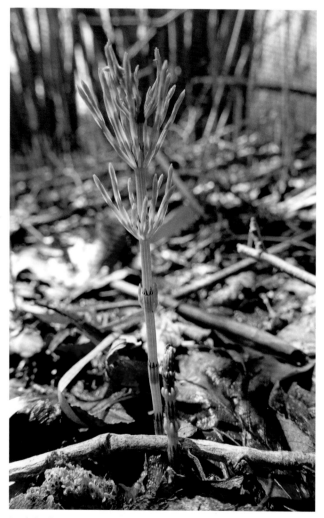

Look for horsetail in watery terrain. Horsetail is a diuretic, having an affinity to the watery terrain of our body, in other words, the urinary tract.

How to Identify

Considered a "living fossil" predating flowering plants, *Equisetum* is an ancient genus of plants native to many parts of the world, with a great concentration native to North America. Horsetail emerges in spring as upright, single-stemmed, grooved, hollow shoots with jointed sections. At the top of the stem is a cone-like structure called a sporophyte. Fertile tan-white stems lack chlorophyll and die back in spring after producing spores, while sterile stems are green and continue to develop through the growing season. As the sterile stems mature they send out fine branches in whorls that emerge from the joints or nodes. The leaves appear as inconspicuous little teeth hugging the nodes. Horsetail spreads by branching rhizomes.

Field horsetail grows up to 3 feet, produces up to twenty whorls per branch, and has four to fourteen dark brown teeth at the top of the sheath-like, joined leaves. Its upright branches are solid and are surrounded by three or four teeth where they are attached to the stem.

Scouring-rush is an unbranching species of horsetail with tan-gray, fringed sheaths at the nodes, each ringed at the bottom by a black band. There may also be a slightly thinner black band at the tops of the sheath, forming a black-tan-black pattern from top to bottom. The common name is thanks to its rough, ridged, silica-containing stem that campers and explorers have used for scrubbing pots and pans.

Where, When, and How to Wildcraft

Horsetail does not mind having its feet wet, often growing in marshes and at the edges of waterways. Field horsetail isn't limited to wet habitats and adapts its appearance according to locale. In wetter areas, the branches appear long and lanky nearer the top of the plant, while on drier land the plants can grow dense and shrubby with branches fringing the base.

Collect the green infertile stems of horsetail from spring to fall using plant shears. Cut your harvest into smaller pieces to use fresh in tincture or vinegar or to dry for infusions.

Medicinal Uses

Through its form, horsetail—pliable, jointed, ancient—speaks to us of strength in the structural elements of the body. Horsetail is rich in silica and imparts the fortifying nature of this element to connective tissue, bones, skin, hair, and nails. Drink a nourishing decoction of horsetail, stinging nettle, red clover, yellow dock, plantain, and mint to prevent or heal from broken bones and to fortify brittle hair and nails. Add a strong decoction of horsetail to baths to aid in mending damaged connective tissue—adding comfrey root and elder leaves and stems bolsters the healing effects.

Akin to the watery environs in which it often grows, horsetail promotes fluid release in the body. In other words, it's diuretic.

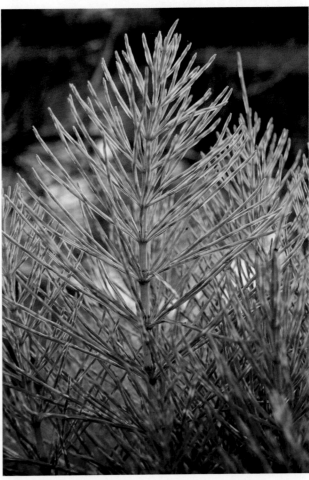

Horsetail dons flexible hair-like branches in whorls up its jointed stem, reminding us of its usefulness for mending weak bones, hair, and connective tissue.

Using horsetail with cranberry, common mallow, and goldenrod can relieve urinary tract inflammation and infection in cases of cystitis or urethritis.

Horsetail tones the urinary tract and can be helpful for preventing bedwetting and incontinence due to a weak bladder.

Apply a horsetail poultice externally on fresh wounds to stop bleeding and aid in healing of skin tissue.

⚠ Precautions

Horsetail uptakes minerals from the earth, including lead. Consider the waterway or soil the horsetail is growing in, and whether it is a place where runoff or industrial waste has settled.

Large doses or extended use of horsetail may potentially lead to thiamine deficiency. To reduce this risk, stick to the recommended doses of this herb and consider an on-again, off-again approach to taking horsetail internally.

Future Harvests

Favor the more widespread species of horsetail—field horsetail and scouring-rush—over other species, many of which are threatened or endangered in parts of the Northeast. Always check your local conservation status before harvesting.

HERBAL PREPARATIONS

Tea
Standard decoction of dried aerial parts
Drink 4 ounces up to 3 times per day.

Tincture
1 part fresh aerial parts
2 parts menstruum (95% alcohol,
   5% water)
Take 5–20 drops up to 3 times per day.

Japanese honeysuckle

Lonicera japonica
PARTS USED flowers, leaves, stems

Japanese honeysuckle is a cooling, blood-cleansing, antiviral, and antibacterial herb that clears toxic inflammation caused by infection.

How to Identify
Japanese honeysuckle is a perennial twining vine with simple, opposite, ovate leaves that are 1½–3 inches in length. Its young stems and flower buds are covered in fine, downy hairs.

Pairs of white tubular flowers bloom in summer, their heady aroma sweetly scenting the air. And like its moniker suggests, honeysuckle tastes sweet, too. Pinch the bottom tip of the flower and slowly pull out the pistil to reveal a honey-sweet gem of nectar. Once you've sampled this delight, then it's time to suck on the bloom to enjoy the rest of the nectar.

Berries appear in fall and are dark purple to black. They are inedible to humans, but birds like them.

Where, When, and How to Wildcraft
Look for Japanese honeysuckle thriving in the sunny to partially shaded edges of

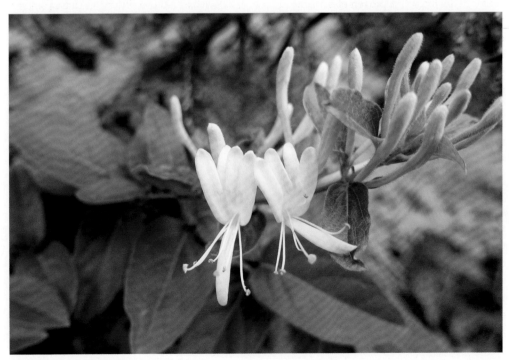

Honeysuckle leaves, flowers, and stems are antimicrobial and used commercially as a natural preservative in cosmetics.

forested areas and climbing on shrubs and along fences. The vine does fine in poor soils and frequently inhabits sandy, coastal areas.

In summer, harvest the white blossoms in the morning or evening to prevent wilting. Sometimes a second flush of blossoms occurs in early fall. Gather leaves and stems from the tops of vines through fall and sometimes early winter.

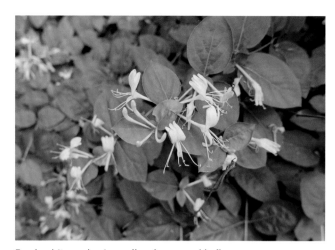

Fresh white and aging yellow honeysuckle flowers appear together, a feature that inspired the name *Jin yin hua*—gold-silver flower—in its native China.

Medicinal Uses

Japanese honeysuckle is primarily used in Chinese medicine to dispel wind-heat or externally contracted infections or toxins, such as *Streptococcus pneumoniae* and *Salmonella* infections. It has proven effective for treating pneumonia and asthma. Drink a cold infusion of the flowers and leaves at the onset of infections that present with flushing, fever, and sore throat. Add forsythia fruit for added cooling and antimicrobial effect.

The divine smell and taste of the blossoms can be captured in elixir or syrup form or infused in honey. This sweet medicine has a particular influence over the spleen and immune system.

Honeysuckle stems are traditionally used to treat arthritic joint pain and relax tight tendons and ligaments. A bath, compress, or poultice would assuage these painful conditions.

Apply Japanese honeysuckle–infused oil to soothe red, hot skin conditions such as acne and boils. Use a cool honeysuckle flower and stem compress to ease headache from overheating, reduce breast tissue inflammation (mastitis), and ease menstrual cramps where the abdomen is hot to the touch.

⚠ Precautions

Japanese honeysuckle may be too cooling for those with a cold constitution. Adding warming herbs such as spruce or pine could help balance out the coolness of honeysuckle.

Future Harvests

Japanese honeysuckle is an introduced, sometimes invasive, vine that grows in abundance. Collecting the leaves, stems, and flowers will not endanger this species. In other words, there's plenty to go around.

HERBAL PREPARATIONS

Tea
Standard or cold infusion of fresh or dried flowers
Drink 4 ounces as needed.

Tincture
1 part fresh flowers
2 parts menstruum (50% alcohol, 50% water)
Take 10–25 drops as needed.

Japanese knotweed

Fallopia japonica (syns. *Polygonum cuspidatum, Reynoutria japonica*)
PARTS USED rhizomes, shoots

Turn to Japanese knotweed as a preventative for cardiovascular disease,
and as an ally in healing from autoimmune conditions and systemic infections,
including Lyme disease.

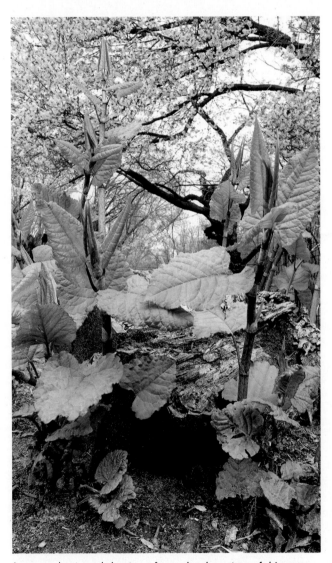

Japanese knotweed shoots up from a hardy system of rhizomes in spring.

How to Identify

Japanese knotweed is an herbaceous perennial that begins its yearly cycle in spring with low-growing (about 1 foot) shoots that can reach up to 10 feet tall by summer. Stems are smooth and hollow with red splotches along their length and prominent red joints. In spring, the shiny green leaves feature a hint of red as they unfold into a sort of shovel shape edged with a subtle wavy outline. As the leaves mature, they lose their luster, becoming thoroughly green and matte in appearance, arranged alternately in a near zigzag pattern down the drooping stem. Tiny creamy white flowers bloom along tall spikes in summer. Papery seeds develop in late summer to early fall. Thick, branching rhizomes are brown on the outside and tan-orange on the inside.

Where, When, and How to Wildcraft

Japanese knotweed is not very particular about where it grows, though it does seem to favor moist soil. You'll most often find it in the edge—in ditches, abutting fences, bordering roadways, and near marshes, lakes, and rivers.

Collect Japanese knotweed shoots in spring while they are juicy and unbranched. You can break them off where they feel tender or use clippers. Peel off the leaves and outer layer of skin, if it's tough, before cooking.

Harvest the rhizomes in the spring just before or as the young shoots begin to emerge or in fall when the plant begins to die back. Look for last year's dried-up, tan-colored stems— they look like bamboo. Be prepared with a variety of digging and cutting implements. Loosen the soil around one of last year's stems with a small garden fork and dig down with a shovel or trowel. Apply pressure to break apart the rhizome. If it's loose enough, you could use the dried stem as a handle to pull up the root.

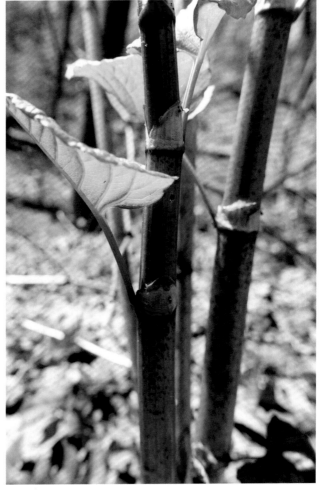

Bright red nodes reflect painful, inflamed conditions in the joints of the body, hinting at what this plant is helpful for.

Medicinal Uses

Japanese knotweed is a poster child for much-despised, hard-to-eradicate weeds. But what if we shift this perspective to appreciate that a versatile, much-needed medicine is in great supply, often right in our backyards? (Thank you, Mother Earth.)

One of the chief applications of Japanese knotweed is for pain and inflammation in the joints, especially related to autoimmune disease or systemic infection. Notice the red inflamed joints of the plant and you'll be reminded of this use. Conditions where this appears include rheumatoid and psoriatic arthritis, ankylosing spondylitis, lupus, and Lyme disease.

Red splotches on the stem of Japanese knotweed are a signature for the blood. The plant contains resveratrol, a polyphenol that imparts antioxidant and cardioprotective benefits. Japanese knotweed stanches bleeding, reduces high blood pressure, improves blood cholesterol, regulates blood sugar, and removes toxins from the blood.

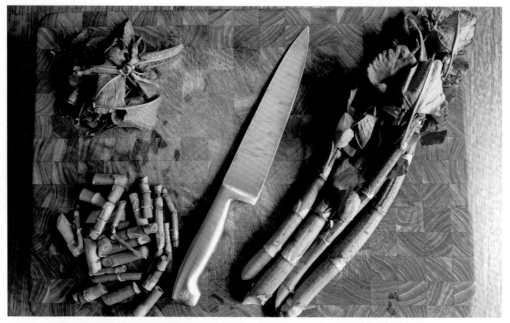

Japanese knotweed shoots are mildly sour and serve as a nutrient-dense, blood-cleansing spring vegetable.

⚠ Precautions

Use caution when using blood-thinning medications, as Japanese knotweed may potentiate their effects.

If you have or think you have contracted Lyme disease (*Borrelia burgdorferi* or related co-infections), see a physician right away. Work with a knowledgeable medical herbalist or physician well-versed in herbs to develop a personalized protocol.

Future Harvests

The Japanese name for this plant, *itadori*, translates as "removes pain." The inverse of that statement describes the tenacity of Japanese knotweed in the landscape—pain to remove. Japanese knotweed spreads by thick, hard-to-remove rhizomes. You could cut down an entire stand of knotweed and it will reappear again just as hardy as before. Harvest at will and give thanks for this abundant plant.

HERBAL PREPARATIONS

Tea
Standard decoction of dried rhizomes
Drink 1 cup up to 3 times per day.

Tincture
1 part fresh rhizomes
2 parts menstruum (65% alcohol, 35% water)
Take 60–90 drops 3 times per day.

Impatiens capensis
orange or spotted touch-me-not
PARTS USED aerial parts

Most folks who know jewelweed recognize it as an antidote to poison ivy rash, though it's best used topically as a preventative.

How to Identify

Jewelweed is an herbaceous self-seeding annual that grows near riparian zones, often neighboring poison ivy. Tender, green, oval-shaped leaves are scalloped and when water droplets collect on the leaves, they appear as little jewels, often rolling right off. Immerse a leaf in water and witness the silvery sheen covering it. Stems are glaucous, meaning they have a cloudy gray-blue coating.

Orange flowers, often spotted, bloom in summer. They are reminiscent of a small pointed cap like a fairy would wear. It's fun to gently pinch the narrow green seed capsules to experience a mini explosion of edible seeds. This is where the name "touch-me-not" comes

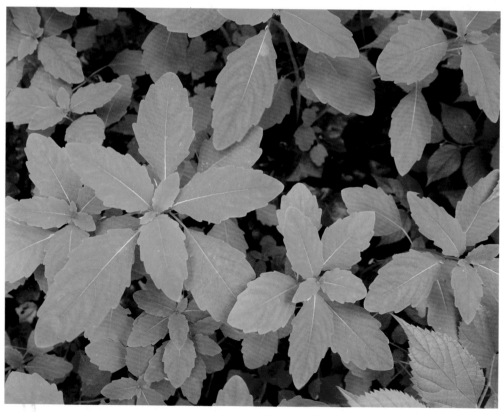

Oblong, scallop-edged leaves radiate from each central stem.

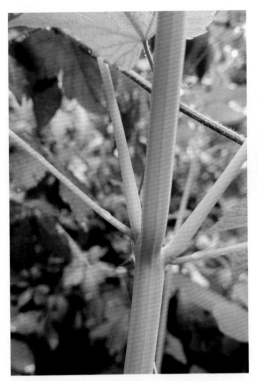

Juicy, semi-translucent stems have a pale blue-green tinge.

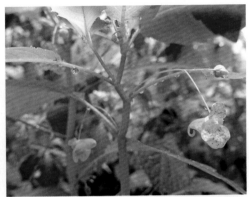

Bright orange blossoms shaped like a fairy's cap are beloved by hummingbirds.

from. After the seeds disperse, the sheath of the capsule curls back into little spirals.

Where, When, and How to Wildcraft

You'll most likely find jewelweed growing in damp earth, in concavities in the soil, or near rivers, lakes, and marshes.

Before heading out on a hike, pick a few leaves and stems. Rub them between your hands to release their juice and then rub this crushed poultice over exposed skin to prevent poison ivy rash. Collect aerial parts from late spring through summer to craft into vinegar or herbal ice cubes.

Medicinal Uses

The most common use of jewelweed is as a preventative for poison ivy rash. For some folks it works well to relieve the rash after exposure, but for others a plantain poultice or mugwort salve works better. Jewelweed preparations also come in handy for nettle stings, heat rash, scalds, and other skin irritations. You could make jewelweed oil, but because of the juiciness of the herb, it's likely to get moldy. A more reliable preparation is jewelweed ice cubes. Blend fresh jewelweed with a splash of water then freeze in ice cube trays.

Future Harvests

Taking about one-third of the aerial parts of a jewelweed patch is a decent harvest that will yield a good amount of medicine without harming the future of this plant. As always, take only what you need and leave enough for the birds, bees, and other pollinating creatures.

HERBAL PREPARATIONS

Infused vinegar

1 part fresh aerial parts

2 parts apple cider vinegar

Add to a spray bottle alone or with other itch-relieving herbs (such as Saint John's wort, mugwort, plantain, or comfrey) to prevent or treat rash.

Larix species
tamarack, American larch, or eastern larch (*L. laricina*),
European or common larch (*L. decidua*)
PARTS USED bark, needles

Warming, energizing, and immune-supportive, larch is a pine family tree that helps relieve symptoms of cold and flu and improve digestive and urinary health.

How to Identify

Larch is a deciduous coniferous tree native to North America, Europe, and Asia. Needle-shaped leaves are arranged in whorled clusters—ten to twenty needles for *L. laricina* and thirty to sixty-five for *L. decidua*—in a spiral around the branch. Unlike other members of the pine family, larch leaves turn yellow and shed in fall. On the tamarack, small red cones, ½–¾ inches long, form in summer turning brown by fall. European larch cones are more than twice as large, 1½–2 inches in length. Larch grows 50–75 feet tall in more alkaline soils, and much shorter in acidic bogs, sometimes only to 30 feet.

Where, When, and How to Wildcraft

Find larch in damp, open areas of forests, parks, and shrublands in the northern range of the Northeast, from northern Pennsylvania and New Jersey into eastern Canada. Native tamarack is more widespread than introduced European larch, though the former tree is critically imperiled in Rhode Island and borderline vulnerable in New Jersey.

In spring, prune young branch tips with hand pruners or a small tree pruning saw.

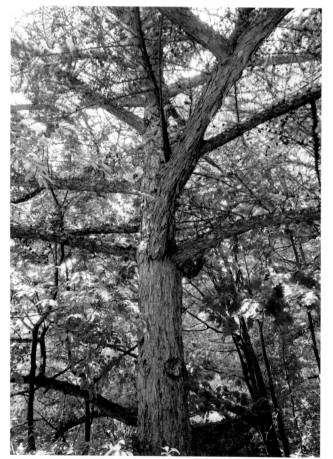

As larch ages, the bark becomes flaky, ridged, and plated.

Your harvest will contain bark and needles, which can be used together or separately. With a sharp knife, shave the outer bark from the branches to reveal the red-brown inner bark. Peel away the inner bark with the knife. Use this fresh in tea, tincture, or honey, or dry it for later.

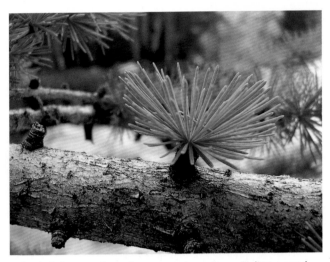

Whorled clusters of needles emerge in spring, spiraling around the branch. In fall, they turn yellow and fall to the ground, a unique trait of this pine family tree.

Medicinal Uses

Larch tones mucous membranes and is a useful remedy for respiratory, intestinal, and urinary afflictions.

Drink an inner bark and needle decoction to relieve airway inflammation and to quell coughs—add honey for its sweetness and soothing qualities. Gargle with a bark and needle decoction or diluted tincture to soothe sore throats and mouth sores.

Larch contains arabinogalactan, a polysaccharide that promotes healthy gut bacteria, improves the health of the intestines, and in turn boosts the immune system. A daily tonic decoction of the inner bark is healing to the gut lining and can help allay symptoms of irritable bowel syndrome and Crohn's disease. The same preparation is helpful for those who have recurring urinary tract infections.

Externally, use the decoction and diluted tincture as a wash, or make a poultice for healing burns, sores, and rashes.

The flower essence bolsters confidence in those who perpetually avoid asserting themselves in anticipation of inadequacy and failure.

Future Harvests

Carefully gathering a few small branches or fallen twigs will not endanger this graceful tree. Keep in mind, however, that tamarack is at risk in some parts of the Northeast, so take only what you need.

HERBAL PREPARATIONS

Tea
Standard decoction of inner bark and/or needles
Drink 2–4 ounces up to 3 times per day.
Use as a wash for rashes, burns, and wounds.

Tincture
1 part fresh inner bark and needles
2 parts menstruum (95% alcohol, 5% water)
Take 15–25 drops up to 3 times per day.

Flower essence
Follow instructions for making flower essences on page 54. Take 3 drops on the tongue or in water 3 times per day or as needed.

lemon balm

Melissa officinalis
Melissa, balm
PARTS USED flowering tops, leaves

Lemon balm lifts the mood, calms the nerves, and evokes an overall sense of well-being with even just a sniff of its cheerful citrus aroma.

How to Identify

Lemon balm is an herbaceous perennial plant in the mint family. Like most other mints, lemon balm has a square stem and opposite toothed leaves. The leaves of lemon balm tend to have a slight yellow tinge, flat base, flat surface with prominent veins, and scallop-toothed edges that point toward the tip. The distinctive lemon aroma is what gives away this plant. When lemon balm flowers in summer, bees happily bumble around its small white blooms.

Where, When, and How to Wildcraft

A garden escapee, lemon balm is likely found at the edges of park trails, abandoned farm fields, and meadows. If you spot some in a community garden or neighbor's yard, ask permission first.

Pinch off the leaves in late spring through early fall before flowering to encourage more leaf growth and to provide your harvest. Harvest the flowering tops in summer. Lemon balm is best used fresh to capture

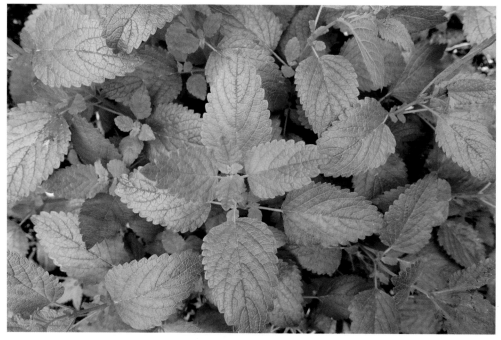

Melissa is the Greek word for "bee," at the root of which is the word for "honey" (*meli*). The honey-sweet energy of lemon balm helps to shift a sour disposition and soothe jangled nerves.

the precious essential oils in cold infusion, tincture, honey, or elixir form.

Medicinal Uses

The word "balm" evokes a sense of soothing and restoring mind, body, and spirit, which sums up the gifts of lemon balm.

Think of those bees buzzing about the flowers of lemon balm and you'll be reminded of some of this plant's uses. Lemon balm eases the buzzing sensation of conditions such as tinnitus and anxiety and relieves the stinging pain from herpes or shingles. The antiviral activity of lemon balm is useful for treating the herpes virus. Drink the cold infusion and use lemon balm-infused oil in a salve or lip balm to reduce the severity and duration of cold sores.

Brew a warm infusion of lemon balm to soothe anxiety-related stomach upset. Combine lemon balm with linden in an infusion or tincture to decrease hyperactivity and lower blood pressure. Lemon balm, catnip, and elderflower make a pleasing infusion for reducing fever that even children will enjoy.

Lemon balm and motherwort are a classic combination for improving hyperthyroidism and rapid heartrate.

Lemon balm has a sweetness that lifts the spirits. Drink a cup of fresh lemon balm infusion to shift a sour mood, help remedy the blues, or cope with nervous exhaustion. Lemon balm helps to focus the mind and calm the body, making it a great aid to meditation.

Apply a cool compress of lemon balm to relieve headache brought on by tension or stress. Use a wash to soothe burns and rashes.

 Precautions

Lemon balm may have inhibitory effects on thyroid hormone production. Conversely, it may improve thyroid health, even in those with hypothyroidism. This is a case where it is important to have an understanding of your body's individual responses and proceed with great attention when using an herb therapeutically. One helpful way of doing this is to document use of all herbs, foods, and supplements and track your body's reactions. Work with an herbalist or healthcare practitioner with herbal experience to determine the best course of action for your unique needs.

Future Harvests

Lemon balm is an introduced plant that easily reproduces by seed. There is no concern of overharvesting this plant.

HERBAL PREPARATIONS

Tea
Standard or cold infusion of fresh or dried leaves
Drink 1 cup as needed.

Tincture
1 part fresh flowering tops or leaves
2 parts menstruum (50% alcohol, 50% water)
Take 15–30 drops as needed.

Infused oil
1 part fresh leaves
2 parts oil
Craft into a lip balm to use on cold sores, following the directions for making salves on page 58.

Infused honey
1 part fresh flowering tops or leaves
2 parts honey
Enjoy by the spoonful.

---

linden

Tilia species
basswood, lime tree
PARTS USED flowers, leaves

*With sumptuous blossoms, mucilaginous leaves, and light bark, linden is a
sensual delight that extends deep healing to the mood, mind, heart, and digestion.*

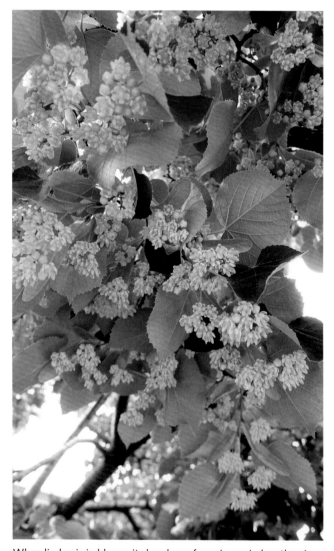

When linden is in bloom, its heady perfume is carried on the air, beckoning bees and humans with its alluring scent.

How to Identify

Linden is a deciduous tree in the mallow family represented by both native and introduced species in the Northeast. They hybridize naturally so it is sometimes difficult to classify species. Luckily, they are all medicinal.

The bark varies a bit by species but tends toward sinewy and gray. Linden leaves are heart shaped and toothed with an asymmetrical base. The leaves of some species (*T. tomentosa*, *T. petiolaris*) are white underneath. Young leaves unfurl translucent in spring, often featuring a red tinge.

From late spring to early summer, fragrant creamy white-yellow flowers bloom in small clusters on pale green, oblong, papery bracts. The flowers are hermaphroditic with both male and female parts and are pollinated by insects—visit a linden and you'll likely see an abundance of bees working diligently to collect pollen and nectar.

Linden provides a large canopy of draping branches

often widespread enough to have a picnic or large gathering under. Standing under linden evokes the feeling that you are being embraced by this nurturing tree. There is an old saying that "lightning never strikes linden." Unlike upright trees like oak that serve as lightning rods, linden has a downward-tending habit. I'm not sure I would test the theory, though I like the visual reminder that differentiates linden from other trees.

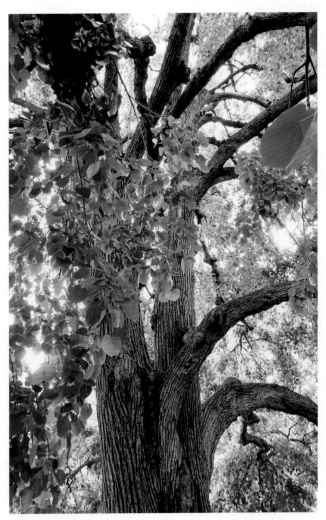

Standing within her feminine circle of branches, linden imparts a motherly quality with an overall feeling of embrace.

Where, When, and How to Wildcraft

You'll most likely see linden in open fields, parks, and meadows. It sometimes grows near the forest's edge or in depressed areas of the soil where it is moist, such as in floodplains.

Collect leaves by hand in spring while they are young, translucent, and edible, or throughout summer as they become opaque and darker green.

Gather flowers when fragrant and heady, typically just as they open, on a dry morning if possible. Collect the entire inflorescence, winged bract and all. Leave enough goodness for the bees and other pollinating insects. Linden honey is a particularly delicious light variety of honey you might be lucky enough to find at your local farmers market.

Medicinal Uses

Cooling and moistening, linden imparts a pacifying quality to irritation in the body. Drinking an infusion of the blossoms is a delightful and effective way to enjoy the medicine of this generous tree. As you pour the infusion into your cup, you'll see that it is slightly viscous, nectar-like, and ambrosial. This mucilage coats mucous membranes alleviating dry mouth, sore throat, and tickling cough.

Sipping the infusion also brings relaxation to tense nerves and anxiety-ridden stomachs. Children who get overstimulated are gently assisted by linden's soothing qualities.

When cold or flu leaves you feeling down and out, linden flower infusion lessens symptoms, reduces fever, and lifts the spirits. Combine linden with lemon balm, valerian root, and skullcap to take the edge off illness and provide comfort to ease into sleep.

Linden's heart-shaped leaves call to mind the heart and indeed linden offers relief for physical and energetic heart ailments. Combine it with hawthorn and rose to reduce hypertension, heart palpitations, and atherosclerosis. This same combination conveys lightness to a heavy, grief-stricken heart.

Linden flower essence helps those who hold onto fear and worry in their bodies, tending toward a constricted state. It brings softness and a sense of opening to the mind and body.

Future Harvests

Gathering flowers, leaves, and twigs from linden will not harm the tree. Just leave enough blossoms for the bees.

HERBAL PREPARATIONS

Tea

Standard or cold infusion of fresh or dried flowers
Drink 4–8 ounces as needed.

Tincture

1 part fresh flowers and leaves
2 parts menstruum (40% alcohol, 60% water)
Take 15–25 drops as needed.

Infused honey

1 part fresh flowers
2 parts honey
Enjoy by the spoonful or add to hot water for a sweet floral tea.

Flower essence

Follow instructions for making flower essences on page 54. Take 3 drops on the tongue up to 4 times per day or as needed.

lobelia

Lobelia inflata
puke weed, Indian tobacco
PARTS USED aerial parts

Balloon-like seedpods give away lobelia's use as a respiratory stimulant for conditions like asthma and chronic bronchitis.

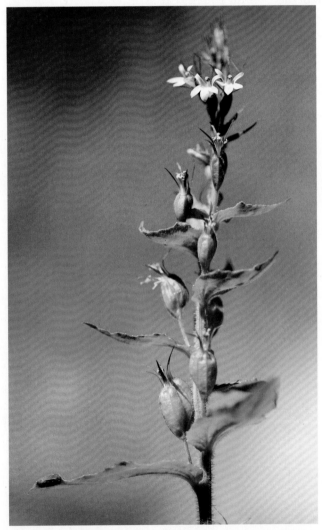

Pale violet flowers bloom from the bottom up, yielding to inflated green fruit. This pattern alludes to the upward and outward energy of this plant's medicine.

How to Identify

Lobelia is an annual herb in the bellflower family with a height varying from just a few inches to about 2½ feet depending on soil conditions. Hairy, toothed, green leaves with an oval to lance shape and pointed tip grow 2–3 inches long and ½–1½ inches wide, alternately arranged up a hairy stem. In summer, small white to pale blue-violet, bilaterally symmetrical, tubular flowers bloom from the bottom up on spikes emerging from leaf axils. They feature three pointed lobes on the lower lip. The flowers are followed by small green balloon-like fruit—this is where the specific name *inflata* derives.

Taste the fresh leaves to get a sense of this plant's medicine. The acidity is like a zap to the tongue. If you've ever dared touch your tongue to a 9-volt battery, it's a bit like that.

Where, When, and How to Wildcraft

Lobelia is a widespread native plant that grows in a range of settings. You might find it growing trailside in a park or in a farm field, on a mountainside, or in a meadow. Maybe even at a riverside or lakeshore in full sun or dappled light.

The best time to harvest is when lobelia has begun to fruit in late summer. At this time, flowers and fruit exist together. If you find an abundant patch, clip the aerial parts of one or two plants. If it seems there aren't that many plants, pluck a few of the fruits and leaves. Lobelia is potent medicine and you won't need much. Leave enough behind to go to seed for next year's harvest. Dry the plant parts or infuse in alcohol- or vinegar-based tinctures, or in oil.

Medicinal Uses

Check out those balloon-like pods on lobelia, a signature for the lungs, air, and breath. Lobelia opens the airways to stimulate respiration in those experiencing airway inflammation. Useful applications for lobelia tincture or infusion include asthma attacks, bronchitis, and whooping cough.

The aerial parts (leaves, flowers, and seedpods) are all utilized for their expectorant properties and for their antispasmodic, nervine, and diaphoretic actions. Take care in using only recommended doses as lobelia is emetic, in other words causes vomiting, in higher doses. This action was once a desired effect, prescribed by First Peoples and early colonial doctors to purge out toxins.

Lobelia is extremely helpful for people seeking to quit smoking tobacco cigarettes. Lobeline, an alkaloid present in the plant, creates a taste aversion to tobacco. Interestingly, lobelia can be smoked with other herbs such as mullein and marshmallow leaf to help with tobacco smoking cessation. You can also take lobelia in a tincture if you don't want to perpetuate the addiction to smoking itself.

The homeopathic remedy can be taken to the same effect.

Craft an oil infused with lobelia to relax muscle spasms, soothe joint pain, or calm restless legs. Combine with crampbark for added muscular relaxation.

⚠ Precautions

Start with small doses until you get to know the potency of this plant. In larger-than-needed doses, lobelia brings on nausea and vomiting.

Future Harvests

Be sure to correctly identify this species as several related species are at risk, including great blue lobelia (*L. siphilitica*). Encourage future harvests by saving the seeds and scattering them in the soil after the frost date for your area has passed.

HERBAL PREPARATIONS

Tea
Standard infusion of dried aerial parts
Drink 2 ounces as needed.

Tincture
1 part fresh aerial parts
2 parts menstruum (50% alcohol,
   50% water)
Take 10 drops as needed.

Infused oil
1 part fresh aerial parts
2 parts oil
Massage into sore muscles or incorporate into a tension-relieving salve.

---

maple

Acer species
sugar maple (*A. saccharum*), box elder (*A. negundo*), silver maple
(*A. saccharinum*), red maple (*A. rubrum*), black maple (*A. nigrum*)
PARTS USED bark, leaves, sap

This emblematic tree of the Northeast provides more than just syrup and
beautiful foliage. Maple bark, leaves, and sap are restorative for the skin,
eyes, lungs, and digestive system.

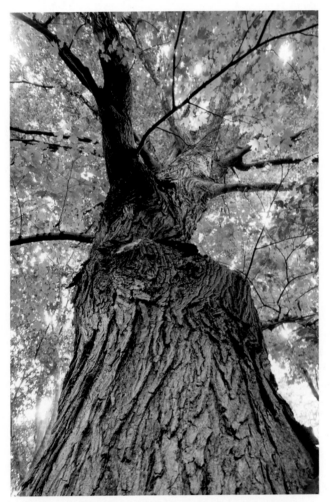

Sugar maple has the highest concentration of sugar content
in its water, making it the most common species tapped for
syrup production.

How to Identify

Maple is a deciduous tree with
an opposite branching pattern.
There are eight native species
of maple in the Northeast, and
at least five introduced species
that are fairly widespread.

With the exception of box
elder, which has compound
leaves, maple leaves are simple
and palmate with three to five
pointed lobes and long petioles
or stalks. In fall these leaves
provide a spectacular display of
colors worthy of its own tourist
industry known as "leaf peep-
ing." Another feature of maple
that makes them desirable is
their sap, which is boiled down
to that deliciously sweet syrup
we like to put on pancakes and
waffles. Some of the species
commonly tapped for this sweet
nectar include sugar, silver, red,
black, and box elder.

Fairly inconspicuous flowers
appear in late winter to early
spring growing in clusters and
ranging from pale green to
red, depending on the species.
These are among the first tree

flowers to appear. By late spring female flowers develop into those fun-to-watch maple seeds (samaras) that have regional nicknames like maple keys, helicopters, polynoses, and whirlybirds.

In winter, identify maples by their opposite branching pattern, gray-brown furrowed bark, and V-shaped leaf scars. The leaf scars also have three dots called bundle scars that resemble a monkey's face.

Where, When, and How to Wildcraft

Maples are shade-tolerant and can be part of the understory in mixed hardwood forests. Some species tend toward moister soil and appear along lakeshores and riversides. Maple trees are also commonly found growing in full sun in parks, meadows, and fields. Introduced species such as Norway maple (*A. plata-noides*)—once planted as street trees because of their moderate tolerance to pollution—find their homes in human-disturbed habitats.

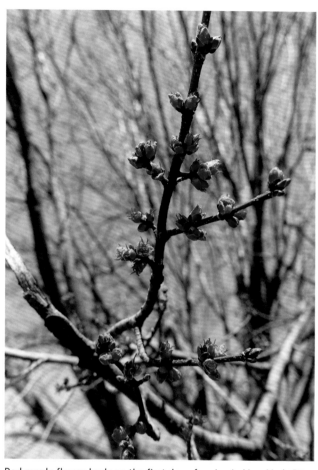

Red maple flower buds on the first day of spring in New York City.

Tap mature maple trees for sap in late winter, when the days are above freezing (32°F) and the nights are below freezing. Choose trees wider than 12 inches in diameter that have good sun exposure. Look to the bark as another sign for tapping readiness and as a key to determining species. Mature sugar maples have bark that is gray-brown and vertically furrowed or plated. Distinguish sugar maples from similar-looking Norway maples by the bark and terminal buds (the buds at the tip of the branch). Sugar maple

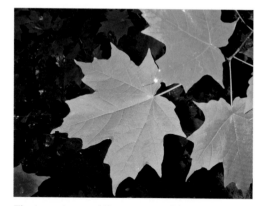

The importance of the sugar maple in North American culture is evident in the Canadian flag with the sugar maple leaf as its most prominent symbol.

has dramatically furrowed, shaggy bark while Norway maple has tighter-knit, modest furrows. Terminal buds of sugar maple are small, brown, and sharply pointed versus the brown-red, plump, overlapping scales featured on buds of Norway maple.

Collect leaves from midspring through early fall to use fresh or dried for skincare applications. Prune branches in early spring when the sap is still flowing. Choose suckers and watersprouts, or branches less than ½ inch in diameter on mature trees.

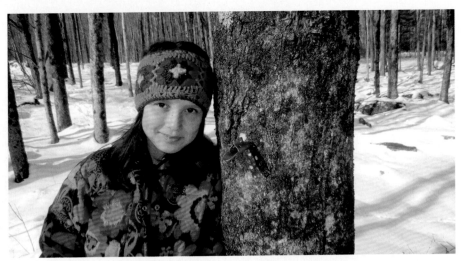

Tapping trees and processing sap into maple syrup can become a yearly ritual to celebrate the gifts of nature and appreciate the effort it takes to make this sweet condensed liquid.

Tapping for Sap and Making Syrup

What a treasure sweet delicious maple syrup is! But this blessing of condensed maple sap doesn't just make itself. First a maple tree has to be mature enough and ready to give up its sap and someone has to tap for it when the conditions are right: days above freezing (32°F) and nights below freezing.

What you'll need:

- Twig or drill and spile
- Lightweight food grade bucket or water bottle
- Cheesecloth or other filter

- Cooking pot
- Heat source
- Candy thermometer
- Storage container

Before starting, make sure all of your equipment is scrubbed clean with hot water, especially the spile (if you are using one) and collecting vessels. There are at least two approaches to tapping:

Medicinal Uses

These days maple is primarily sought after for its sweet sap, thanks to the ingenuity, technology, and long-standing traditions of First Peoples. Aside from the sweet reward of syrup, maple has been a source of healing for its astringent and expectorant properties.

Astringent and cleansing, maple bark has a history of use for wound care and current research suggests leaves collected in summer and fall have cosmetic benefits for skin.

Twig tap method: This method is slower than drilling, but it's kinder to the tree. Find a sturdy twig that measures about 2–3 inches long and ¼ inch in diameter. The twig can be solid or you can hollow out a thin elder or sumac branch that's ½ inch thick or thinner. Whittle down the end of the twig to an angled point with a pocketknife. Using a hammer or rock, tap the pointed end of the twig into the bark at an upward angle, about 1 inch deep. Just under the twig, tie a bucket around the tree with rope or cut a hole into the side of a plastic bottle to fit over the twig. The sap will start flowing along or through the twig into your vessel. If you've used a solid twig and the sap flows down the bark of the tree instead, carve a channel in the top of the twig to direct the flow of sap. Keep checking back daily to note your yield and change out the bucket or bottle if it fills.

Drill and spile method: Depending on the size of your spile, select either a ⁵⁄₁₆ or ⁷⁄₁₆ drill bit. Drill a hole into the trunk of the tree about 3 feet up from the ground and about 2 inches deep, either level or at a 10-degree angle upward. For trees 21–27 inches in diameter, drill two holes. For trees wider than 27 inches, drill three holes. Gently tap the spile in and place the collection bucket under it on a hook.

Filter the sap you've collected via either method through a fine-mesh sieve or cheesecloth and store it in the refrigerator or outside (if the temperature is below 40°F) until you are ready to boil it down. When you've collected enough sap, it's time to boil. How will you know how much is enough? To give a sense of yield, 40 pints (5 gallons) of sap from a sugar maple could result in about 1 pint of syrup. For other maples, the ratio could be about 80:1.

You'll want to boil the sap outside as the process produces a lot of steam. Over an outdoor gas range or fireplace, pour small amounts of sap into one or more shallow open pots. Fill the pan with a few inches of liquid and try to maintain that amount, adding a little bit at a time. Don't let the liquid in the pot get too shallow as it can scorch and don't pour too much in as it can boil over.

Once the sap starts to condense and darken, you can consolidate it into one pot and bring the operation indoors. Continue boiling until the syrup reaches a temperature of 7.1°F over water boiling, which varies depending on your elevation and the barometric pressure. A simple way to do this without a special calculator or complicated equations is to take the temperature of the sap just as it begins to boil. That's your baseline temperature. Once it gets to 7.1°F above that, the syrup is ready. Store in the refrigerator for up to 1 year. It will keep longer in the freezer, but I'm going to guess you'll use it all up before too long.

After the stagnation of winter, maple sap provides a mildly diuretic, nourishing tonic with several essential minerals such as manganese, calcium, potassium, and iron. The sap or inner bark decoction is traditionally used as a wash for sore eyes. A decoction of the inner bark also relieves coughs, measles, and dysentery.

Use maple syrup as a sweet preservative for cough syrups. Its preserving power is not as potent as that of honey or vegetable glycerin, so store your syrup in the refrigerator and use within 3 months.

⚠ Precautions
Box elder (*A. negundo*) bark is traditionally used as an emetic so proceed with caution when using this species internally.

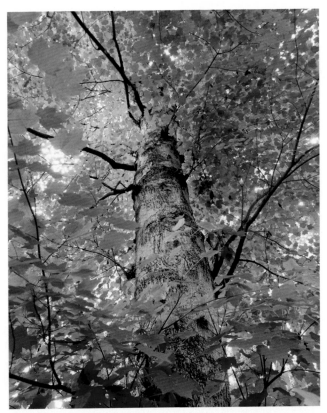
Maple trees don't mind a little shade and are often found in the understory of mixed hardwood forests.

Future Harvests
Climate change has already altered the conditions for maple sap production. Sugaring seasons have dramatically shifted to begin earlier and end more than a week sooner than in the 1960s.

The Asian longhorned beetle is also a threat to maples and other hardwood trees. If you see borer holes in the trunk large enough to stick a pencil in, it's a sign that the tree is infested. Do not harvest from infested trees and do not move the wood. If the tree isn't already in a quarantine area, report it to the USDA Animal and Plant Health Inspection Service.

Black maple (*A. nigrum*) is at risk of endangerment in several states and Canadian provinces. While gathering a few leaves from this tree is okay, it's best to avoid tapping it for sap.

HERBAL PREPARATIONS

Tea
Standard infusion of fresh or dried leaves
Use as a wash for wounds, add it to baths, or apply to the face as a toner.
or
Standard decoction of fresh or dried bark
Take 2 ounces as needed. Use as a wash.

Filipendula ulmaria
queen of the meadow, meadow dropwort
PARTS USED flowers, leaves

Meadowsweet is known for its sweet aroma, and its anti-inflammatory and pain-relieving properties, which are useful for treating joint pain and gastric ulcers.

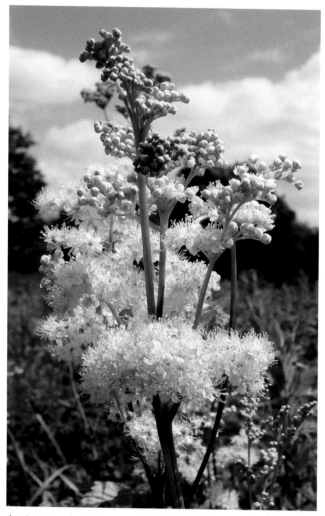

Ancient people of Europe and the British Isles used meadowsweet to flavor mead, an alcoholic honey-based beverage. With this herb's anti-inflammatory properties, it's a bit like a hangover preventative infused right into the boozy brew.

How to Identify

Meadowsweet is a perennial herbaceous plant in the rose family introduced to North America from Eurasia. It grows in an upright habit to a height of 3–6 feet. The compound pinnate leaves sport seven to nine larger leaflets with intermittent tiny ones, dark green on top and downy white beneath. The specific name *ulmaria* derives from the resemblance of the leaves to those of elm.

By the middle of summer, fragrant clusters of tiny, five-petaled, white (sometimes pink) flowers bloom up the red to purple stem. Bees collect the pollen from the beautifully delicate blossoms.

Where, When, and How to Wildcraft

As the name suggests, meadowsweet grows happily in the full sun of meadows. This plant doesn't mind having its feet wet and grows just as well in ditches as in well-watered flower gardens. Meadowsweet has naturalized throughout the

Northeast, represented in every state and province in the region.

By hand or with clippers, collect the leaves and flowers of meadowsweet in summer when they are just blooming. These can be used fresh or laid on a screen to dry for later use.

Medicinal Uses

Meadowsweet is a dynamic herb with a range of medicinal applications. Cooling and astringent, it balances gastric acidity and tones the mucosa. Meadowsweet infusion is particularly useful for healing hyperacid conditions of the gastrointestinal tract including heartburn, gastric reflux, and peptic ulcers. The astringency meadowsweet provides is applicable to afflictions of the lower GI tract, calming diarrhea and dysentery.

Meadowsweet contains salicylic acid, the key ingredient in aspirin, which consequently was named after *Spirea*, this herb's original genus label. Unlike aspirin—which is pain relieving yet poses a risk of gastrointestinal (GI) bleeding—meadowsweet reduces pain and inflammation while protecting and even healing the GI tract. This is one of those cases where isolating a chemical constituent from a plant undermines the beautiful balance that plants maintain in their whole and natural state.

Meadowsweet is antimicrobial and has effect in diphtheria and pneumonia. The diaphoretic action of meadowsweet is useful for sweating out a fever.

Meadowsweet is an anticoagulant and improves blood flow, removing built-up uric acid and other toxins. This is useful for those

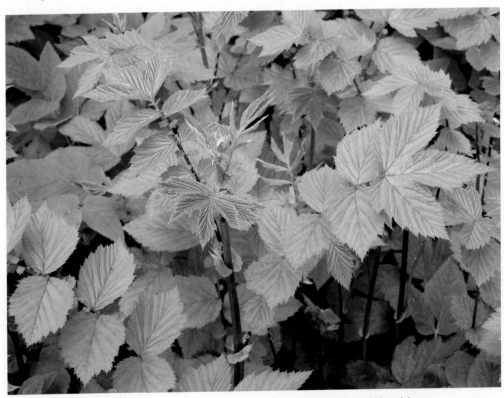

The species name *ulmaria* refers to the leaflets, which are reminiscent of elm (*Ulmus*) leaves.

with gout and arthritic conditions. Take the tincture or infusion internally and apply meadowsweet-infused oil to soothe sore muscles and painful joints. Run a warm bath and add a strong meadowsweet infusion for the same effect.

Meadowsweet was traditionally used as a strewing herb for its sweet fragrance and cleansing properties. Tie a bundle of dried meadowsweet flowers to hang by your front door to invite in feelings of wellness and abundance. Burn the herb as incense to attract love in all its forms. Meadowsweet flower essence restores a feeling of wholeness, connection, and self-acceptance.

Precautions

Do not use meadowsweet if you have an allergy to aspirin.

Children under 16 with fever or recovering from viral infection should avoid meadowsweet for the risk of Reye's syndrome, a rare but serious condition induced by salicylates.

Meadowsweet may stimulate bronchial spasms in those with asthma, so it's best to avoid if you have this condition.

Consult with your healthcare provider if you are taking blood-thinning medication, as meadowsweet might potentiate anticoagulant effects.

Future Harvests

Meadowsweet is an introduced plant that readily self-seeds. There is no concern over its future in the Northeast.

Queen of the prairie (*F. rubra*), a related plant native to the Northeast, is critically imperiled in New Jersey and Pennsylvania. The pink color of the flowers distinguishes this plant from introduced meadowsweet.

HERBAL PREPARATIONS

Tea
Standard infusion of dried flowers and leaves
Drink 1 cup as needed.

Tincture
1 part fresh flowers and leaves
1 part vegetable glycerin
2 parts menstruum (50% alcohol, 50% water)
or
1 part dried flowers and leaves
1 part vegetable glycerin
4 parts menstruum (50% alcohol, 50% water)
Take 30–60 drops as needed.

Infused oil
1 part fresh flowers and leaves
2 parts oil
or
1 part dried flowers and leaves
4 parts oil
Massage into tender spots to relieve pain and inflammation.

Flower essence
Follow instructions for making flower essences on page 54. Take 3 drops on the tongue up to 4 times per day or as needed.

mimosa

Albizia julibrissin
Persian silk tree, albizia
PARTS USED bark, flowers

Mimosa is a gentle mood restorative that supports the processing of grief, anger, and stress. It restores focus and restful sleep in cases of memory loss and insomnia due to tension.

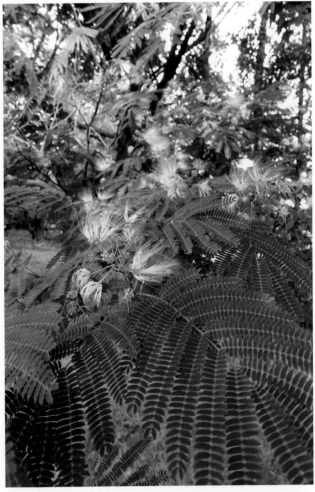

Mimosa blossoms have a dreamy, silky quality, especially when blown by a breeze. The specific name *julibrissin* is a corruption of the Farsi (Persian) word *gul-i abrisham* meaning "floss silk," referring to the flowers.

How to Identify

Mimosa is a fast-growing, short-lived deciduous tree in the bean (Fabaceae) family. Emerging from a slender, branched trunk, mimosa has a spreading canopy of feathery compound leaves that are twice divided, or bipinnate. There are ten to twenty-five primary pinnae or divided leaflets, each with forty to sixty tiny leaflets of their own. The leaflets fold in when darkness falls or when rain is imminent.

Whimsical, fragrant, pink (sometimes red or white), pompom-shaped flowers bloom in summer. These are followed by brown, flat beans or seed-pods that decorate the tree through winter.

Where, When, and How to Wildcraft

Mimosa is mainly present in the southern part of the Northeast, reaching only as far north as Massachusetts. It is an introduced pioneer species that easily self-seeds in soil that's been disturbed by human activity.

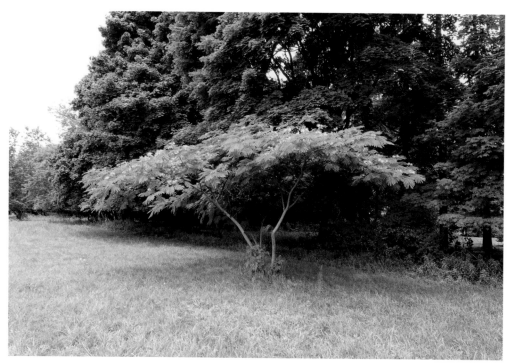

Mimosa trees create an elegant canopy of feathery leaves in open spaces or human-disturbed soils.

Some folks plant it as an ornamental, which is received with mixed reviews. While it is a beauty, mimosa has a fairly short life span and is prone to wilt fungus and mimosa webworms (*Homadaula anisocentra*). Despite these problems, mimosa is a wonderful medicine tree.

Collect the flowers in summer to use fresh in tinctures and cold infusions. Dry them on a screen or in a paper bag for later use.

Since mimosa grows so fast, it can do with a regular pruning. Use a pruning saw to prune mature branches (about 2 inches or wider in diameter) in spring and early summer. Carefully peel away the outer bark with a knife and strip the tan inner bark away from the branch. Alternately you can cut a lengthwise strip from the branch and peel away both layers of the bark. Cut the inner bark into pieces and dry on a screen for later use or add it fresh to the flowers in tincture.

Medicinal Uses

Just sitting with the mimosa tree gives me a sense of laid-back ease. The pink pompom flowers with their fine filaments call to mind the nervous system. Mimosa flowers and bark reduce pain and tension and come to the rescue when we are restless, insomniac, and irritable due to unprocessed emotions.

Sipping the flower infusion encourages breath where there is constriction, like a gentle sigh of relief. When we are tense, angry, and resentful we tend to hold our breath, gripping in the chest and abdomen. Mimosa sends a sweet breath of relaxation through these held places of tension.

If taking the flowers alone makes you feel ungrounded, add the bark or incorporate a grounding herb such as burdock or dandelion root, which can also aid in releasing pent-up anger and tension. For support when processing grief, consider combining mimosa with violet, hawthorn, and linden. To treat insomnia exacerbated by discursive thoughts, add motherwort and skullcap. This combination would also serve as a helpful preparation for meditation.

Mimosa bark is specific in Chinese medicine for regenerating connective tissue. Combine with horsetail and elder for greater effect in healing physical trauma to the bones, tendons, and ligaments.

Combine mimosa bark with dandelion leaf and forsythia fruit in a decoction applied topically to quell the pain and inflammation of abscesses.

Precautions
Mimosa is not recommended during pregnancy due to its blood-circulation stimulating effects.

Future Harvests
No need to worry about gathering flowers and bark from mimosa. This introduced species readily self-sows wherever there is an opening in the landscape.

HERBAL PREPARATIONS

Tea
Standard or cold infusion of fresh or dried flowers
Drink 4–8 ounces 3 times per day or as needed.
or
Standard decoction of fresh or dried bark
Drink 1–2 cups 3 times per day or as needed. Use as a wash or compress for abscesses, boils, and connective tissue injuries.

Tincture
1 part fresh bark and flowers
2 parts menstruum (50% alcohol, 50% water)
Take 60–90 drops 3 times per day. If using just the flowers, reduce this dosage by half.

Mentha species

American wild mint (*M. canadensis*), apple mint (*M. suaveolens*), peppermint (*M. ×piperita*), spearmint (*M. spicata*), water mint (*M. aquatica*), wild mint (*M. arvensis*)

PARTS USED aerial parts

Mint is a stimulating, cooling herb used as a catalyst and flavoring agent for herbal blends. It is helpful as a fever reducer, a digestive aid to calm colic, and a mild pain reliever for headache.

How to Identify

There are at least ten species of mint growing in the Northeast with introduced garden escapees outnumbering native mints. All mints described here have square stems and opposite, toothed, aromatic leaves.

Where, When, and How to Wildcraft

Look for mints in moist soil in the edges and along trails or forested areas, growing in dappled light or full sun.

The only tool you need is your fingers to pinch off the tops of the plants, either

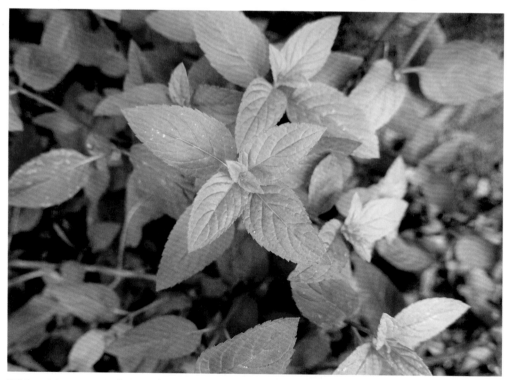

While mints are generally interchangeable, they do have their nuances. Particularly, peppermint tends toward pungent and enlivening while spearmint is earthy and mellow.

before or during flowering from spring through fall. Use fresh or dry in hanging bundles for later use.

Medicinal Uses

Mint is a handy herb for your home apothecary. On its own it has a good variety of medicinal qualities—working as a stomach soother, fever reducer, and itchiness remedy. But it really comes in handy as a catalyst in herbal formulations. Mint has a way of opening the channels so the body can more readily receive the medicine of other herbs.

To relieve digestive upset, including gassiness and colic, add mint to chamomile, lemon balm, and catnip in a tea or tincture. If giving this to a child, spearmint or apple mint would be gentler choices versus invigorating peppermint.

Add mint to blends for nervous tension and anxiety, such as hops, skullcap, and lemon balm. For an herbal pick-me-up, drink an infusion of peppermint, stinging nettle, and chicory. To treat cold and flu symptoms while reducing fever, a classic combination is elderflower, yarrow, and mint.

For topical applications, mint combines well with plantain and chickweed to soothe itching and mild pain from scrapes and insect bites. Add the tincture or infused oil to salves for muscle and joint pain with oils infused in Saint John's wort, comfrey, and eastern cottonwood.

⚠ Precautions

Avoid peppermint in pregnancy as it can be too stimulating to the uterus in large doses. Small doses of spearmint are safe as a complementary herb in blends with other prenatal supportive herbs such as stinging nettle, raspberry leaf, and red clover.

Future Harvests

Mints are fairly prolific reproducers and sometimes considered weedy. Harvesting the tops of mint plants just as they go into flower encourages leaf growth and you can continue to harvest from the same plants throughout the growing season.

HERBAL PREPARATIONS

Tea
Standard or cold infusion of fresh or dried aerial parts
Drink 4–8 ounces as needed. Use as a wash for skin irritation and muscle pain.

Tincture
1 part fresh aerial parts
2 parts menstruum (50% alcohol,
  50% water)
or
1 part dried aerial parts
5 parts menstruum (50% alcohol,
  50% water)
Take 10–30 drops as needed. Makes a nice addition to summer cocktails.

Infused vinegar
1 part fresh aerial parts
2 parts apple cider vinegar
Take by the teaspoonful or splash in sparkling water for a refreshing beverage.

Infused honey
1 part fresh aerial parts
2 parts honey
Take by the spoonful or add to tea.

---

motherwort

Leonurus cardiaca
PARTS USED flowering tops

There's a lot in a name. Motherwort has been known for centuries as a tonic to allay women's health issues, from menstrual cramps to hot flashes. And like the best loving mother, this herb calms the nerves and strengthens the heart.

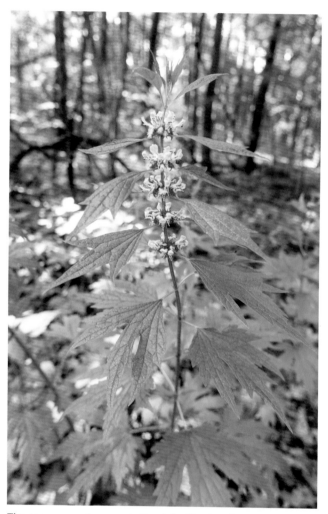

The genus name *Leonurus* is Greek for "lion's tail"—after the way the leaves look emerging from the fuzzy flower whorls. The specific name *cardiaca* speaks to the long use of motherwort as a heart tonic.

How to Identify

Motherwort is an herbaceous perennial that grows 2–4 feet tall. It is recognizable as a mint family plant by the characteristic square stem, opposite leafing pattern, and tubular flowers. The leaves are three-lobed and as you look down the stem, you'll notice the lower leaves are larger than the upper and feature deeper lobes. Lanky and graceful in maturity, the outspread pairs of leaves remind me of a succession of wings with groups of fluffy pale pink-purple flowers tucked in between at the leaf axils. Once the flowers wilt away, whorls of spiky fruit are left behind, each bearing four nutlets.

Where, When, and How to Wildcraft

Motherwort is an introduced plant that finds its home at the edges of forests, along roadsides, and in meadows and fields.

Gather the top third of the plant in summer when in flower. Tincture fresh or dry for later use. Motherwort doesn't make the tastiest tea, but you can combine it with sweeter herbs or infuse in honey.

Medicinal Uses

When left feeling irritable, out of sorts, and anxious to the point of palpitations, motherwort provides a sense of release and expansion. A few drops of the tincture are often enough to calm nerves, aid in relaxation, and reduce jumpiness brought on by stress, or in some cases hormonal imbalance as in hyperthyroidism. The bitter taste can bring on a shuddering sensation that is consistent with other relaxing nervine herbs. This action reflects a sort of "shaking off" of stress and tension from the body. The bitterness also signifies the herb's action on the liver and digestive system. Taking the tincture can help release trapped gas from the abdomen, a symptom frequently brought on by nervous tension.

The species name *cardiaca* is a clue to motherwort's historical and current use as a restorative heart tonic. Motherwort strengthens the heart, particularly in functional, stress-related heart conditions such as white-coat hypertension.

Motherwort is a boon to women's health issues, useful at every stage, from maiden to crone. Take a few drops of the tincture to relieve menstrual cramps. Use the tincture before and during labor to strengthen uterine contractions. The tincture also comes in handy for coping with the pressures of motherhood. Combine motherwort with passionflower and hops to assuage menopausal insomnia and hot flashes.

⚠ Precautions

Avoid during pregnancy, except in the 4 weeks before full term.

Take care with blood-thinning medications as motherwort may have anti-clotting effects.

Future Harvests

Harvesting the aerial portions from healthy stands of motherwort will not endanger this fairly widespread introduced plant.

HERBAL PREPARATIONS

Tea
Standard infusion of dried flowering tops
Drink 2–4 ounces as needed. Sweeten with honey or add to blends with aromatic herbs.

Tincture
1 part fresh flowering tops
2 parts menstruum (50% alcohol, 50% water)
or
1 part dried flowering tops
5 parts menstruum (50% alcohol, 50% water)
Take 3–30 drops as needed.

---

mugwort

Artemisia vulgaris
cronewort
PARTS USED flowering tops, leaves

Mugwort is a bitter, stimulating nervine that brings flow to digestion, circulation, the uterus, and the mind.

How to Identify

Mugwort is a shapeshifter. In early spring, look for ground-hugging, deeply divided, light green leaves that are downy white on the underside. In late spring, the plant grows to a few inches tall and the leaves darken, reminding some people of parsley—at least when seen from the top. The key is to look under the leaves at the silvery white undersides. Mugwort has an unmistakable spicy, earthy, slightly camphoraceous scent—the crushed leaves can smell a bit like a cross between mushroom, mint, and cinnamon.

As mugwort ages, the stem becomes woodier and sometimes purplish. The upper leaves can come to a single point or have three points

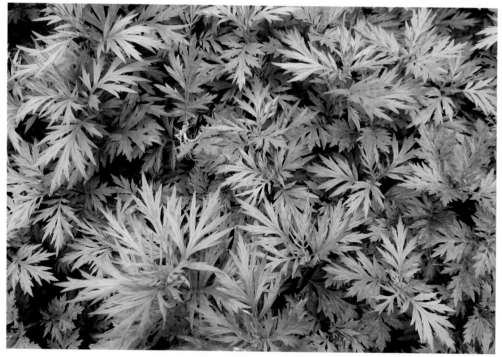

Mugwort predates hops as the bittering agent in beer and it is thought that the name mugwort comes from a "mug" of beer. While in some accounts mug is an adaptation of the Old Norse word *muggi* meaning "marsh" or the Old English word *moughte* for "moth" as the plant has been used for centuries to repel moths. "Wort" derives from Old English *wyrt*, meaning root, herb, vegetable, or spice.

or more and grow to about 1 inch. The lower leaves have a shape reminiscent of a flame (which speaks to some of its applications) and are broader with multiple points. Mugwort blooms in late summer to early autumn in long clusters of small green flowers, sometimes with a purplish color at the tips.

The plant usually grows in large stands and can grow up to about 5 feet. In fall, you might find mugwort leaves that have changed to brilliant shades of red and purple.

There are perhaps fifteen *Artemisia* species present in the Northeast, though not all ubiquitously. Two very common introduced species that are used somewhat interchangeably with mugwort are sweet annie (*A. annua*) and wormwood (*A. absinthium*).

Where, When, and How to Wildcraft

Mugwort grows in the edge, in disturbed soils, between forest and field, along roadsides, and near waterways. In the spring, pinch the tops off young mugwort plants to add to salads and vinegars. In summer, harvest the top third of the plant by bending the stem back and forth above the leaf node (this gets easier as the season progresses) or with a knife or small clippers. By the time mugwort is in flower, this is the easiest time to harvest by hand, without any tools.

Medicinal Uses

Artemisias are named after Artemis, Greek goddess of the wild hunt, childbirth, and the moon. This allusion is apropos in that mugwort stimulates the uterus to bring on delayed menses—also called the moon cycle—and eases menstrual cramps. It also aids in inducing vivid and lucid dreams. One may place a piece of fresh mugwort near their bed, fill a sachet with dried leaves or flowers, or drink or smoke the dried plant before bedtime.

Artists may find mugwort a pleasant companion for shifting perception and stimulating creative flow. Bundles of mugwort can also be tied together, dried, and burned to purify a space or to shift one's senses.

Traditionally, mugwort was placed in the shoes of weary travelers, and a strong infusion of mugwort makes a lovely bath tea for sore and tired muscles. Acupuncturists and Chinese medicine practitioners use dried mugwort (moxa) in a ground-up ball of fluff burned on top of needles, or in wand or stick form burned directly on or above the affected area to stimulate circulation.

The bitter quality of mugwort tells us that it is useful for stimulating digestive flow, aiding in digestion and elimination. Mugwort can be useful for relieving both constipation and diarrhea, as well as bloating and flatulence. It is used in cooking in Japan, Korea, and China, likely for the aforementioned purpose. The herb can be added to a bitters blend to take before or after meals.

Another name for mugwort is cronewort, referring to

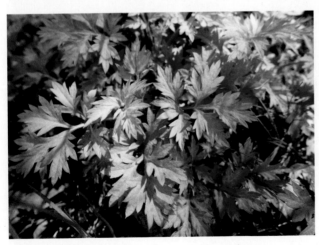
Young leaves of mugwort in spring resemble parsley.

women in perimenopause as it can help ease the entry into this phase of life.

Mugwort helps combat the effects of urushiol, the component of *Toxicodendron* species plants (poison ivy, poison oak, and poison sumac) that instigates a rash. One would simply rub the fresh leaves together in their hands and massage onto affected areas or make a poultice or compress with the leaves to apply to the skin.

Taking a cup of hot mugwort infusion can help stimulate sweating in case of fever.

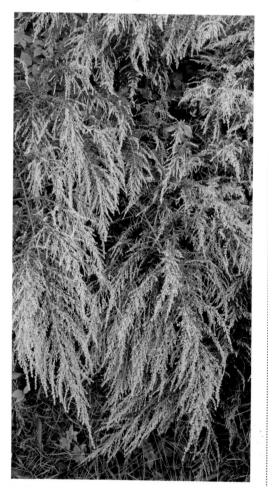

By late summer to early fall mugwort is in full flower and reaches up to about 5 feet in height or, in this case, falls over with the weight of its blooms.

⚠ Precautions

Mugwort stimulates the uterus so it should not be used during pregnancy.

People who are allergic to plants in the aster family may want to avoid mugwort. Contact dermatitis has been reported in some people.

Mugwort can uptake heavy metals so do not harvest from abandoned lots or contaminated sites.

Future Harvests

Mugwort is a hardy perennial and considered invasive so, in most cases, there is plenty to go around.

HERBAL PREPARATIONS

Tea
Standard or cold infusion of dried leaves and/or flowering tops
Drink 4–8 ounces up to 3 times per day.

Tincture
1 part fresh leaves
2 parts menstruum (50% alcohol, 50% water)
or
1 part dried leaves
5 parts menstruum (50% alcohol, 50% water)
Take 10–30 drops as needed.

Infused oil
1 part fresh flowering tops and/or leaves
2 parts oil
or
1 part dried flowering tops and/or leaves
4 parts oil
Use as a massage oil or to anoint the third eye before meditation or sleep.

Morus species

white mulberry (*M. alba*), red mulberry (*M. rubra*)

PARTS USED fruit, leaves, root bark, twigs

Cooling, soothing mulberry stimulates circulation of fluid through the body removing stagnation from the joints, reducing hypertension, and bringing relief to cold and flu symptoms.

How to Identify

Two species of mulberry (*Morus*) grow in the Northeast, both deciduous trees that reach 35–50 feet tall. Both trees, when young, can feature a variety of leaf shapes—heart-shaped, roughly mitten-shaped, and three-lobed. As the trees mature, more so in red mulberry, the leaves will tend to one leaf shape, primarily heart-shaped. The leaves are toothed and grow alternately on the branch. White mulberry leaves are shiny on top while red mulberry leaves are dull. Sometimes the two hybridize in the wild so it may be difficult to determine the species.

The bark starts out with vertical orange intersecting lines covering a greenish gray

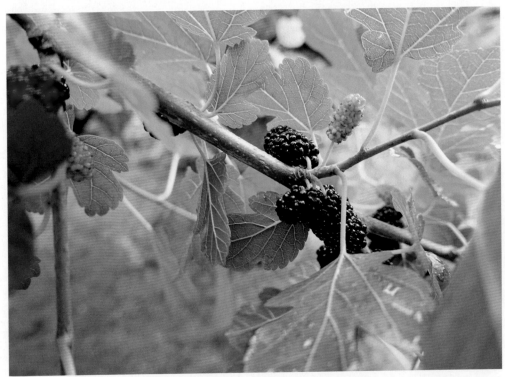

Being host to the silkworm, white mulberry was introduced to North America for silk production. Unlike the hardy tree, the industry never took root.

background, but as it ages it darkens and becomes more furrowed and sometimes platy. In the case of red mulberry, it can even be shaggy looking.

Mulberry trees can be dioecious (distinct male and female trees) or monoecious (male and female flowers on the same tree). In early spring, small yellow-green flowers bloom. In late spring to midsummer, female flowers develop into sweet, edible, cylinder-shaped fruits that look like blackberries. On white mulberry, ripe fruit can be white, pink, dark red, or purple to black.

White mulberry is a host tree to the silkworm (*Bombyx mori*) and was brought to these shores in hopes of developing a silk industry. While the North American silk trade did not take off, white mulberry certainly did. It is considered weedy and invasive in most

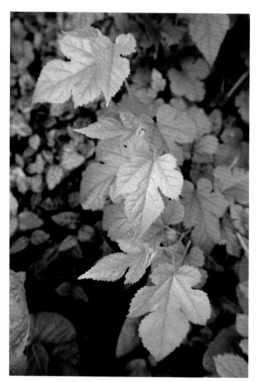

Mulberry leaves are inconsistently formed, from heart- to mitten-shaped.

places, particularly when it volunteers as a street tree. While its berries are delicious, edible, and medicinal, some folks aren't too keen on how they litter and stain the sidewalk.

Where, When, and How to Wildcraft

White mulberry is a pioneer species that fills the gaps in disturbed soils. Red mulberry is more often found in the understory of forests and in damp soil, along waterways, and in floodplains.

Gather fruit in summer to use fresh in jam, pie, juice, and syrup. You can also dry the berries in a low temperature oven or dehydrator. The traditional time to harvest leaves is in fall after the first frost. They can be tinctured fresh or dried for use in tea. Prune young twigs in spring before the energy of the tree goes into the fruit. These can be dried or tinctured fresh.

Harvest roots of young white mulberry trees in winter before the ground has frozen or as it thaws toward springtime. Chop them with pruning shears to dry for later use.

Medicinal Uses

Just about every part of the mulberry tree has been used medicinally in China for thousands of years. In general, the root bark, twigs, leaves, and fruit are cooling in nature, influence blood circulation, and have antimicrobial properties.

Drink mulberry leaf infusion to relieve hot, dry respiratory infections categorized by dry, burning sore throat; cough with dryness or thick yellow mucus; and red, dry eyes. The root bark is used similarly, though it is more suitable for coughs with thick phlegm. The leaves are also traditionally used to stop nose bleeds and coughing up of blood. Use the leaf infusion as a wash or compress on the eyes to reduce puffiness, soothe dryness, and clear up infection.

The fruit is nourishing, blood building, tonic—and tasty. It's certainly one of the more delicious forms of herbal medicine and is used traditionally for iron-deficient anemia and premature graying of hair. Eating the fruit or taking the berry syrup can help relieve constipation in those who tend to have dry constitutions.

Mulberry twigs are diuretic and impart an antispasmodic and pain-relieving effect on rheumatic conditions, especially those due to fluid build-up in the joints. Considering it is also useful for numbness and itching in the limbs through its ability to move and nourish fluid in the body, it may be useful for restless legs syndrome, specifically when it is due to mineral deficiency. The twig tincture would be useful for this purpose, as well as in cases of hypertension.

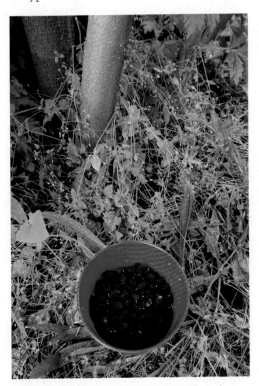

Mulberry trees yield a good amount of fruit that can be harvested from late spring to early summer.

Future Harvests

Red mulberry is endangered in four states (Connecticut, Massachusetts, Pennsylvania, and Vermont) and one province (Ontario). While collecting twigs, leaves, and fruit will not likely harm the tree, it's still a good idea to know from which tree you harvest. White mulberry, on the other hand, is considered weedy and invasive. Take advantage of the prolific reproductive abilities of white mulberry by harvesting the roots of this species.

HERBAL PREPARATIONS

Tea
Standard infusion of dried leaves
Drink 1 cup 3 times per day. Use as a wash or compress for dry, irritated eyes.
or
Standard decoction of root bark and/or twigs
Drink 1–2 cups 4 times per day.

Tincture
1 part fresh leaves, root bark, and/or twigs
2 parts menstruum (50% alcohol, 50% water)
Take 60–90 drops up to 4 times per day.

Syrup
Using the berries, follow instructions for making herbal syrups on page 52. Take 1 tablespoonful up to 3 times per day.

mullein

Verbascum thapsus

PARTS USED flowers, leaves, roots, stalks

Mullein fills many roles in the herbal apothecary as an ally for respiratory ailments, a lymphatic fluid remover, an earache soother, and an anti-inflammatory pain reliever. As a dream-enhancing herb, it also lights the way through liminal spaces.

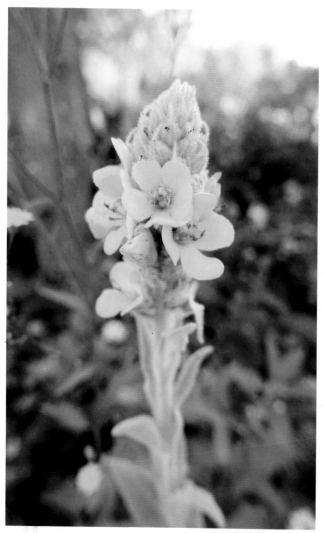

Mullein flower essence assists us in standing upright and confidently in truth, shedding light on where we might not be completely honest with ourselves.

How to Identify

Mullein is a fuzzy biennial herbaceous plant that begins its cycle as a basal rosette of ovate- to lance-shaped, gray-green leaves covered entirely in down that's both soft and itchy. Some compare the texture of the leaves to flannel and this feature inspired one of its lesser-used common names, flannel plant. In its second year, mullein sends up an erect stalk of alternating leaves which get progressively smaller toward the top. At the apex is a long spike of creamy yellow, five-petaled flowers. This spike kind of reminds me of an ear of corn with the flowers exploding open into buttery popped kernels. The plant can reach heights of 7 feet, though this varies depending on habitat. Mullein plants can appear singly, in pairs, triads, or whole families in the landscape. Roots are thin and tan and can have a bit of a hairy appearance.

Where, When, and How to Wildcraft

Mullein tends toward open spaces and is happy to establish

itself in poor, rocky soils along train tracks, tucked back from roadsides, or just out in a field. However, railroad right-of-ways are often heavily sprayed with weed killers, so it is not a good place from which to collect mullein. Don't count on it to be in the same place year after year like some other weedy plants. Mullein seems to pop up wherever it chooses.

Gather the leaves from the first- or second-year plant whenever they are fresh. It's nice to pick both, compare, and note if you experience any differences with their taste, energetics, and actions.

Pick the flowers by hand in summer to infuse in oil, tincture, or to make a flower essence.

Dig the root of the first-year plant in mid-fall through winter or the second-year plant in early spring before it sends up its stalk. Tincture directly or dry it for later use.

Alternately, you can harvest the entire plant when in flower to dry and use in tincture, tea, and oil.

Medicinal Uses

At least as far back as the first century CE, mullein was considered a lung tonic. Its origins are Mediterranean, but once European colonists brought it to the Americas, it became part of the healing repertory of First Peoples. Mohegans steep mullein in molasses to ease coughs. Other tribes smoke the leaves to relieve wheezing or use the mashed roots for respiratory complaints.

Mullein leaf has a pleasant, mild taste, slightly sour and astringent with a hint of sweetness and bitterness. Its overall softness as a plant translates into a gentle yet powerful medicine for the respiratory and nervous systems. Mullein leaf infusion and tincture

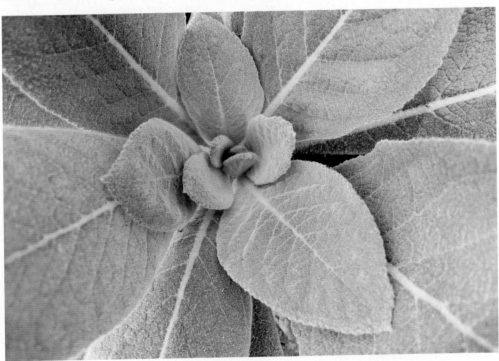

Beware the hairs! Be sure to double filter mullein leaf infusion (or use a coffee filter) to eliminate irritating hairs.

helps loosen and expel mucus from the lungs in unproductive coughs. Combine with coltsfoot and wild cherry bark to soothe dry hacking coughs that keep you up at night.

Mullein leaves are used in dreaming teas, smoking blends, and in dream pillows to enhance lucid dreaming.

Those who suffer from asthma find relief in both short and long courses of the medicine. For short-term relief of asthma attacks, use the tincture in small, frequent doses. Alternatively, the leaf can be burned, and the smoke inhaled to relieve acute lung spasms. Take the infusion or tincture daily over the course of weeks or months to strengthen and tone the lungs.

Internally and externally, mullein leaf can help move fluid build-up from swollen glands. Make a mullein poultice by dipping a whole leaf in the heated infusion and placing it on the affected area. The poultice also helps relieve pain and injury of the joints and connective tissue.

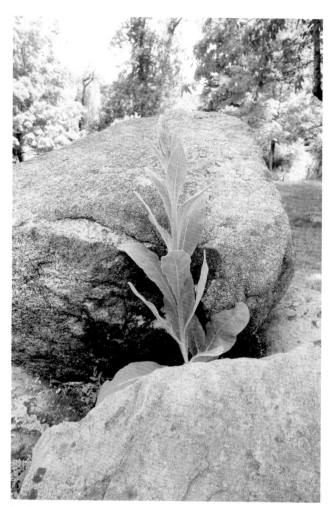

Mullein happily grows in poor soils, even wedged between rocks!

The root is earthy and more astringent than the leaf. Chew it to relieve tooth pain and inflammation. The roots and stalks are sedative, antispasmodic, and lubricating to the joints. Some herbalists use mullein root to relieve kinked neck and back vertebrae and to realign broken bones. If you look at the plant in its second year with its remarkably tall flower stalk, does it perhaps resemble a spine? At times the flower stalks grow crookedly, sending out multiple stalks off the main one, appearing disjointed and out of whack. This signature lets us know that mullein can help us come back into alignment, physically and mentally.

The root is also used in cases of urinary incontinence, especially when caused by swollen prostate or weakness of the trigone sphincter at the base of the bladder. It benefits those with chronic or recurrent cystitis, and has been known to help stop bedwetting.

Use mullein flower oil in cases of recent injury or when an old injury flares up. Old breaks and sprains that cause intense pain can be relieved both externally with the oil and by taking mullein flower tincture internally. Oil infused with mullein flower and fresh garlic is a classic remedy for earache and infection. If you suspect the eardrum is ruptured, do not put oil or any other drops in the ear.

Mullein flower essence helps one be in alignment with the truth, especially when there's a sense of not being honest with oneself.

⚠ Precautions

When making mullein leaf infusion, use a coffee filter to eliminate irritating hairs.

Future Harvests

Mullein is a fairly widespread introduced plant that spreads by seed. Still, give a moment of thanks when harvesting the whole plant as this reduces mullein's ability to reproduce in the wild.

HERBAL PREPARATIONS

Tea

Standard infusion of dried leaves
Drink 1–2 cups as needed.
or
Standard decoction of fresh or dried roots
Drink 4 ounces as needed.

Leaf tincture

1 part fresh flowers and/or leaves
2 parts menstruum (50% alcohol, 50% water)
or
1 part dried flowers and/or leaves
5 parts menstruum (50% alcohol, 50% water)
Take 20–40 drops as needed.

Root tincture

1 part fresh roots
2 parts menstruum (95% alcohol, 5% water)
or
1 part dried roots
5 parts menstruum (60% alcohol, 40% water)
Take 20–40 drops as needed.

Infused oil

1 part fresh flowers
2 parts oil
Use as ear drops or as a massage oil.

Flower essence

Follow instructions for making flower essences on page 54. Take 3 drops on the tongue up to 4 times per day or as needed.

New England aster

Symphyotrichum novae-angliae
PARTS USED flowers, leaves

This late summer beauty benefits respiratory constriction and congestion, and can be taken as a tea, tincture, steam inhalation, or smoked to relieve, relax and open the airways.

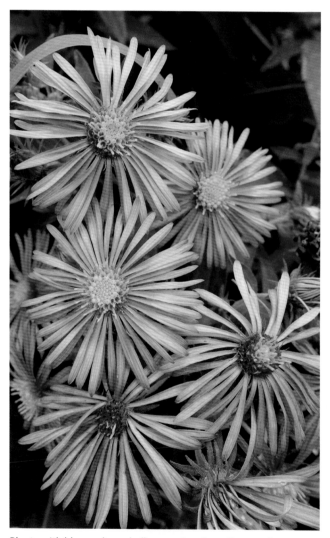

Plants with blue and purple flowers signal an effect on the nervous system. Antispasmodic and sedative, New England aster serves as a good example for this signature.

How to Identify

New England aster is a perennial plant in the aster family that can grow up to 6 feet but tends to be closer to about 4. Simple, narrow, ovate leaves with three prominent veins grow alternately, clasping the stem. Eye-catching, fragrant, pale to dark-purple ray flowers with yellow centers bloom in late summer, signaling autumn's imminence.

Where, When, and How to Wildcraft

Find New England aster gracing fields and meadows throughout the Northeast. It especially prefers moist soil in sunny open areas and edges. You'll often see it growing alongside its fellow late-blooming aster family plant, goldenrod. The vibrant colors of the two together—purple and golden yellow—are striking and evoke a sense that fall is around the corner.

Clip the top third of the plant in late summer when in bloom. Strip off the leaves and flowers and snip up the stems with clippers or scissors. It's best to tincture the flowers fresh or dehydrate immediately as they dry to seed fluff after picking.

Medicinal Uses

New England aster is primarily used as a relaxing antitussive herb for asthma, allergies, and coughs. Combine New England aster flowers with goldenrod in tincture or tea for respiratory infections that feature a drippy nose. To the flower infusion, add plantain leaves for their demulcent, moistening quality for dry coughs. Make a steam of New England aster flower infusion to help clear sinuses. Inhaling the smoke of the flowers and mullein leaves can help quell an asthma attack, bringing relaxation to airway spasm.

Drink a hot cup of flower infusion, with the addition of mint and elderflower if desired, to open the pores and induce sweating in case of fever.

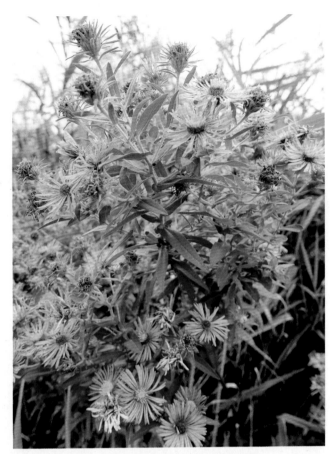

New England aster has hairy stems and leaves a sticky residue on the fingers when crushed.

An infusion of the flowers and leaves has a carminative effect, relieving tightness, gassiness, and bloating in the abdomen.

New England aster was used topically by Eclectic physicians for skin rashes caused by poison ivy or poison sumac.

Future Harvests

Gather the flowering tops from a few plants in abundant stands of New England aster, leaving the lower stems and roots intact. Spare plenty—at least 80%—of the flowering plants for the bees and butterflies, and so the plant can self-seed and produce future harvests.

HERBAL PREPARATIONS

Tea
Standard infusion of dried flowers and leaves
Drink 2-4 ounces as needed.

Tincture
1 part fresh flowers and leaves
2 parts menstruum (50% alcohol, 50% water)
Take 10-25 drops as needed.

Quercus species

PARTS USED bark, leaves, flowers, nuts (acorns)

Rich in tannins, oak is primarily employed for its drying astringent powers.

How to Identify

Oaks are deciduous trees that range from stately, upright, and lush to scraggly, lanky, and sparse. There are two main categories of oak, red and white. Red oaks tend to have leaves with pointed lobes and deeper sinuses (the space between lobes). They usually produce smaller acorns as well. White oaks generally have wide, curvy leaves with several rounded lobes. Some oaks don't seem to fit either category, by their leaves at least, with narrow, toothed, unlobed leaves that resemble holly. The dried, brown leaves of some oaks remain throughout the winter, a phenomenon known as marcescence. I love to stand under these oaks when the wind blows for the transportive rattling sound the leaves make when scraping together.

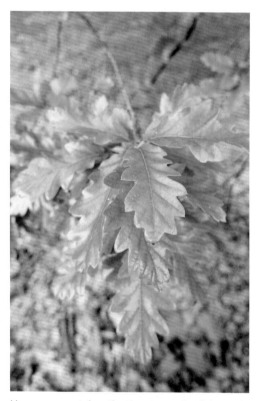

Have you ever taken the time to smell oak leaves? Some are enticingly fragrant. Next time you are near an oak tree, take a sniff.

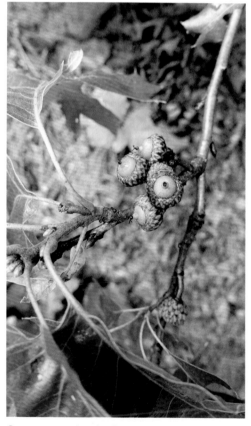

Green acorns ripening in summer.

In spring, very inconspicuous female flowers grow on their own little twigs. Hanging below the newly unfurling wing-like leaves are the dangling green male flowers or catkins. These litter the ground once they dry up and are released by the tree.

The nuts we call acorns develop from the fertilized female flowers. They take all summer to ripen, going from green to brown by late summer to fall. Acorns are all generally round or egg-shaped and sport detachable caps or cups that vary from shaggy to scalloped.

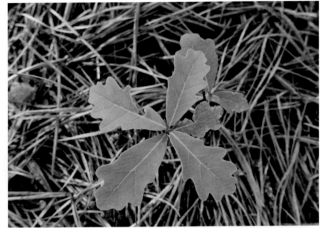

Young white oak emerging out of pine leaves. Oaks acidify soils due to their high tannin content.

Where, When, and How to Wildcraft

Oaks are fairly well distributed throughout the Northeast and vary in habitat, from floodplain to forest. They are often planted as street trees, especially pin oak (*Q. palustris*) for its sturdiness, fast growth, and pollution tolerance.

Gather male flowers in spring as they begin to fall. You could probably stand under a tree with a bowl to collect them as they drop.

The easiest and most sustainable way to gather bark, twigs, and leaves is to look for fallen branches after storms. Collect acorns when they fall in, well, fall. All parts dry pretty readily if left out on a screen indoors.

Medicinal Uses

All parts of oak, even the galls formed by tiny wasps (*Callirhytis* spp.), have been used traditionally as medicine around the world for thousands of years. Oak is known for its astringency and is used primarily to tone tissue and dry up excess fluids. Taste a bit of oak tea and you'll feel this for yourself.

The taste and mouthfeel might remind you of drinking black tea, which also contains those tightening tannins. Just don't drink too much, as it is extremely drying, and can cause headache and abdominal pain in excess. Drinking the tea in small doses or taking a bit of the tincture is beneficial for halting diarrhea and dysentery.

Make a mouthwash of oak infusion to heal mouth ulcers and tighten gums to shore up loose teeth. Add plantain and echinacea for added effect.

Oak leaf and bark decoction—combined with plantain, raspberry leaf, and mugwort—used as a vaginal steam or wash clears up discharges and tightens tissues. The infusion or decoction is useful as a sitz bath for hemorrhoids, particularly if they are bleeding.

A bath, wash, or compress of oak infusion helps soothe rashes, burns, and bruises. It tones varicose veins and can help reduce muscular pain and mild injury from overexertion.

Oak flower essence benefits those who think their energy is unlimited and keep pushing through pain and exhaustion only to have an utter collapse.

⚠ Precautions

All parts of oak are very drying. Reserve oak for short-term use and don't overdo it when taking internally. The astringency of the tannins causes headache and stomach cramping.

Future Harvests

We think of oak as hardy and abundant, so it may be surprising to note that at least 12 native species of oak are at risk in the Northeast. Despite this, harvesting the leaves, twigs, and acorns of these oaks will not do widespread or lasting harm to these much-revered trees.

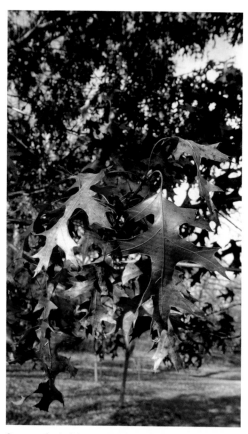

Some oaks hold onto their leaves in winter in a phenomenon known as marcescence. I love the way the sound of the leaves rattling together in the wind has a transportive, energy-shifting quality.

partridgeberry

Mitchella repens

PARTS USED fruit, leaves, stems

Long used in the Northeast as a women's herb, partridgeberry facilitates healthy contractions during childbirth and eases menstrual cramps.

How to Identify

Partridgeberry is an evergreen, prostrate (low-creeping) vine that rarely reaches 1 or 2 inches off the ground. Small, smooth, egg- or slightly heart-shaped leaves grow oppositely along the stem. Leaves are often bisected by a markedly pale green-yellow vein.

Abundant clusters of partridgeberry plants feature stems that root at the nodes, branching off in several directions, carpeting the forest floor.

White (to barely pink), fragrant, trumpet-shaped flowers bloom in pairs in early spring.

Each pair of flowers gives way to one bright red berry featuring two dimples, a sort of imprint of the former blooms. Berries are edible but most humans find them bland. Birds, and likely other forest dwellers, enjoy them.

Where, When, and How to Wildcraft

This is one of those times where looking down at your feet may reward you. Look for partridgeberry creeping low to the ground in moist, acidic forest soils, often growing through or alongside moss.

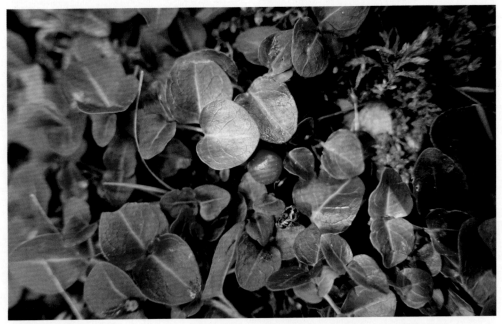

While the berries aren't commonly used in herbalism today, they are traditionally used by the Haudenosaunee to ease labor pains. The Innu (Montagnais) make a jelly with them to treat fevers.

Gently snip the ends of long unrooted stems and leaves from plentiful colonies. I like to use baby nail scissors for this kind of work, or you can carefully pinch the stems with your nails. Take care not to pull up the rooted nodes.

Collect a few berries to nibble on or incorporate fresh into tinctures.

Medicinal Uses

Partridgeberry leaf and stem decoction is cooling and astringent with a subtly sour taste, hinting at its vitamin C content. This or the tincture is primarily used to promote women's health, particularly during and after pregnancy, and during the menstruating years. Partridgeberry stimulates and eases childbirth, brings on delayed menstruation, reduces excessive bleeding, and assuages menstrual cramps. Some herbalists use partridgeberry to prevent miscarriage. Craft a lotion with barberry decoction to soothe sore nipples. Make a compress with the addition of honeysuckle and rose to reduce mastitis. Partridgeberry is energetically clearing and can be infused in baths or washes for pregnant women who experience worry, emotional upset, or relationship woes.

The herb is also diuretic and can be used in combination with antiseptic herbs such as barberry and goldenrod to clear up urinary tract infections. Pair with mullein root tincture to prevent bedwetting. Combine with nettle root and beggarticks to ease the symptoms of benign prostatic hyperplasia.

⚠ Precautions

Partridgeberry may be too drying for those who tend to have a dry constitution (think dry skin, dry mouth, etc.). In these cases, combining partridgeberry with mallow or other mucilaginous herbs would reduce the drying effect.

Future Harvests

Partridgeberry is fairly stable in the Northeast, though changing climate and shifting ecosystems as well as habitat loss are putting it at risk. To encourage future harvests, propagate by clippings in spring. Use 6- to 12-inch cuttings from the leading tip of well-established plants. Gently pull up any rootlets without damaging them. Replant the ends about 1 inch into the soil. Check back in a few months to see if these babies are taking off.

HERBAL PREPARATIONS

Tea
Standard decoction of dried leaves and stems
Drink 1 cup 3 times per day.

Tincture
1 part fresh leaves and stems
2 parts menstruum (95% alcohol, 5% water)
or
1 part dried leaves and stems
4 parts menstruum (60% alcohol, 40% water)
Take 40–60 drops 3 times per day.

Lotion
Follow instructions for making lotions on page 60. Use partridgeberry decoction in place of the water component in the recipe. Use for minor skin irritations and to relieve sore nipples.

peach

Prunus persica

PARTS USED flowers, fruit, leaves, pits, twigs

Cooling and moistening peach soothes irritation and inflammation triggered by a range of causes, including allergens, anxiety, external heat, respiratory ailments, and digestive distress.

How to Identify

Peach is a deciduous tree in the rose family cultivated for its juicy delicious fruit. It has alternate branching and ovate to lanceolate leaves with fine teeth and a pointed tip that reach up to 5 inches long. Five-petaled pink to white flowers bloom in early spring before the leaves appear.

It's likely you know what the fruit looks like. Orange-colored, fuzzy-skinned, roundish fruit with juicy yellow-white to orange flesh ripen in mid- to late summer. Inside is a single dimpled reddish tan pit.

Peach trees hail from Asia and Persia, hence the species name *persica*.

Where, When, and How to Wildcraft

Where peach trees grow wild is a direct reflection of human activity. You'll find them in fields or sunny edges that were either the

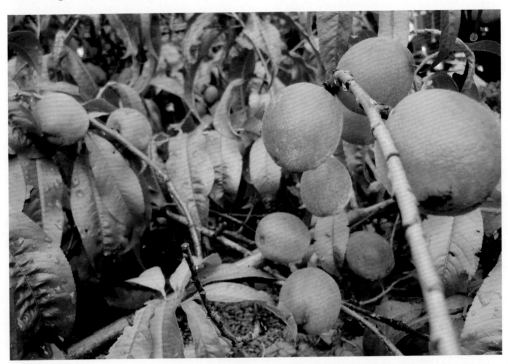

Thinking of the fuzzy skin and blush color of peaches calls to mind a rosy-cheeked overheated person, hinting at the ability of peach to cool heat and reduce inflammation.

site of old orchards or where someone tossed the pits.

Collect flowers and young twigs in early spring to tincture fresh or dry for later use. Pick leaves in spring and summer—use them right away or dry for later use in teas and topical applications. Take care to choose leaves that are not wilted. Like its relative, wild black cherry, peach leaves and pits contain cyanogenic glycosides that become concentrated as the leaves wilt.

Enjoy eating the fruit when it's juicy and ripe in summertime. Clean and dry the pits then tincture them or save for use in cold infusions.

Medicinal Uses

Peach is an excellent cooling, moistening remedy for redness, irritation, and inflammation in the body and on the skin. The leaves, flowers, twigs, and pits have a relaxing effect on overactive immune responses and on the nervous and digestive systems. Use the tincture or tea in small frequent doses to quell an allergy attack. The tea or tincture is also helpful for autoimmune flare-ups in conditions like psoriasis, rheumatoid arthritis, and inflammatory bowel disease.

Sip peach leaf and flower tea—infused hot or cold—before bedtime to facilitate sleep if you are overstimulated or overheated. The addition of rose and linden would make a lovely tea to cool you off and induce restful slumber.

Small doses of peach leaf tea or glycerite can help reduce nausea and vomiting in children and in pregnancy (never use the pit during pregnancy). Peach fruit or juice can be enjoyed for the same effect.

Use the leaves topically in a poultice or compress to relieve insect stings and bites and hypersensitivity reactions to allergens.

Peach pit is used in Chinese medicine to break up stagnation in the blood, particularly in the uterus, intestines, and lungs. It is useful for constipation due to dryness in the intestines, a common condition in elders or those who are bedridden.

⚠ Precautions

Use the leaves fresh or fully dried. Leaves that are wilted contain the highest concentration of cyanogenic glycosides. The fresh leaves and pits also contain these glycosides, though when taken in appropriate doses, peach is a useful medicine with limited unwanted effects.

Do not use peach pits during pregnancy due to their potential teratogenic effects.

Future Harvests

Harvesting the twigs, leaves, flowers, and fruit of peach trees will not imperil this introduced, cultivated tree.

HERBAL PREPARATIONS

Tea
Standard or cold infusion of dried leaves
Drink 4 ounces up to 3 times per day. Use as a wash for bites, stings, and other skin irritations.

Tincture
1 part fresh twigs and leaves
2 parts menstruum (50% alcohol, 50% water)
Take 10–20 drops as needed or up to 3 times per day.
or
1 part pits
4 parts menstruum (40% alcohol, 60% water)
Infuse for 10 days. Take 20 drops up to 3 times per day.

Vinca species
lesser periwinkle or myrtle (*V. minor*), greater periwinkle (*V. major*)
PARTS USED flowers, leaves, stems

*Periwinkle is a garden escapee that stimulates circulation to
the brain and reduces internal and external bleeding and discharges.*

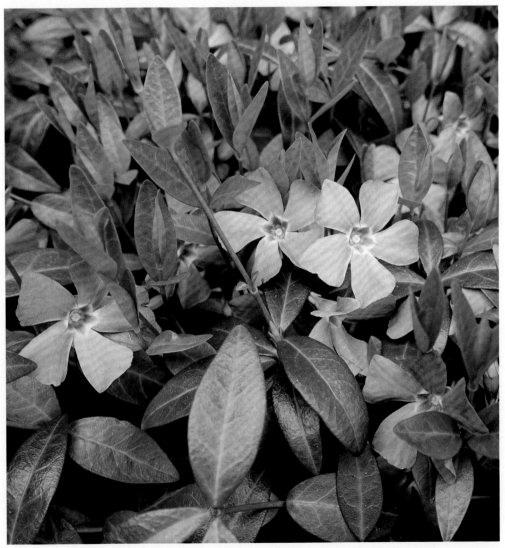

Blue-purple flowers are a signature for the sedating, antispasmodic, and brain-stimulating qualities
of periwinkle.

How to Identify

Periwinkle is an herbaceous plant, sometimes appearing as a prostrate shrub, with long trailing stems, giving it a vine-like appearance. Its evergreen leaves are shiny, ovate, opposite, and come to a point. Tubular, five-petaled, blue-purple flowers bloom in spring, sometimes with a second bloom in late summer to fall. On closer inspection, you'll see the center of the bloom has a white star-shaped outline.

Where, When, and How to Wildcraft

Periwinkle is an introduced plant commonly used as ground cover in gardens. You'll find it growing in the sun-dappled edge in parks, in gardens, and along wooded trails. Lesser periwinkle is more widespread than greater periwinkle; the two species look fairly similar to one another, but everything on greater periwinkle is larger.

Snip the ends of vining branches throughout the year to use fresh or dried. Craft a flower essence from the blooms in spring.

Medicinal Uses

Periwinkle has a bitter, acrid taste that makes it more fitting to take in tincture form. The leaves dilate blood vessels and stimulate circulation to the brain. Modern applications of the plant include treatment of dementia, arteriosclerosis, and hypertension. Combine periwinkle with ground ivy and ginkgo to reduce tinnitus related to poor circulation.

Styptic and astringent, periwinkle is useful for internal and external hemorrhages and discharges, including excessive menstrual bleeding. Apply a poultice of the leaves to wounds to promote healing and stop bleeding. Place a cotton ball or cloth soaked with periwinkle infusion in the nostrils in case of nose bleed. Periwinkle is also used homeopathically for uterine bleeding, eczema, acne, and skin ulcers.

Add a dropperful each of periwinkle, wild bergamot, and cinquefoil tinctures to 2 ounces of water to make a wash for mouth sores or gargle for sore throat.

Periwinkle is sedating and antispasmodic. Combine periwinkle, catnip, mugwort, and lemon balm in a slumber-inducing, dream-enhancing tea to sip before bedtime.

Periwinkle flower essence helps us apply learnings from past experiences to new projects and phases of life.

⚠ Precautions

Do not use periwinkle in pregnancy, due to its influence on the blood.

Avoid use in constipation and in those with low blood pressure.

If you are taking medication for high blood pressure, closely monitor your levels as dose adjustment may be warranted. Consult with your healthcare practitioner.

Future Harvests

Periwinkle is a fast-growing ground cover that thrives in gardens and disturbed soils. Collecting the leaves, stems, and flowers will not endanger this introduced plant.

HERBAL PREPARATIONS

Tea

Standard infusion of dried leaves and stems
Drink 2-4 ounces as needed. Use as a wash, poultice, or compress for wounds.

Tincture

1 part fresh flowers, leaves, and stems
2 parts menstruum (50% alcohol, 50% water)
Take 5-15 drops as needed, up to 3 times per day.

Pinus species
eastern white pine (*P. strobus*), pitch pine (*P. rigida*)
PARTS USED bark, needles, pitch, pollen, twigs

*Pine has a peaceful and energizing energy, with applications for the immune,
nervous, reproductive, urinary, and respiratory systems as well as the skin.*

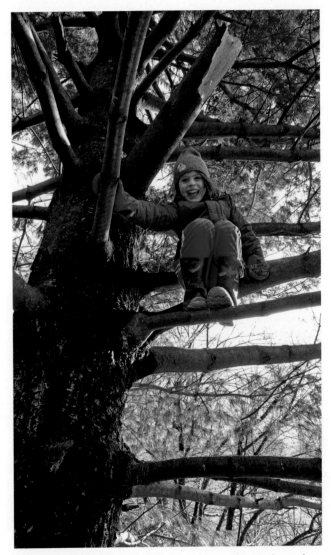

The whorled branches of pine form a ladder, making it the perfect
climbing tree.

How to Identify

Eastern white pine is an
evergreen tree with a
whorl-patterned branching
habit. In older trees, the
branches extend well above
arms reach. The leaves are
delicate, soft needles in groupings of five. Bark is platy and
ranges from gray to dark brown.
Small, curved, pollen-bearing
male catkins appear in clusters
in spring, each one about 1 inch
long and yellow-orange in color.
The slender, elongated female
cones are 3–8 inches long.
Where the tree is wounded
or has dropped a branch,
sticky white pitch exudes. The
fragrance of pine, sweet and
resinous, urges one to breathe
deeply, instilling a feeling of
peace in the mind and body.

Pitch pine features rigid needles in groupings of three. The
habit of pitch pine varies greatly
depending on its environment.
In mountainous regions, pitch
pine is a low-growing shrub
reaching only about 1 foot high.
In winter, you'll find a wide
variety of birds nibbling at the
seeds in pitch pine cones.

The stout, roughly pyramid-shaped cones are 1–3½ inches long.

Where, When, and How to Wildcraft

Eastern white pine is found in parks, in or at the edges of forests, and near swamps.

Pitch pine is common in coastal areas and is the dominating species of pine barrens, often growing alongside oak.

Pines often drop their branches after windy days, making it easy to gather bundles of medicine, leaves, twigs, and inner bark. If you don't find fallen branches, prune young stems, about ¾-inch wide or smaller. With a sharp knife, cut a line lengthwise down the brown outer bark to reveal the white to green inner bark. Peel off the outer bark and scrape the knife downward along the stem to separate the inner bark. It'll come off in shreds. To give a sense of how much you'll get, five stems about 6 inches in length yield

about 2 ounces of inner bark. It's messy work but it's worth it. Rinse your hands with alcohol or simply exercise patience—the pitch will eventually wear away. I kind of like the stickiness of the pitch on my fingers, and once it wears off I find my fingers feel softer and smoother.

You won't always find it, but if you do, the pitch alone is valuable medicine. Collect it by gently scraping it from the bark with a knife without damaging the outer bark of the tree. Scrape the pitch into a jar to tincture right away or save for use in salve or honey.

In early spring, collect the male catkins for their pollen. There's no need to remove the pollen from the catkins, just process them right away in tincture.

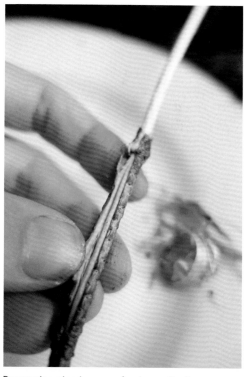

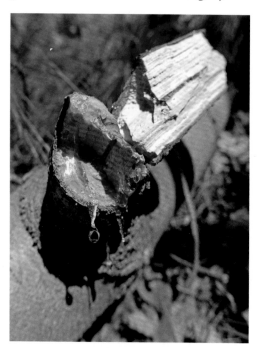

Waiting for nature's invitation to gather pitch inspires a feeling of gratitude for Earth's generosity.

Processing pine is messy business. Peeling away the outer bark from twigs leaves a persistent sticky residue on the fingers, hands, arms, and anywhere else it touches.

Wear old clothes when harvesting and working with pine, as the pitch pretty much sticks to clothing indefinitely. Turpentine or mineral spirits will dissolve the pitch, though be sure to wash your hands well after using these strong solvents.

Medicinal Uses

Walking through a grove of pines is medicine in and of itself. Pine scent signals us to inhale deeply, and the dried fallen needles dampen sounds of the forest and invoke a sense of peace. With its breath-inspiring action, it's no surprise that pine needles, inner bark, and pitch—in tea, tincture, or honey—clear the lungs of congestion, alleviating sticky coughs. The needles and inner bark contain vitamin C and help reduce cold symptoms and soothe sore throats. Historically, the needles were used to prevent scurvy, or severe vitamin C deficiency.

Applied directly to wounds and splinters, pine pitch acts as a drawing agent that heals, protects, and removes irritation from the skin simultaneously.

The long slender needles of pine are a signature for the nerves and the whorled branches growing rhythmically up the tree for the heart and spine. Pine is a pain-relieving circulatory stimulant. Applied externally and taken internally pine needles, bark, and twigs relieve pain in the muscles, joints, and back. Make a salve with oils infused with pine, Saint John's wort, and mugwort to massage into sore muscles. Add pine needle and bark decoction to a hot bath to ease the pain and swelling of rheumatic conditions.

Pine pollen is a valuable source of amino acids, vitamins, and minerals. The pollen in tincture form boosts testosterone and increases vitality and stamina, which in turn remedies depletion-related conditions such as erectile dysfunction. In China, the pollen in powder form is used as a longevity tonic.

Pine is diuretic and antimicrobial. Use the twigs or inner bark with goldenrod and

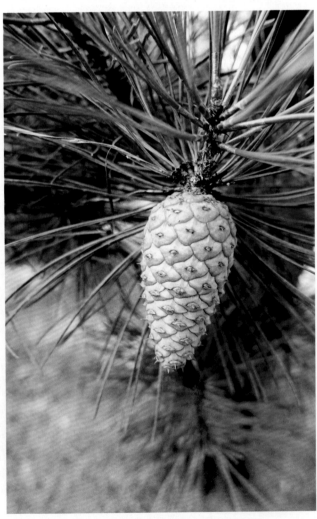

The immature cone of pitch pine is green and tightly closed.

horsetail to reduce pain, inflammation, and infection in the urinary tract.

Pine flower essence helps us move on from self-blame or self-inflicted guilt from past events, whether or not we were in error. It instills freedom to move past self-limits.

⚠ Precautions

Pine pollen tincture is indicated for men over 30 years old with reduced androgen levels. Pine pollen powder does not increase androgen levels and most people can take it safely. Start with small doses in case you are allergic to the pollen.

Future Harvests

The easiest, most sustainable way to gather pine medicine is to collect from freshly fallen branches. If these aren't readily available, mindfully prune small branches from mature trees.

HERBAL PREPARATIONS

Tea
Standard infusion of fresh or dried needles
Drink 2–4 ounces as needed.

Tincture
1 part fresh bark, needles, and pitch
2 parts menstruum (95% alcohol, 5% water)
Take 10–30 drops as needed.
or
1 part pollen
5 parts menstruum (70% alcohol, 30% water)
Take 30 drops 2 times per day. Hold the tincture under the tongue for 60 seconds or so before swallowing.

Infused honey
1 part fresh needles
2 parts honey
Take 1–3 teaspoons as needed.

Infused oil
1 part fresh bark, needles, pitch, or twigs
4 parts oil
In a double boiler, gently warm the oil and pitch together to incorporate. Use for sore muscles and frazzled nerves, or in a chest rub for cough.

Flower essence
Follow instructions for making flower essences on page 54. Take 3 drops on the tongue up to 4 times per day or as needed.

pipsissewa

Chimaphila umbellata
prince's pine
PARTS USED flowers, leaves

Warming, astringent, and anodyne, pipsissewa dries up discharges, helps clear
infection, and relieves pain. It has an affinity with the blood and urinary tract.

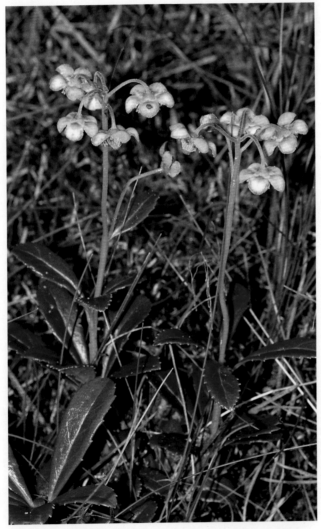

Pipsissewa is said to come from a Cree word, *pipisisikweu*, that
translates as "it breaks into small pieces," speaking of its efficacy
in breaking up stones in the urinary tract.

How to Identify

Pipsissewa is a native evergreen
plant related to wintergreen—
the leaves when crushed have
a similar scent. Leaves are
shiny, thick, toothed, and
grow in grouped pairs that
look like whorls. Woody stems
grow 4–12 inches in height.
In late spring, these brownish
stems sport small umbels of
tiny white to pink five-petaled
flowers with prominent green
ovaries. Round seed capsules
follow the flowers and remain
through winter.

Where, When, and How to Wildcraft

Pipsissewa is primarily found in
healthy forests as an understory
plant. Gather leaves (mindfully)
throughout the year. Tincture
fresh or dry the leaves on
screens in a well-ventilated area.

Medicinal Uses

The First Peoples of North
America traditionally use pipsissewa for a variety of health
complaints, from blisters to
coughs. Several tribes of the
Northeast employ it as a blood

purifier, sometimes in combination with plants such as elder and mallow.

The wintergreen scent reveals the presence of methyl salicylate, one of the components that lend this plant its pain-relieving properties. Coupled with its astringent nature, this makes a good medicine for internal bleeding in the case of ulcers or postpartum hemorrhage.

Pipsissewa is utilized most often in cases of urinary tract infection, especially where other remedies have been unsuccessful. The leaves dry up discharges, soothe pain and inflammation, and stanch bleeding. Use in combination with cranberry and mallow to aid in the healing process of the urinary tract.

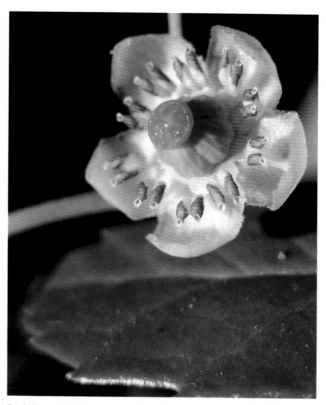

Each flower features a prominent green ovary at its center.

Pipsissewa flower essence brings clarity and releases worry, facilitating decision-making in those who don't trust their own choices.

Future Harvests

Take care not to trample or disturb the soil surrounding pipsissewa plants. They do not take well to soil compaction. Pipsissewa is difficult to cultivate and is at risk due to habitat loss, habitat disruption, and overharvesting. If you find pipsissewa in abundance, mindfully harvest only one or two leaves from a few plants. If making a flower essence, use the no-pick method.

HERBAL PREPARATIONS

Tea
Standard infusion of dried leaves
Drink 2–4 ounces 3 times per day.

Tincture
1 part fresh leaves
2 parts menstruum (95% alcohol, 5% water)
or
1 part dried leaves
5 parts menstruum (70% alcohol, 30% water)
Take 10–30 drops 3 times per day.

Flower essence
Use the no-pick method described on page 55. Take 3 drops on the tongue up to 4 times per day or as needed.

Plantago species
broadleaf plantain (*P. major*), narrowleaf plantain (*P. lanceolata*)
PARTS USED leaves, roots, seeds

Plantain has a wide range of internal and external uses. It's both astringent and moistening and works to draw out foreign matter from the blood, mucosa, and skin.

How to Identify

Plantain consists of a humbly growing basal rosette of leaves with parallel prominent ribs, tall seed stalks, and tan fibrous roots. Broadleaf plantain has wide, rounded, ovate leaves. Its upright seed stalk is covered almost entirely with tightly packed seeds from top to bottom. Narrowleaf plantain has long lanceolate leaves and its stalks are topped with a green to bluish cone-like seedhead that, when in bloom, is circled by a ring of yellow-white stamens. The way the stalks emerge from the ground and move with the breeze resembles a snake rearing up into a striking pose (one of this plant's signatures).

Both of the species featured here are introduced from Europe and grow abundantly in the Northeast. There are several

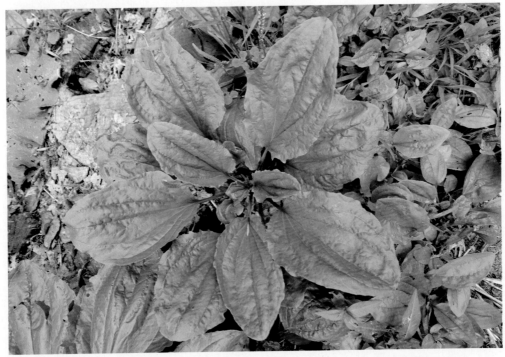

Planta is Latin for "sole of the foot." This can refer to the shape of the leaf as well as this plant being commonly underfoot. The introduced species of plantain (*P. major* shown here) are known as white man's footstep by First Peoples of North America, alluding to its ease of reproduction and distribution.

native species that are fairly analogous medicinally. One of these, heartleaf plantain (*P. cordata*) is a water-loving plant that is endangered across North America. It is an indicator species that is sensitive to changes in water quality; its presence or absence reflects the health of ecosystems.

Where, When, and How to Wildcraft

It's usually not too hard to find narrowleaf and broadleaf plantain. They grow in lawns and parks, and through

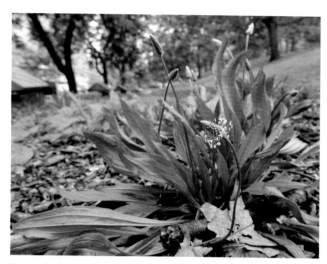

Narrowleaf plantain wears a crown of creamy white stamens when in bloom.

cracks in the sidewalk (though you wouldn't want to harvest those). Narrowleaf plantain is inclined to grow more toward the edge whereas broadleaf often prefers open spaces. Broadleaf plantain also tends toward depressed wet areas in fields. It doesn't mind compacted soil one bit. Both species can be used pretty much interchangeably.

Gather leaves almost year-round, whenever you see them growing. Dig roots anytime as well, from spring through fall. In summer, snip seedheads off broadleaf plantain and strip the seeds to add to smoothies and baked goods.

You really could dig up the entire plant to use all parts as medicine. Tincture the entire plant or its parts, depending on the type of medicine you are looking for. It all dries well, too, for use in teas, poultices, compresses, baths, and washes.

Medicinal Uses

Plantain is alterative, anodyne, anticatarrhal, antihistaminic, anti-inflammatory, antimicrobial, antipruritic, antitussive, aperient, astringent, demulcent, diuretic, emollient, hemostatic, mucilaginous, styptic, tonic, and vulnerary. In other words, plantain clears congestion and coughs, reduces allergic reactions, tightens and tones tissue, moistens mucous membranes, relieves constipation, eases pain and inflammation, draws out toxins, and stops bleeding. Not too bad for a humble weed.

Plantain leaf is a great remedy for cuts, scrapes, and bruises. Infuse oil with plantain leaves to incorporate into wound-healing salves. Plantain is traditionally used to treat snakebite. Take plantain root and leaf internally with echinacea and white horehound to cleanse the blood and apply this mixture to the bite as a poultice to draw venom out from the wound.

A classic application of plantain leaves is as a spit poultice. Simply chew up a leaf, spit it out, and place it on a bite, wound, or bee sting. It will relieve stinging, itching, irritation, and inflammation, and draw out toxins. Keep applying until the symptoms have abated.

Drink plantain leaf infusion for coughs, cold, flu, and throughout allergy season to reduce symptoms.

The seeds are especially mucilaginous and serve as a bulking agent that relieves constipation due to dryness, immobility, and stagnation. The leaf infusion works to relieve conditions of the gastrointestinal tract, including diarrhea, ulceration, hemorrhage, and irritable bowel syndrome. Combine with witch hazel, blackberry leaf, and violet in a sitz bath or suppository to relieve hemorrhoids. Plantain can also help alleviate cystitis, especially in combination with antiseptic herbs with an affinity for the urinary tract, such as barberry.

Future Harvests

Many consider broadleaf and narrowleaf plantain to be weeds. Gathering leaves and seeds will not imperil these prolific producers. However, always be mindful when gathering the roots of any plant, as you are taking that being's life.

Distinguish common broadleaf from endangered heartleaf plantain by the shape of the leaves, which as the name suggests, are more heart-shaped in the latter species.

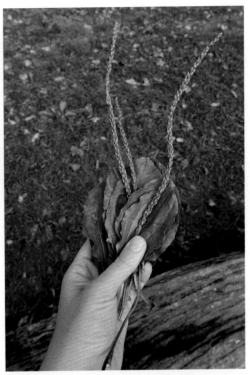

With its broad range of applications, plantain is an essential herb for every home apothecary.

HERBAL PREPARATIONS

Tea
Standard infusion of dried leaves
Drink 1 cup up to 3 times per day. Use as a wash for wounds, bites, or stings.

Tincture
1 part fresh leaves roots, and seeds
2 parts menstruum (50% alcohol, 50% water)
Take 30–60 drops 3 times per day.

Infused oil
1 part fresh leaves
2 parts oil
Use in wound-healing salves or to draw out stings and splinters.

poke

Phytolacca americana
pokeweed, inkberry
PARTS USED fruit, roots

Considered by many to be dangerous to consume due to its toxicity, in the right doses poke is a valuable plant to have in your medicine chest for preventing full-blown illness, moving stuck fluid in the lymphatics, and relieving arthritic symptoms.

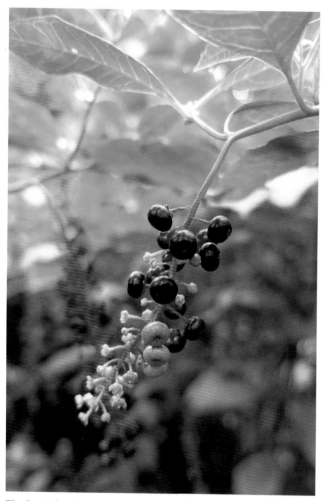

The fruit of poke can be taken one ripe berry at a time in short courses to reduce pain and swelling of rheumatic and arthritic conditions. Consult with an experienced herbalist to determine the dose that's right for you.

How to Identify

Poke is a native perennial herb that emerges in spring as thick, fleshy, light green stems poking out of the ground. Crinkly ovate-lanceolate leaves unfold in an alternate pattern from the stem. As the season rolls on, poke begins to branch, and the stem turns magenta-purple. Small white five-sepaled flowers grow on racemes, yielding to unripe green fruit that ripens to deep purple by the end of summer. Poke grows 4–10 feet tall spreading out to as wide as 5 feet. Older plants develop a shrub-like appearance by summertime.

Where, When, and How to Wildcraft

Poke is most often found in partial shade at the edges of paths and along roadsides and waterways.

If you are really familiar with a patch of poke, visiting it yearly, you can get a rough sense of its age. Dig roots from plants that are at least 3 years old in autumn or early spring when the energy of the plant is closer to the earth. Dry or tincture fresh.

Gather berries in late summer to fall by collecting whole clusters with mostly ripe, undamaged berries. These can be frozen, dried, or made into tincture right away. The berries make an excellent dye yielding a pretty pink color—the genus name *Phytolacca* is Greek for "red dye plant."

Medicinal Uses

Poke root and berries stimulate the immune system and get fluid moving through the lymph nodes. A few drops of poke root tincture come in handy when you start to feel the inkling of a cold or flu coming on—marked by tender or swollen glands, headache, and a general sense of achiness and malaise. It's good to have on hand when traveling, especially if prone to illness in new environments. Again, the dose is just a few drops. Poke is potent medicine and is toxic in large doses.

Poke is anti-inflammatory, antiviral, and pain-relieving. The berries can be taken (swallowed whole) one or two per day every other day for a week to relieve swelling and pain in the joints that accompanies arthritis and rheumatic conditions.

Infuse the root in oil to use topically on swellings of the glands and joints. It is a specific for mastitis and nursing moms can use it homeopathically and externally to relieve sore breast tissue. Just be sure to wash off the

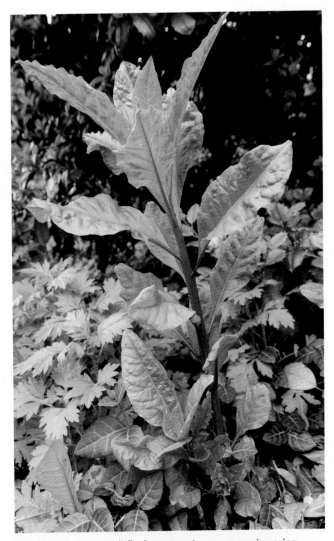

Young poke plants with fleshy green stems emerge in spring. By summer, the stems are magenta-purple and branching.

infused oil before baby latches on.

Blend the infused oil into a lotion to use on acne prone skin, and to dissolve cysts and boils.

Precautions

Poke is toxic in larger than therapeutic doses, so use only small doses in short courses, no more than a few drops of tincture and no

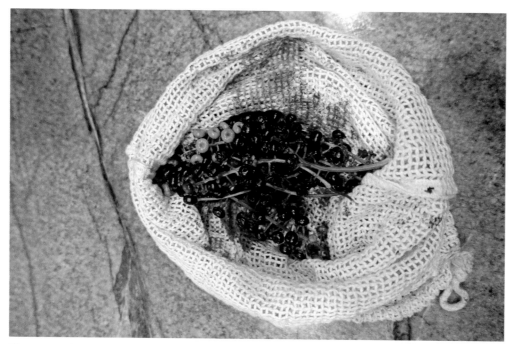

The name poke derives from the Algonquian words *poughkone* and *pocan* meaning "dye plant." The purple berries impart a lovely pink color on fabric.

longer than 1 week at a time. Discontinue if you experience nausea, abdominal pain, diarrhea, or disorientation.

Do not use poke during pregnancy or in children.

Poke may be unsafe for people with compromised immune systems or those who are underweight. Consult an experienced herbalist to determine whether poke is an appropriate choice.

If you aren't comfortable using the herb, try the homeopathic form (*Phytolacca*).

Future Harvests

Poke is fairly widespread. Birds eat the berries and distribute the seeds pretty widely. As with any plant, take pause when gathering the roots, knowing that you are taking the life of the plant.

HERBAL PREPARATIONS

Tea

Cold infusion of 10 fresh or frozen berries muddled in a quart of water

Drink 1–2 ounces every other hour over the course of a day. Discontinue if nausea, abdominal pain, diarrhea, or disorientation ensue.

Tincture

1 part fresh roots
2 parts menstruum (95% alcohol, 5% water)
or
1 part dried roots
5 parts menstruum (50% alcohol, 50% water)
Take 1–5 drops 3 times per day.

prickly ash

Zanthoxylum americanum
common prickly ash, northern prickly ash, toothache tree
PARTS USED bark, fruit

*Warming, stimulating, pain-relieving prickly ash is a traditional
remedy for toothache, joint pain, sore throat, and cough.*

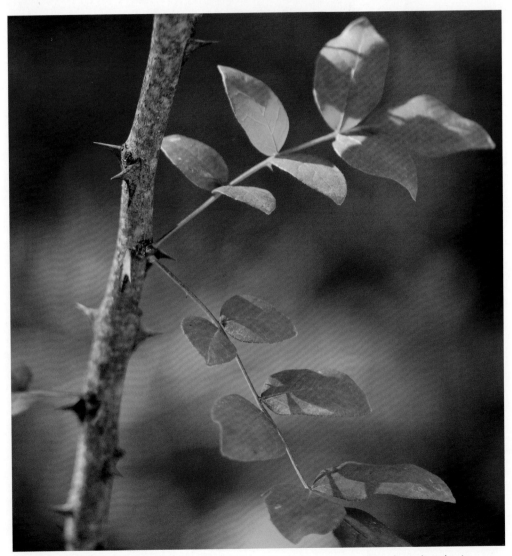

Prickles on plants are a signature for use in stabbing pain. Prickly ash is used to relieve dental pain,
and the pain and inflammation of arthritis.

How to Identify

Prickly ash is a small tree in the citrus family that ranges from a shrubby 4–8 feet to a more tree-like 25 feet in height. Sharp prickles grow at the nodes along the trunk and stem. Fragrant greenish blossoms grow in clusters in the axils in spring.

Pinnately compound leaves with five to eleven small ovate leaflets grow alternately on the stem. The dark green leaflets have tiny translucent glands that look like pinholes against the light.

In fall, small, red, citrus-scented fruit develop, each filled with one or two shiny, round, brown-black seeds.

The taste of the bark and fruit is pungent and aromatic, and imparts a numbing, tingling feeling on the tongue and lips. The tree is related to the species from which Sichuan peppercorns are harvested— *Z. simulans*, *Z. piperitum*, and *Z. bungeanum*. You can cook with the fruit of American prickly ash in the same way.

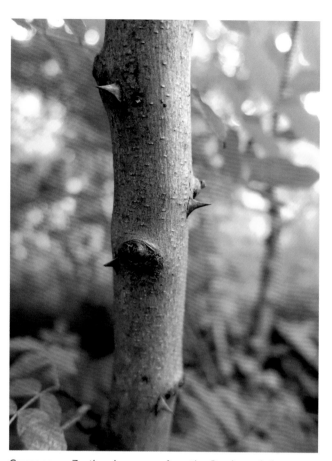

Genus name *Zanthoxylum* comes from the Greek words for "yellow" (*xanthos*) and "wood" (*xylum*).

Where, When, and How to Wildcraft

Find prickly ash growing in a range of conditions, from dry rocky ledges to low-lying moist forest soils. Look for it at the edge of disturbed soils, along fields and meadows, and in thickets and shrublands.

Prune small branches and twigs in spring. It's a good idea to wear long sleeves and thick gloves and pay special attention to the prickles as you harvest. Pick the fruit in fall when it is red and ripe. All parts can be dried or used fresh in tincture or tea.

Medicinal Uses

Prickly ash bark and fruit are warming, stimulating, and numbing. These features make prickly ash a helpful pain-relieving herb, traditionally used for oral pain, including mouth sores and toothache. Dilute the tincture of prickly ash and consider combining it with astringent and antiseptic herbs, such as blackberry root and echinacea, to use in mouthwash to tighten lax gum tissue and relieve dental pain. This can also be gargled to cleanse and numb sore throat due to infection. Sucking on a bit of the bark works, too.

Make a topical wash of prickly ash for use on sore muscles and joints.

Add prickly ash–infused oil to a chest rub salve for cough, with the optional additions of pine, wintergreen, and cottonwood.

Prickly ash can be used as a catalyst in herbal formulas to warm and open the body to receive the other herbs in the blend.

Precautions

Prickly ash causes nausea and vomiting when taken in large doses. Avoid this by using primarily as a topical remedy, mouthwash, or gargle. If you do take it internally, start with small doses and back off if it instigates nausea.

Do not use in pregnancy as prickly ash is stimulating to the uterus and has a history of use as an abortifacient.

Future Harvests

Selectively and mindfully pruning small twigs and branches from mature trees in dense thickets of prickly ash is a sustainable way to harvest. A little bit goes a long way with this medicine, so you really don't need much.

Be mindful not to harvest branches hosting butterfly eggs and caterpillar larvae— giant swallowtail (*Papilio cresphontes*) and other butterflies lay their eggs on the leaves. Gathering fruit will not compromise the tree.

Prickly ash is endangered in New Hampshire.

HERBAL PREPARATIONS

Tea

Standard decoction of fresh or dried bark
Use as a topical wash, mouthwash, or gargle for sore throat.

Tincture

1 part fresh bark and/or fruit
2 parts menstruum (65% alcohol, 35% water)
or
1 part dried bark and/or fruit
5 parts menstruum (65% alcohol, 35% water)
Take 10–20 drops 3 times per day.

Infused oil

1 part fresh bark or fruit
2 parts oil
Use as massage oil for sore muscles and joints. Add to chest rub formulas to relieve cough.

Ambrosia species

common or annual ragweed (*A. artemisiifolia*), giant or great ragweed (*A. trifida*), perennial ragweed (*A. psilostachya*)

PARTS USED flowers, leaves

Ragweed is mostly known as a source of seasonal allergy symptoms. What most folks may not realize is that ragweed can also reduce these symptoms, and work as an antidote in those allergic to the pollen.

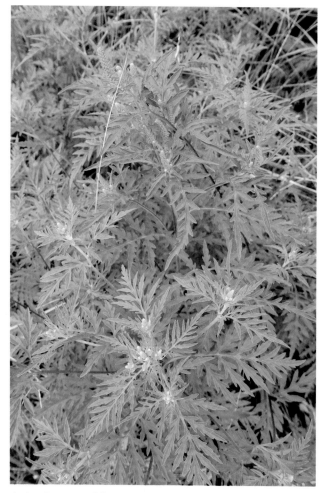

Ambrosia artemisiifolia, or common ragweed, is so named because of the resemblance of its leaves to those of *Artemisia vulgaris*, or mugwort.

How to Identify

Ragweed is a self-sowing annual plant in the aster family. The two most common species of ragweed in the Northeast are common ragweed and giant ragweed. On both, opposite, symmetrical, deeply lobed leaves grace multiple branches on upright hairy stems.

The leaves of common ragweed, *A. artemisiifolia*, have more divisions than giant ragweed, looking a bit like the leaves of *Artemisia vulgaris*, after which the species name derives. A tightly packed upright raceme of yellow-green flowers blooms in late summer. The plant is overall more diminutive than giant ragweed. In compacted edges it grows only a few inches off the ground. If it has more room to grow, it reaches up to 3 feet or so.

The opposite leafing pattern of giant ragweed is more obvious with its large three- to five-lobed leaves. Standing over the plant in its early stages you get a real sense of its

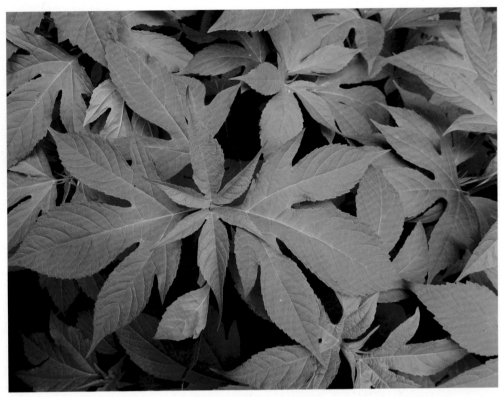

The symmetrically leafed giant ragweed.

symmetry. An interrupted raceme of dangling yellow-green flowers full of windborne pollen bloom in late summer. Once it reaches its apex in late summer—sometimes up to 14 feet—giant ragweed towers over everything around it, save most trees.

Ragweed is native to North America and may have been cultivated as a food crop for its protein- and fat-rich seeds. The seeds are an important pre-winter fattening food source for birds.

Where, When, and How to Wildcraft

Ragweed tolerates compacted soils and a bit of shade—it's most often found in the edge or in ditches along roadsides, near wooded areas, and along paths near fields or meadows.

Some herbalists harvest ragweed leaves before flowering in late spring to midsummer and others collect the flowering tops with the leaves in later summer to fall to tincture as an antidote to this allergen-producing plant. If you choose the latter, strain the tincture through a coffee filter to catch the pollen grains.

Medicinal Uses

Ragweed is synonymous with fall allergies. When viewed through a microscope, ragweed's windborne pollen is spherical and spiky, and easily irritates eyes and the respiratory tract. Interestingly, ragweed is antihistaminic and taking ragweed tincture leading up to fall allergy season can prevent allergic reactions to its pollen. Start with 1 drop and see how your body reacts. If you tolerate 1 drop, increase the dosage to 15–20 drops up to 4 times per day.

Ragweed tincture clears up a dripping runny nose brought on by colds as well as pet and dust allergens.

The astringent nature of ragweed helps stop diarrhea and dysentery.

Applied topically, ragweed leaf is anti-inflammatory and can bring relief to insect bites and minor scrapes. Make a spit poultice with ragweed and plantain to soothe skin irritations.

⚠ Precautions

Ragweed acts as a bioremediator of toxic soil by readily uptaking lead into its roots. Be sure you know the soil from which you harvest is not a former industrial site. The best way to know is to have it tested. A quick search online will yield your local soil testing service.

Wear long sleeves and gloves if harvesting this plant as an antidote for allergies, especially if you are the one who is allergic. Add a mask if the plant is flowering. Some folks who are extremely sensitive to aster family plants may experience a rash just from rubbing against ragweed.

Future Harvests

Ragweed is considered a noxious weed in most places, despite it being native to North America. It spreads easily by seed. Harvest away!

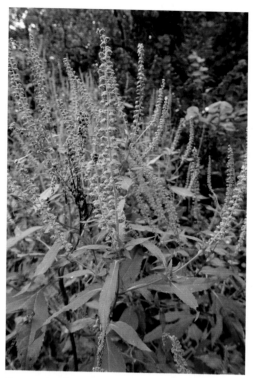

Ragweed pollen is a common source of seasonal allergies in late summer to fall. One antidote is to take a few drops of the tincture internally leading up to the season when it blooms.

HERBAL PREPARATIONS

Tincture
1 part fresh flowers and leaves
2 parts menstruum (50% alcohol, 50% water)
Take 15–20 drops up to 4 times per day.

raspberry

Rubus species

black raspberry (*R. occidentalis*), purple-flowering raspberry
(*R. odoratus*), red raspberry (*R. idaeus*), wineberry (*R. phoenicolasius*)

PARTS USED flowers, fruit, leaves, roots

*Herbalists depend on raspberry for its astringent quality, helping to halt
hemorrhages and diarrhea. It has an affinity with the uterus and remedies
a variety of women's health conditions.*

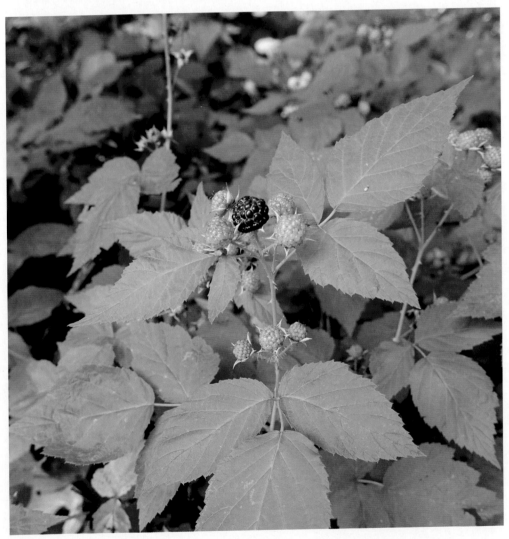

Black raspberry ripening in summer.

How to Identify

Raspberry is a prickly cane or bramble plant in the rose family. The leaves of most species are pinnately compound with three to seven toothed, ovate leaflets, with the exception of purple-flowering raspberry's maple-like leaves. The undersides of leaves are usually downy white. Flowers are typically white and five-petaled, with the exception again being purple-flowering raspberry, which has, you guessed it—purple flowers. Or rather magenta, depending on who you ask.

Where, When, and How to Wildcraft

Raspberry is famous for taking over disturbed patches of soil in forested places and along paths. Gather the leaves in spring before flowering. Tincture or infuse in vinegar directly, or dry completely for use in infusions. Collect flowers in midspring to early summer for use in flower essence.

The variety of raspberry species in the Northeast offers a perpetual harvest through summer. Black raspberry fruit ripens at the beginning of summer, purple-flowering raspberry in the middle of summer, and wineberry and red raspberry closer to summer's end. Enjoy as a trail snack or add to tinctures to increase their nutrient content.

Wear thick gloves and long sleeves when collecting roots so as not to scratch yourself on the prickles. Early spring or fall are the easiest times to gather. The roots are threadlike and thin so you may need to harvest a few of the plants to yield a strong tincture. Or, you can combine them with the leaves and fruit for a whole-plant tincture.

Medicinal Uses

Raspberry leaf makes a pleasant, nourishing tea with astringent, cooling, and toning properties. The nutrient-rich and

Nourishing Mama-To-Be Tea

During pregnancy, it's generally best to follow the less-is-more approach when it comes to taking herbs. Except in the case of nourishing herbs. The aim here is to build the blood and nourish the mom so she can feed the growing baby. When I was pregnant with my son, I drank this infusion daily. It instilled a feeling of health and well-being throughout the pregnancy.

What you'll need:

- 2 parts stinging nettle leaf
- 2 parts raspberry leaf
- 1 part dandelion root
- ½ part red clover
- ¼ part rosehips
- ¼ part spearmint

Combine the herbs in a mixing bowl and store the blended herbs in an airtight container. Measure out approximately ½ cup of herb mixture per quart of water. Add the herbs to a glass quart jar or French press, fill the jar to the top with boiling water, and let infuse for an hour or more. I like to let mine steep overnight. Strain and drink 3 cups to 1 quart throughout the day. You can drink it every or every other day. Leave out the red clover if you have a history of miscarriage due to hormonal imbalance or have a bleeding disorder.

progesterone-balancing leaves are most commonly known for their effectiveness as a women's or mother's herb, from pre-conception to postpartum. Taking raspberry leaf infusion daily or every other day prepares the body for conception, toning the uterus for implantation. Raspberry leaf has been used traditionally to prevent threatened miscarriage. During pregnancy it reduces nausea in morning sickness, strengthens the tone of the uterus for childbirth, and nourishes the mother and baby in utero. For childbirth, it increases the effectiveness of contractions and placenta delivery, tones the pelvic floor muscles, and reduces postpartum bleeding. And to top it off, raspberry leaf infusion encourages milk production and fortifies breastmilk.

The root, leaf, and berries are all used in cases of stomach upset, queasiness, and diarrhea. The astringency of the plant helps to stanch internal bleeding and cease cramping and diarrhea. Combine raspberry leaf with aperient and mucilaginous herbs—such as plantain seed and leaf, violet, and mallow—to relieve constipation.

Make a wash with raspberry leaves to heal mouth sores and to speed healing of weeping wounds on the skin.

Raspberry flower essence increases compassion and empathy in those who are harboring resentment or holding on to past hurts.

Future Harvests

In general, gathering leaves, flowers, and fruit will not endanger raspberry. Keep in mind, though, that when you collect the flowers, you are taking the fruit. If you find an abundant bramble that looks as-yet untouched by birds, lucky you. Take only what you really need and leave behind plenty for our feathered and furred friends.

Gathering roots is another story. Though *Rubus* plants are generally prolific producers, several native species are at risk due to habitat loss and disturbance. Choose roots from a large bramble, or from one of the introduced species such as wineberry or red raspberry. You can also propagate raspberry plants by stem or root cuttings to ensure future harvests.

HERBAL PREPARATIONS

Tea
Standard infusion of dried leaves
Drink 4–8 ounces up to 3 times per day.
or
Standard decoction of roots
Drink 4 ounces up to 3 times per day.

Tincture
1 part fresh fruit, leaves, roots, and/or
    stems
2 parts menstruum (50% alcohol,
50% water)
Take 20–30 drops up to 3 times per day.

Flower essence
Follow instructions for making flower essences on page 54. Take 3 drops on the tongue up to 4 times per day or as needed.

red clover

Trifolium pratense
PARTS USED flowering tops

Sweet, cooling, moistening, nourishing, and estrogen-balancing red clover is an important herb for regulating hormones for fertility and during menopause. It's also a powerful blood-cleansing agent when taken over extended periods, from weeks to months at a time.

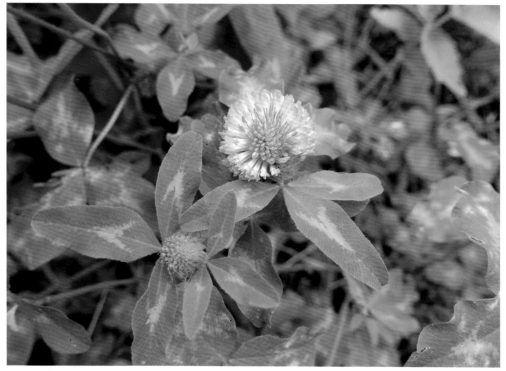

To the ancient Druids of Ireland, Britain, and Europe, the three leaflets of the clover represented earth, sky, and sea.

How to Identify

Red clover is a perennial ground cover plant in the bean family. Leaves are alternate and compound with three oval leaflets, often with a white chevron on each one. Leaflets either have tiny teeth in the margin or no teeth at all. Stems are covered in a fine hair.

The centerpiece of red clover is the pink- to magenta-colored globe-shaped flower that blooms in summer. The flower is made of a tightly packed cluster of individual nectar-filled tubular florets. Surrounding the bloom is a pair of opposing compound leaves. Honeybees and bumblebees are a big fan of these flowers.

Like other plants in the bean family, red clover fixes nitrogen in the soil, making it a good cover crop or green manure. It's also used as animal fodder.

Where, When, and How to Wildcraft

Red clover is at home in open fields and meadows, a farm fugitive that's spread across North America. It blooms from late spring through summer. Collect the flowering tops, stem and all, and dry them for tea or add them fresh to tincture. They make a great addition to baked goods. Select dry, brightly colored, wilt-free blossoms. Red clover decomposes quickly and picking wet or brown blooms will not make for good medicine.

Medicinal Uses

Just as red clover enriches the soil, so it nourishes the human terrain as well. Red clover contains several minerals and vitamins, including calcium, magnesium, zinc, potassium, vitamins A and C, and B vitamins. While it fortifies it also gently detoxifies, blocking environmental pollutants (xenoestrogens) from accumulating in the body. It is a very gentle alterative that works profoundly when taken over a long period of weeks or months.

Red clover contains isoflavones that act as estrogen in the body. This benefits those with low fertility due to low estrogen levels and makes it helpful for mitigating symptoms that arise with menopause, when estrogen levels drop.

For a bone-building, blood-cleansing brew, blend red clover with other mineral-rich herbs—nettle, raspberry leaf, horsetail, elder, and burdock.

Red clover works well with other moistening herbs such as violet and mallow to remedy dry cough. It is a lymphatic herb that helps dissolve benign cysts and soothe swollen glands. Drink a cool red clover tea to treat dry mouth.

Taken internally or applied in a poultice or compress, red clover infusion soothes dry, sensitive skin and helps clear up eczema and acne.

Red clover flower essence encourages a calm disposition, particularly in situations where panic and chaotic thought forms are present.

⚠ Precautions

Do not use red clover if taking blood-thinning medications, as the herb may enhance their effects. Discontinue use 2 weeks prior to surgical procedures.

Red clover is not recommended in those with bleeding disorders.

Red clover may stimulate estrogen receptor–positive breast cancer cells, so there is some concern over its use in estrogen-sensitive cancers. This evidence is based on in vitro (test tube) studies and has not been demonstrated in humans.

Future Harvests

Red clover is a very common introduced plant that is used in farms as a cover crop. It easily escapes cultivation. There is no concern over the future of this plant.

HERBAL PREPARATIONS

Tea
Standard infusion of dried flowering tops
Drink 1 cup up to 3 times per day.

Tincture
1 part fresh flowering tops
2 parts menstruum (50% alcohol, 50% water)
Take 30 drops up to 3 times per day.

Flower essence
Follow instructions for making flower essences on page 54. Take 3 drops on the tongue up to 4 times per day or as needed.

red root

Ceanothus americanus
New Jersey tea
PARTS USED leaves, root bark

When things are stuck, physically and creatively, red root breaks up stagnation, restores flow, and returns tone to lax tissues.

How to Identify

Red root is a densely packed, woody, deciduous shrub in the buckthorn family that grows to about 3 feet tall. Finely toothed, ovate leaves with a pointed tip are pubescent and feature three main veins. Tiny, fragrant white flowers bloom in ball-shaped clusters on long stalks in late spring. In summer, triangular capsule fruit ripen to a dark purple-black.

The woody roots of this plant, as the name suggests, are red, sometimes tan-brown. The plant is deeply rooted, making it drought and fire tolerant—and a challenge to harvest.

Red root leaves and seeds are an important food source for deer, turkey, quail, and the spring azure butterfly (*Celastrina ladon*).

Where, When, and How to Wildcraft

Red root prefers dry soil and is found in sunny open woodland meadows and slopes.

Harvesting the root takes a bit of work. Spring or fall is the best time to do it, when

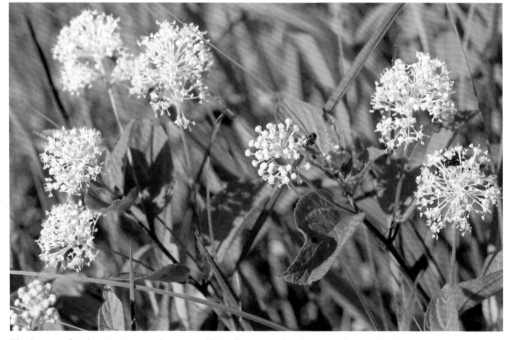

The leaves of red root were used as a tea (*Camellia sinensis*) substitute during the American Revolutionary War, hence the name New Jersey tea.

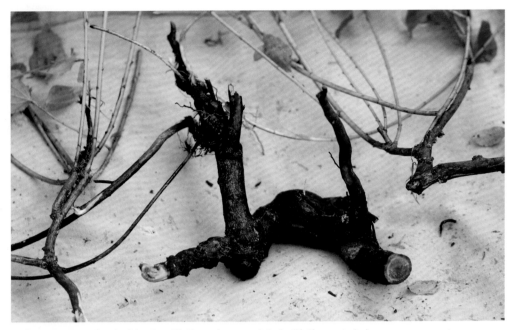

Red is a signature for the blood and is the color associated with the root chakra or energy center. Red root dissolves stagnant or coagulated blood and has a mild blood pressure–lowering effect.

the plant is clear of foliage. Examine the periphery of the plant for branches that root down. Remove the soil and check for horizontal growth. Once you find a horizontal root, use a saw or lopper to prune it from the crown. Cover the hole you've made in the soil and mulch with leaf and branch debris that may have been removed in the process of unearthing the root. Clean and chop the root up outside. Strip off the root bark to tincture fresh or dehydrate in an oven or dehydrator set to the lowest setting.

Collect the leaves in spring or summer to make your own New Jersey tea.

Medicinal Uses

Thick, heavy, cold, damp conditions are resolved with the help of red root. The root bark is astringent and fluid-regulating. It tones tissues while breaking up congestion in the lymph nodes and moving stuck, stagnant blood. A warm decoction reduces swelling in

the glands, soothes sore throat, and clears a lingering cough.

Sluggish digestion or diarrhea caused by cold, damp foods is improved by red root tincture or decoction, especially when paired with warming herbs such as elecampane, sweetfern, and spicebush.

Red root has an affinity with the spleen and benefits those with Epstein-Barr (mononucleosis), parasitic infections, and other conditions that would cause an enlarged spleen.

Apply a compress of red root decoction to bumps and bruises to restore blood flow, reduce inflammation, and dissolve coagulated blood.

When I'm feeling stuck or my creative juices aren't flowing, I make a red root chai with warming, stimulating spices like ginger, cinnamon, and black pepper. This mix invigorates the root and sacral energy centers, instilling courage and confidence and inspiring newfound creativity.

⚠ Precautions

Do not use red root if you are taking medications with blood-thinning or blood-clotting actions.

Avoid use in pregnancy as red root acts as an emmenagogue and potential abortifacient.

Future Harvests

Red root is threatened in Maine, Rhode Island, and Québec, warranting replanting efforts in these areas. Red root can be propagated by cuttings.

To ensure the continued success of this plant in the wild in your region, harvest outer root sections of well-established plants while leaving the majority of the shrub intact.

HERBAL PREPARATIONS

Tea
Standard decoction or overnight cold infusion of fresh or dried root bark
Drink 2–4 ounces 3 times per day.

Tincture
1 part fresh root bark
2 parts menstruum (75% alcohol, 25% water)
or
1 part dried root bark
5 parts menstruum (50% alcohol, 50% water)
Take 10–30 drops 3 times per day.

Rosa species

multiflora rose (*R. multiflora*), beach rose (*R. rugosa*)

PARTS USED flowers, hips, leaves, prickles, roots, stems

All parts of rose are astringent and antioxidant. The fragrant blooms are calming and mildly sedating, the hips are useful as a vitamin C supplement, and the roots and leaves are excellent for reducing diarrhea and discharges.

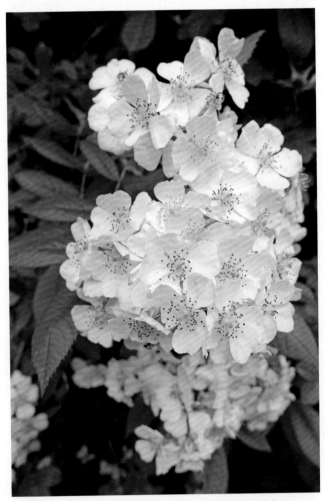

Multiflora rose is a widespread, introduced plant that forms dense thickets. It was planted as a farm field border or hedgerow but is now considered invasive in the Northeast. It's a great rose species to harvest in abundance.

How to Identify

A true wild rose has compound leaves with an odd number of toothed leaflets (most of the time) and five-petaled flowers (except for one or two species native to China with four). Those cultivated roses we give to sweethearts on Valentine's Day are mutants, flowers within flowers or what is called "double-flowered" where the stamens develop into petals. They're still quite lovely and many of these adulterated cultivars are prized for their fragrance and medicinal qualities. Wild roses range from white to dark pink and every shade in between.

Contrary to pop songs and poems, roses have prickles along their stems, not true thorns like their cousin hawthorn. The round- to egg-shaped red fruit of the rose is what we call a hip, though actually these house the tiny fruits inside we call seeds (though they aren't seeds). Those seed-like fruits are called achenes, each one carrying its own single seed. As confusing as the rose may be, she is much beloved by most humans the whole world over.

Birds and other wild creatures enjoy the fruit of rose throughout winter.

Where, When, and How to Wildcraft

Rose is typically an edge-grower found in sun-dappled, open forest areas or in the full sun of a meadow or field. Multiflora rose, recognized by its abundant clusters of small white to pink blooms, is a common invasive plant that volunteers in disturbed habitats. Beach rose is a hardy seaside species prized for its large hips.

Gather the flowers from late spring into summer to tincture fresh, make flower essence, distill rosewater, infuse in vinegar or honey, or dry for cold and hot infusions. The hips are traditionally harvested in late fall and winter after the frost, which makes them softer and sweeter. You can mimic mother nature by harvesting ripe red hips and freezing them for 24 hours before using them. Dig roots in spring or fall, before or just after leaf development. Collect leaves for tea from spring through early fall.

Medicinal Uses

What flower evokes the feeling of love more than the rose? The scent alone has the power to turn us on, lift us out of dark emotions, and tame feelings of frustration. With its mild bitter quality, rose has a gentle action on the liver, the seat of anger and where we process hormones and toxins. Rich in antioxidant vitamin C, rose is cooling and cleansing to the blood. Rose tincture or infusion regulates reproductive hormones and curbs premenstrual symptoms.

Rose is a perfect complement to what is known in Ayurvedic medicine as a pitta constitution, one that leans toward heat, excitation, and inflammation. Overheated from

the summer sun? Make a cold infusion of rose petals for the ultimate summer cooler. Rose-infused vinegar is an excellent sunburn remedy and skin toner. Spritz yourself with rosewater to tame inflamed breakouts and rashes.

Rose roots are the most astringent part of the plant and help control diarrhea. Rose petals, leaves, and root help balance intestinal flora and normalize the gut. Combine with mallow, violet, and burdock for irritable bowel syndrome.

Incorporate rosehips into cold and flu formulas. They work well with elderflower, lemon balm, chamomile, and mint.

While most people who know rose think of it mostly as an herb for the heart, rose has a strong association with the eyes and vision, both inner and outer. Drinking rose tea before bedtime is said to induce prophetic dreams.

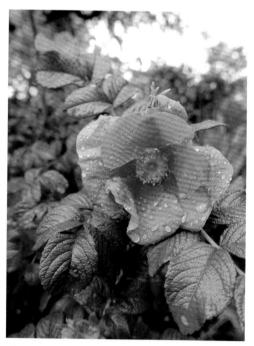

The typical pink or red color of rose blooms is indicative of its effectiveness for reducing redness and inflammation.

Do-It-Yourself Rosewater

Making hydrosols (plant or flower waters) is a fun and simple way to extract the delicious aromas of plants. Rosewater is just one kind of hydrosol you can make with this method. Other plants that would make good hydrosols include elderflower, honeysuckle, mint, or sweet clover. For this recipe you're going to make a home distiller with a few common items.

What you'll need:

- Heatproof bowl or measuring cup
- Flat, sturdy, heatproof object for elevating the bowl or measuring cup
- Large pot with lid
- 2 cups dried rose petals, or 4 cups fresh rose petals
- Filtered or distilled water
- Ice

Place your flat, sturdy, heatproof object in the bottom of the pot. You can use a clean brick covered in aluminum foil, a heatproof plate, or a shallow metal food storage container (as I've done). On top of the flat object, place a heatproof bowl or measuring cup. Add the rose petals to the pot. Fill with enough filtered water to cover the rose petals. Place the pot on the stove. Flip the lid of the pot upside down and place it over the pot, making sure it creates a seal. Add ice to the top of the upturned pot lid.

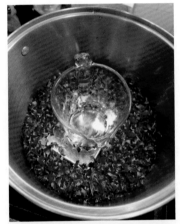

Turn on the heat. Once the water begins to boil, turn down the heat so that it is gently steaming. Replace the ice on the pot lid as it melts. I use a baster to remove any accumulated water and then add more ice. After 30 minutes, turn off the heat. Carefully remove the lid so as not to spill ice water into the pot. Remove the bowl or measuring cup that now has the distilled rose water inside. Pour into a dark glass spray bottle and label. Spritz and enjoy!

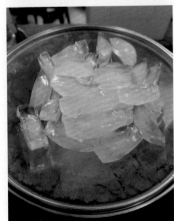

Taking the whole plant tincture, including the prickles, helps establish healthy energetic boundaries.

The flower essence of rose allows us to give and receive love openly and unconditionally. It instills a deeper connection to ourselves, to spirit, and to the world around us.

 Precautions

Rose may be too cooling for some people. For those with cold constitutions, blend rose with warming herbs—pine, spicebush, cinnamon, or ginger.

Future Harvests

Favor the roots of introduced species of rose, such as multiflora and beach rose. There are several species of native rose that are endangered or threatened throughout the Northeast. Harvesting a modest amount of leaves, petals, prickles, and fruit from these species is a sustainable way to enjoy native roses.

HERBAL PREPARATIONS

Tea
Standard or cold infusion of dried flowers
  or hips
Drink 4 ounces as needed. Use as a wash or compress for conjunctivitis, sore eyes, rashes, and burns.

Tincture
1 part fresh flowers, prickles, and stems
2 parts menstruum (40% alcohol,
  60% water)
or
1 part dried flowers, prickles, and stems
5 parts menstruum (40% alcohol,
  60% water)
Take 10–30 drops as needed.

Infused honey
1 part fresh rose petals
2 parts honey
or
1 part dried rose petals
4 parts honey
Savor by the spoonful. Use topically as a facial treatment.

Infused oil
1 part fresh rose petals
2 parts oil
or
1 part dried rose petals
4 parts oil
Whip into lotions, mix into salves, or use for a sensual massage.

Infused vinegar
1 part fresh rose petals
2 parts apple cider vinegar
Makes a great treatment for sunburn. Use as a skin toner to reduce redness.

Elixir
1 part fresh rose petals
1 part honey
1 part spirit of choice
Follow instructions for making elixirs on page 51. Enjoy in sparkling water as a refreshing summer cocktail.

Saint John's wort

Hypericum perforatum

PARTS USED flowering tops

Saint John's wort is way more versatile than its reputation as a depression herb. It's a powerful ally as a restorative for the nervous, immune, and digestive systems and a potent wound healer, to boot.

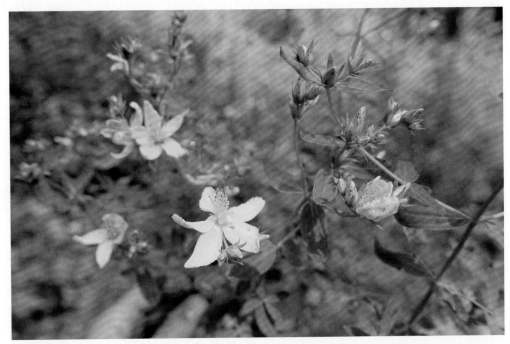

One interpretation of the genus name *Hypericum* derives from the Greek words *hyper* and *eikon* meaning "exceeding any imagination" or "beyond compare" referring to the potency of the plant. The species name *perforatum* refers to the translucent glands on the leaves that look like little holes or perforations.

How to Identify

Saint John's wort is a perennial herbaceous plant, upright and with many branches. Leaves are small, elliptical, and opposite with a unique feature. Hold a leaf up to the light to reveal pin-prick size translucent glands that give the leaves a perforated look. Delicate, five-petaled, yellow flowers with prominent yellow stamens and tiny black dots in the margins of the petals bloom through the summer, with their traditional peak falling on Saint John's Day or the pagan midsummer, June 24.

The flowers you want to collect are the ones that leave a red stain on your fingers when you pinch them, revealing the presence of hypericin, a constituent with antimicrobial effects.

Where, When, and How to Wildcraft

Saint John's wort is often found in the partially shaded edge, though sometimes in full sun, of fields, meadows, and disturbed areas.

On a dry summer day, gather flowering tops with not-yet-opened or just-opened blooms that exude red stain when squeezed. Infuse the flowering tops—stems, leaves, blooms and all—fresh in tincture and oil. You'll notice the infusions turn a rich red over time. For tea, you can dry the flowering tops.

Medicinal Uses

One way to express the benefits of Saint John's wort is to say it restores feeling and feelings. The infused oil or salve soothes nerve pain and heals minor nerve damage. Take the tincture and use the oil topically to alleviate muscle and menstrual cramps and rheumatic conditions. To lift mood in mild depression and seasonal affective disorder (SAD), reduce anxiety, and encourage restful sleep in these conditions, take the tincture daily for 4 weeks or more.

Combine with elder and anise hyssop in tea or tincture to take the edge off cold and flu symptoms, particularly malaise and spasmodic cough.

Saint John's wort is antiviral and coupled with its nervine actions is particularly useful for reducing the severity of shingles. Use the tincture internally and the oil or salve externally—it pairs well with lemon balm for this and other herpes infections.

A salve made with the infused oil is healing to wounds. Dilute 40 drops of tincture in 2 ounces of water to wash the wound before applying the salve. Unlike comfrey that can heal and seal in bacteria in deep wounds, Saint John's wort is a safe healer for puncture wounds. (Interesting how the leaves look like they have tiny punctures in them.)

While Saint John's wort taken internally may cause photosensitivity (increased risk of sunburn), the oil applied externally works as a mild sunscreen and soothes the pain and redness of sunburn. I love the complexity and often paradoxical nature of herbs.

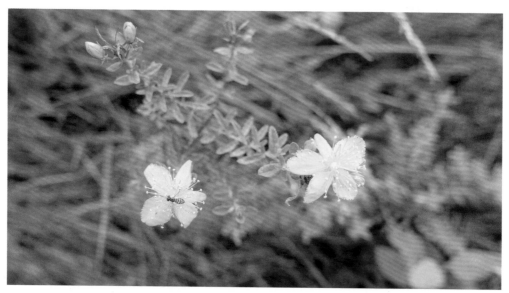

Saint John's wort has a strong association with the sun and the Greek gods Hyperion and Helios. The herb and flower essence strengthen the solar plexus chakra.

Taken as tea or tincture, Saint John's wort supports the solar plexus energy center and gut brain. It facilitates better decision making and instills self-trust. The herb is restorative to the digestive system, tones lax intestines, and facilitates blood cleansing through the liver and kidneys. Saint John's wort also strengthens the bladder and helps curb bedwetting and stress incontinence.

Similar to the herb's effects, the flower essence restores a stronger sense of self, assists in establishing healthy boundaries, helps us face fears, and strengthens the will.

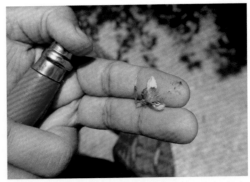

The sign of a fresh, potent blossom is the red stain it leaves on your fingers when you pinch it, revealing the hypericin content.

⚠ Precautions

Saint John's wort may cause photosensitivity in some people, which shouldn't be a problem if you use the herb for SAD in winter. However, it may increase risk of sunburn if taken spring through fall.

Do not use Saint John's wort during pregnancy or breastfeeding.

Saint John's wort should not be taken concomitantly with a wide range of prescription medications, including but not limited to the following: medications affecting the CYP450 pathways, HIV/AIDS medications, immunosuppressants, anticonvulsants, oral contraceptives (potentially), psychotropic and antidepressant medications, and triptans used to treat migraines. Consult with a healthcare professional before using Saint John's wort if you are taking prescription medication.

Future Harvests

Picking the flowering tops of Saint John's wort does not put this introduced species at risk. Keep in mind that several species of *Hypericum* endemic to the Northeast—with a history of medicinal use by First Peoples—are threatened or endangered. Harvesting primarily from the introduced species

(*H. perforatum*) is one way to safeguard the future of these rare gems. Another way to protect them is to fight for wild spaces by stewarding the land and pushing for conservation efforts.

HERBAL PREPARATIONS

Tea
Standard infusion of dried flowering tops
Drink 4–8 ounces as needed. Use as a wash or compress for bruises and wounds.

Tincture
1 part fresh flowering tops
2 parts menstruum
Take 20–40 drops up to 3 times per day.

Infused oil
1 part fresh flowering tops
2 parts oil
Use as massage oil for sore joints and muscles. Craft a salve for wound care and sunburn.

Flower essence
Follow instructions for making flower essences on page 54. Take 3 drops on the tongue up to 4 times per day or as needed.

Sassafras albidum
PARTS USED leaves, root bark

Sassafras is best known as a spring tonic that cleanses and moves the blood after the stagnation of winter.

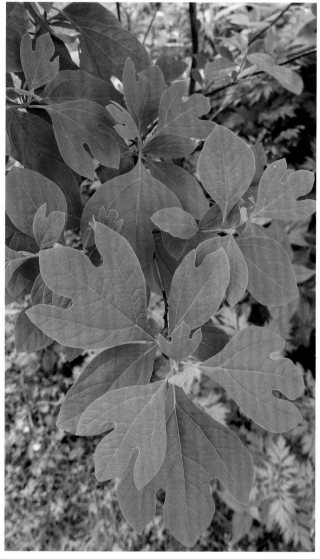

Sassafras has three leaf forms: oval-shaped, mitten-shaped, and three-lobed.

How to Identify

Sassafras is a deciduous shrub or tree in the laurel family. It features three different leaf shapes: an unlobed oval, a mitten, and one with three lobes. Leaves are waxy and highly mucilaginous. Young trees and shrub forms have greenish bark that is covered with orange-brown fissures. Mature trees have reddish brown, thickly plated bark.

The leaves and roots have a spicy-minty-floral aroma and flavor. Once you smell the roots you'll recognize the scent as root beer—sassafras root was once used as an ingredient in that beloved beverage.

Clusters of tiny, six-petaled, fragrant flowers that are greenish yellow to creamy yellow-white bloom in spring before the leaves emerge. These develop into bluish black, oval-shaped fruits that ripen in fall.

A variety of birds depend on the fruit and serve as seed-dispersers. Many mammals rely on the fruit, bark, and wood for food, including black bears, beaver, and rabbits.

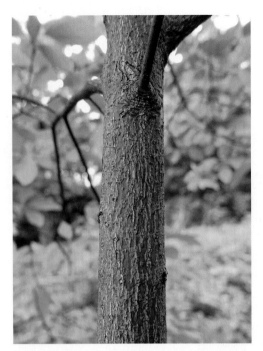

Young trees have green bark covered with orange-brown fissures.

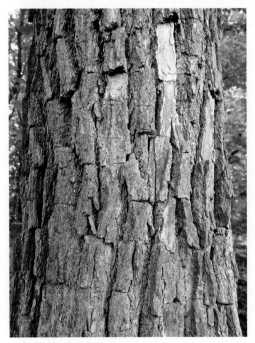

The bark of mature trees is deeply ridged, platy, and reddish brown.

The leaves and twigs are an important forage for deer.

Where, When, and How to Wildcraft

Sassafras is a pioneer species that fills a niche in disturbed soils. Look for it along paths, roadsides, in fields, and young woodlands.

Wildcraft leaves from spring through fall. Use them fresh or dry them. Powdering the leaves is traditional and known as filé powder in Creole circles, originating from the Choctaw people in the South. Use the powder topically for injuries or in culinary preparations to thicken sauces, soups, and stews (think: gumbo).

Look for saplings or suckers in full shade of abundant sassafras groves. They likely won't make it to adulthood. They're fairly easy to pull up out of the ground after a little light digging with a hand trowel. You can also find the roots that connect mature mother trees to the saplings and dig some of those. Start with the sapling and unearth it, following the root closer to the mother tree. Gather when the ground is soft, from spring through fall. Small roots can be used as is. For larger roots, strip off the outer layer and simmer the inner bark to make tea or syrup.

Medicinal Uses

Sassafras is a renowned spring cleansing tonic. Combine it with cleavers, nettle, and birch in a decoction to sip into springtime. This blend nourishes and stimulates circulation of blood and lymphatic fluids; detoxifies the liver; encourages healthy digestion, assimilation, and elimination; tones the urinary tract; reduces inflammation in the joints; and helps mitigate seasonal allergies.

The stimulating warmth of sassafras aids the body in kicking colds and other respiratory infections. Pine, white horehound, and wild bergamot would all be good partners to sassafras for facilitating healing of cough, sore throat, and the general ickyness of viral and bacterial infection. As a fever reducer, sassafras works well with boneset and mint. Use sassafras as a gargle for tonsillitis and lesions of the mouth and gums. Add self-heal, wild bergamot, and echinacea for added effect.

Sassafras root makes a nice addition to a warming bitters blend with other digestive herbs like elecampane, black walnut, and chicory.

Although sassafras is warming, it also has a cooling effect via its blood-thinning powers. This comes in handy during the summertime, acting as a refrigerant in our bodies, making the heat more tolerable.

Apply the mucilaginous leaves or a poultice of the inner root bark as a soothing poultice for sprains, bruises, burns, and bites. Dust on the powdered leaf to clear up weepy wounds and poison ivy rash.

⚠ Precautions

Do not use sassafras if you are taking medications with blood-thinning or blood-clotting actions.

Sassafras should not be used during pregnancy due to its blood-thinning effects.

In a mid-twentieth-century study, safrole—a constituent isolated from sassafras leaves and root—given in high concentrations to rats was shown to be carcinogenic, in rats. Safrole is also found in cinnamon, nutmeg, basil, and anise. Safrole is not water soluble, and on top of that, I don't know anyone taking safrole on its own without the rest of the sassafras leaf or root. In short, drinking moderate amounts of the decoction or infusion of sassafras is perfectly safe.

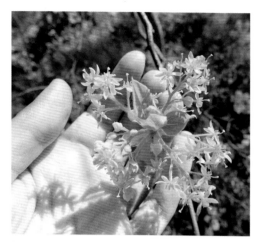

Fragrant yellow-green flowers bloom in spring.

Future Harvests

Sassafras is a native species that is threatened in Maine and Vermont. Mindfully collecting the leaves will not harm the tree. In healthy stands of sassafras, saplings are the easiest and most sustainable to harvest. Be mindful to take only what you will use.

HERBAL PREPARATIONS

Tea
Cold infusion of fresh or dried leaves
Drink 1 cup as needed. Use as a wash or poultice for wounds and bites.
or
Standard infusion or decoction of root bark
Drink 1 cup as needed. Apply as a poultice to bruises and sprains.

Syrup
Reduce root decoction by half and add equal parts honey or maple syrup. Enjoy with seltzer in homemade soda or cocktails.

self-heal

Prunella vulgaris
heal all, common selfheal
PARTS USED aerial parts in flower

This common lawn dweller packs medicinal punch in a tiny package.
As the name suggests, this herb is a consummate wound healer, as well
as a time-honored remedy for afflictions of the throat.

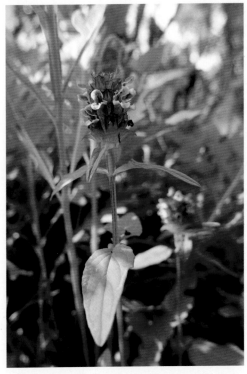

In the edge, self-heal gets the chance to grow up to about 1 foot tall.

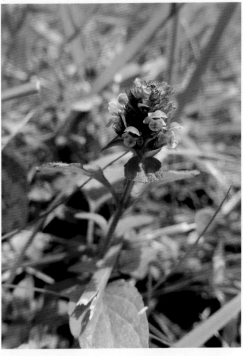

In lawns and regularly mowed fields, self-heal is more diminutive, reaching only a few inches off the ground.

How to Identify

Self-heal is a low-growing perennial plant in the mint family, native to North America and Eurasia. From a square stem emerge pairs of opposite lanceolate leaves (up to 3½ inches long) with very finely serrated or smooth margins. Sitting atop the stem is a densely packed, cone-like flower spike composed of overlapping hairy bracts. Many tiny, purple, tubular, two-lipped florets like open mouths bloom throughout summer. Beneath the flower spike are a pair of opposing, stalkless leaves that look a bit like wings.

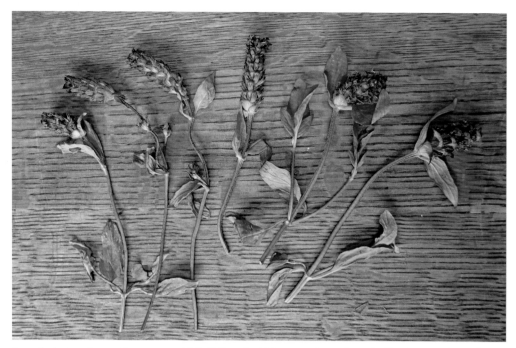

Prunella derives from a German word "die Bräune," which somewhere along the line became "brunella." Both are synonyms for quinsy, a type of throat infection where pus builds up behind the tonsils, for which self-heal is a remedy.

The plant can grow up to 1 foot tall in places with less human traffic, like the edge. It's more often shorter, reaching only a few inches high in lawns where mowing and trampling keeps it short.

Where, When, and How to Wildcraft

Self-heal likes space to spread out and is found in lawns, fields, and meadows across the entire continent. You'll also find it growing in a weedy edge and sometimes in riparian or lakeside zones.

Collect the entire aerial portion of the plant when in bloom to tincture fresh or dry for later use.

Medicinal Uses

Self-heal is astringent, mucilaginous, cooling, and dispersing. It's useful for inflammation and infection, as well as skin and mucous membrane injury. In all parts of the Northern Hemisphere where this plant grows, it has been used traditionally to heal wounds and reduce fever.

Those little open-mouthed flowers gracing the top of self-heal are a signature for use in afflictions of the throat. Drink the infusion to soothe sore throat and swollen tonsils. Alternately gargle with tincture or infused honey diluted in warm water or warm rose infusion with a pinch of sea salt.

In Chinese medicine, self-heal is used for swollen glands and goiter and modern research demonstrates its efficacy for cancer based on traditional Chinese formulae. Some studies point to the ability of self-heal to target thyroid cancer in particular.

The two-lipped flower is also indicative of the two sides of an open wound. Combine self-heal with meadowsweet and mallow in an infusion to heal ulcers in the gastrointestinal tract. Apply the poultice to stop bleeding, reduce pain and inflammation, and prevent infection in fresh cuts and scrapes. Use the poultice or compress with chickweed to shrink inflamed boils. Craft a salve or lotion with self-heal–infused oil to promote the regeneration of healthy skin.

Self-heal reduces blood pressure and liver inflammation, helping to quell outbreaks of anger and frustration. Apply a cool compress of self-heal and rose to treat heat- or tension-induced headache.

Self-heal flower essence aids those who have a hard time distinguishing their own inner voice from other people's voices and opinions. It allows them to make positive lifestyle choices based on their own inner compass.

Future Harvests
Self-heal is a prolific self-sower and spreads underground by runners. It's a tough little plant that readily pops back up after repeated mowing.

HERBAL PREPARATIONS

Tea
Standard infusion of dried aerial parts in flower
Drink 4–8 ounces as needed. Use as a wash for wounds or compress for headache.

Tincture
1 part fresh aerial parts in flower
2 parts menstruum (50% alcohol, 50% water)
or
1 part dried aerial parts in flower
5 parts menstruum (50% alcohol, 50% water)
Take 30–60 drops 3 times per day.

Infused honey
1 part fresh herb
2 parts honey
Enjoy by the spoonful. Dilute in warm water with sea salt as a gargle for sore throat.

Infused oil
1 part fresh aerial parts in flower
2 parts oil
Add to wound-healing salves or lotions to promote healthy skin.

Flower essence
Follow instructions for flower essences on page 54. Take 3 drops on the tongue up to 4 times per day or as needed.

Capsella bursa-pastoris
PARTS USED aerial parts in flower

The heart-shaped fruits of shepherd's purse hint at its circulatory stimulating effects and its use for internal and external bleeding.

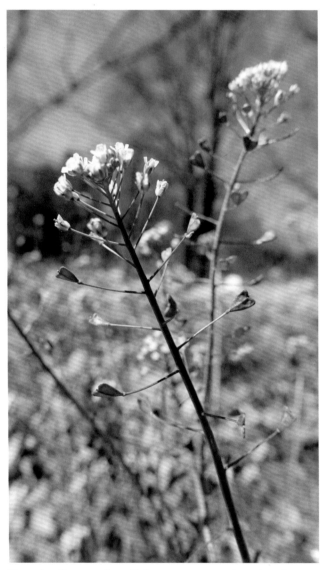

The scientific name *Capsella bursa-pastoris* translates literally as shepherd's purse.

How to Identify

Shepherd's purse is an introduced annual or biennial herb in the mustard family, native to Eurasia and naturalized around the world. It starts as a basal rosette of oblong-lanceolate leaves, often with deep lobes. The plant grows up to 18 inches, a thin stem graced with alternating heart-shaped fruit or seed capsules (the shepherd's purse) that's topped with four-petaled, white-pink to white-green flowers growing in a clustered raceme.

Where, When, and How to Wildcraft

Shepherd's purse grows in fields, meadows, and lawns where the mower blades don't reach. Like other introduced species, it tends toward the edges, either in full or partial sun, and doesn't mind poor soil quality. It is well distributed across the continent.

Collect the aerial portions in flower in spring to add fresh to tincture. You can dry it for tea, though it's best used fresh or within a few months of drying. The fresh leaves, flowers, and seedpods are a tasty, mildly peppery addition to salads.

Medicinal Uses

Astringent, circulatory-stimulating shepherd's purse halts internal and external hemorrhages. Taking the tincture or infusion stanches bleeding from the organs and tissues, including the stomach, lungs, intestines and urinary tract. It has long been used as a remedy for uterine hemorrhage, especially following childbirth and to reduce excessive menstrual bleeding.

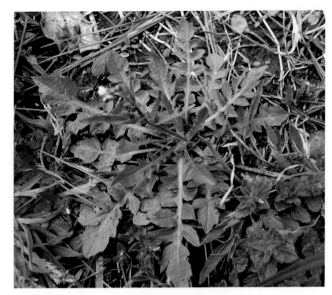

The deeply lobed basal rosette of leaves.

Apply a poultice of shepherd's purse, with the optional addition of plantain and chickweed, to treat scrapes and cuts. To treat a nose bleed, soak a cotton ball in the juice or infusion and place it in the affected nostril.

For gastric and duodenal ulcers, combine shepherd's purse with chamomile and licorice. To assist in healing from ulcers, avoid food triggers—alcohol, caffeine, and gluten—and incorporate stress-reduction practices.

Shepherd's purse tones the bladder and helps resolve bedwetting.

⚠ Precautions

The internal use of shepherd's purse is not recommended during pregnancy. Use with caution in those with low blood pressure or those taking concomitant blood-thinning medications.

Shepherd's purse accumulates toxins from the soil—know the land's history of use and potential for contamination before harvesting.

Future Harvests

Harvest away—shepherd's purse is prevalent across the globe and is considered a weed in these parts.

HERBAL PREPARATIONS

Tea
Standard infusion of dried aerial parts in flower
Drink 2–4 ounces as needed.

Tincture
1 part fresh aerial parts in flower
2 parts menstruum (50% water, 50% alcohol)
Take 30–60 drops as needed, up to 4 times per day. Take in more frequent doses for postpartum bleeding, 20–40 drops directly under the tongue as needed.

Polygonatum species

PARTS USED flowers, rhizomes

Solomon's seal is a sweet and moistening tonic for dry or debilitated constitutions and a chief remedy for musculoskeletal ailments.

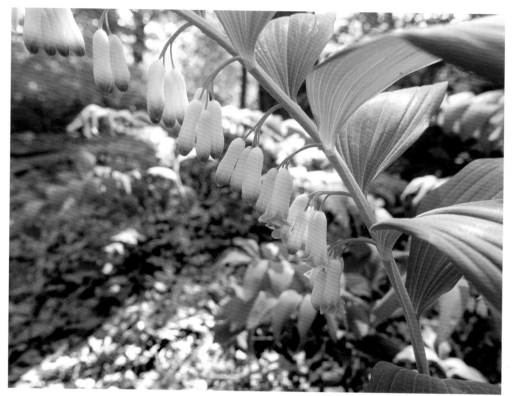

Creamy white to yellow-green flowers hang down like little bells, blooming from bottom to top.

How to Identify

A graceful understory perennial, Solomon's seal emerges in spring from a thick, creamy white rhizome that looks a bit like a segmented worm. Its round scars indicate the previous year's stem growth. Some liken the rhizome to the intestines and look to it as a signature for its use there. Another interpretation is that the roots look like bones and joints. The genus name *Polygonatum*

translates as "many knees" and Solomon's seal is an important remedy for the musculoskeletal system.

Solomon's seal emerges in early spring as an upright shoot of tightly furled leaves. Alternate, ribbed, smooth-margined, ovate leaves unfold from a long, arching, subtly zig-zagging stem that reaches 1–3 feet in length. Dangling down like little bells, small clusters of creamy white to yellow-green

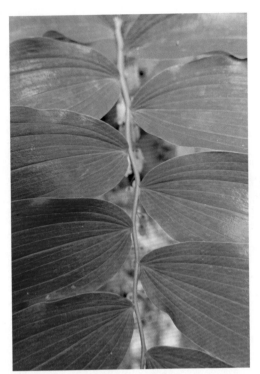

Stalkless leaves emerge from a subtly zig-zagging stem.

flowers bloom from the bottom to the top. Once fertilized these become round black-blue fruit that ripen in late summer to fall.

Where, When, and How to Wildcraft

Solomon's seal tends toward moist soil in dappled light to shade, at the edges of forest paths and roadsides.

Look for abundant patches to harvest from in the fall. You can harvest the rhizome from the previous years' growth by finding the root at the base of the plant with your fingers and tracing back a few inches across and under the soil. Take care not to disrupt the aboveground portions of the plant. Using a small trowel or knife, penetrate the rhizome to sever it from the newer growth. If you find a rhizome that's connecting two shoots you can harvest the section in between them. Count the knobby joints

to determine the age of the plant. Clean off the rhizome and tincture or infuse in oil fresh, or cut it up and dry it for use in decoctions.

Medicinal Uses

Sweet, earthy, moistening, and nourishing Solomon's seal rhizome aids dry conditions. It facilitates elimination in cases of dry constipation, soothes a dry cough, and reduces inflammation where there is a lack of lubrication in the joints and connective tissue. It's this last application that Solomon's seal has become best known for in Western herbalism.

Take Solomon's seal internally as a tincture or decoction for a variety of musculoskeletal ailments, such as tendon and ligament injury, sprains, herniated discs, broken bones, and arthritic conditions. Sometimes small doses, a few drops of tincture for instance, taken for a few days or a week or two is enough to facilitate healing and relief (and sometimes more may be required for longer periods of time). The good news is Solomon's seal is nourishing with little to no contraindications. Solomon's seal combines well with other herbs for pain and inflammation, including mullein root and stalk, Saint John's wort, and horsetail internally and comfrey root externally. Solomon's seal also works externally as poultice, liniment, or an infused oil for injury.

Solomon's seal is considered a yin tonic in Chinese medicine—the signature is flowers blooming from the bottom up and the way the flowers hang down from below the bending stem. Combine with burdock to build strength when recovering from illness, injury, or stressful circumstances. This pairing is also beneficial for building up healthy gut bacteria after a round of antibiotic treatment.

Solomon's seal is also useful as a sexual restorative tonic. It tightens the tissues around the uterus in case of prolapse, reduces excess menstrual flow, and restores vaginal moisture. It complements burdock and milky oats in cases where erectile dysfunction stems from stress and fatigue.

The flower essence is used for protection and increasing synchronicity. It helps nurture partnerships and aids in developing discernment and wise decision making.

Carry a slice of the dried rhizome as an amulet of protection and for helping make wise choices in relationships and career.

Future Harvests

Polygonatum biflorum is endangered in Vermont and *P. biflorum* var. *commutatum* is endangered in New Hampshire and borderline vulnerable in New Jersey.

Only gather rhizomes from abundant colonies of Solomon's seal. Collecting sections of the rhizome that aren't directly attached to the growing portion is a fairly sustainable way to harvest, within reason. Don't harvest from the same patch year after year and consider repopulating this valuable plant ally in a forest garden. Solomon's seal is fairly easy to propagate by rhizome division. If this plant is in a happy spot—partial to full shade and moist soil—it will proliferate.

Also keep in mind that the animal community depends on this native plant for food.

HERBAL PREPARATIONS

Tea
Standard decoction of dried rhizomes
Drink 4 ounces as needed.

Solomon's seal tincture
1 part fresh rhizomes
2 parts menstruum (95% alcohol, 5% water)
or
1 part dried rhizomes
2 parts menstruum (60% alcohol, 40% water)
Take 5–30 drops as needed, up to 3 times per day. Use as a liniment for musculoskeletal injury.

Infused oil
1 part fresh rhizomes
2 parts oil
Apply to injured or inflamed muscles, tendons, ligaments, or joints.

Flower essence
Use the no-pick method described on page 55. Take 3 drops on the tongue up to 4 times per day or as needed.

spicebush

Lindera benzoin

PARTS USED fruit, leaves, twigs

Just as the name suggests, spicebush has spice. The warming, stimulating qualities of this native shrub are helpful for dispelling fever and easing aches and pains from rheumatic conditions.

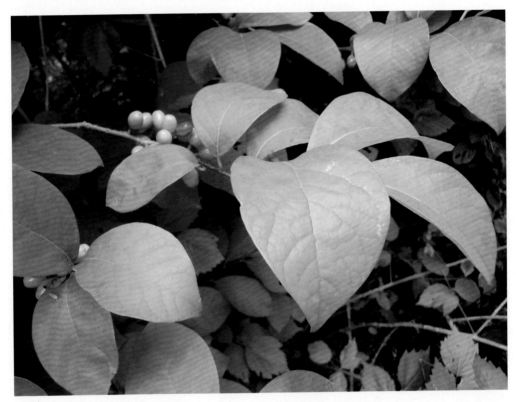

Fruit ripens from late summer to fall.

How to Identify

Spicebush is a woody shrub in the laurel family with a wide rounded habit that grows 6–12 feet tall. Deliciously fragrant, tiny, yellow-green flowers hug the branches in spring before the leaves emerge. Just a little later in spring, the smooth-edged, broadish ovate leaves with a prominent tip that very subtly curves to one side emerge, growing alternately on the branch. They release a lovely spicy scent when crushed. Female plants pollinated by a nearby male will develop small (less than ½ inch), red, egg-shaped fruit that taste and smell like allspice.

Birds and insects depend on spicebush for food, including the spicebush swallowtail butterfly (*Papilio troilus*), which eats the leaves.

Where, When, and How to Wildcraft

Find spicebush in the moist understory, in ravines, and along streams.

Collect the green leaves in summer by pinching here and there off the branch. Dry them or steep them fresh in sun tea or cold infusion. Graze over the shrub to look for choice twigs to prune. Cut 2–3 inches at the tip, above an outward pointed leaf node. These can be dried or tinctured fresh. Gather berries (technically drupes) as they ripen in late summer to fall to freeze, dehydrate, or tincture fresh.

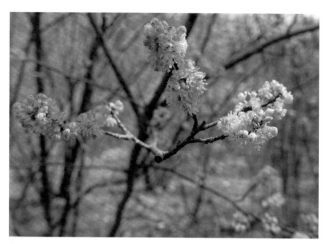

Citrus-floral-spice is one way to describe the scent of spicebush flowers. If only this book had a scratch-and-sniff feature.

Medicinal Uses

Spicebush is a warming circulatory stimulant that brings relief to gastrointestinal upset, cold and flu symptoms, and the aches and pains of rheumatic conditions. It has been used traditionally to eradicate intestinal parasites.

Drink a warm infusion of the fruit, leaves, and twigs, and then crawl under the blankets to sweat out a fever.

Spicebush eases flatulence and abdominal bloating. Take a tincture of the fruit to facilitate healthy digestion of fatty meals. Add hawthorn berries, sassafras, and lemon balm to make a tasty digestive blend.

Infuse the twigs and fruit in oil to craft a salve for bruises and sore muscles and joints. Saint John's wort–, pine-, and cottonwood-infused oils would make a nice addition.

⚠ Precautions

Avoid taking spicebush during pregnancy as it may be too stimulating to the uterus.

Future Harvests

Harvesting a few twigs, leaves, and berries for medicinal use is generally okay as long as you note which shrubs you've harvested from and pay attention if someone else was harvesting before you. Spicebush is considered vulnerable in Maine and Vermont, so pay extra heed in those parts to not overtax this native shrub.

HERBAL PREPARATIONS

Tea
Standard or cold infusion of fresh or dried fruit, leaves, and/or twigs
Drink 2–4 ounces as needed.

Tincture
1 part fresh fruit
2 parts menstruum (50% alcohol, 50% water)
Take 10–20 drops as needed.

Infused oil
1 part fresh fruit and twigs
2 parts oil
Use as a massage oil to warm cold extremities and stimulate blood flow to sore spots.

spotted Joe Pye weed

Eutrochium maculatum (syn. *Eupatorium maculatum*)
gravel root
PARTS USED flowers, leaves, roots, stems

Reflective of the wet environs it inhabits, spotted Joe Pye weed stimulates fluid release through its diuretic and diaphoretic effects. It's most often used for urinary tract complaints.

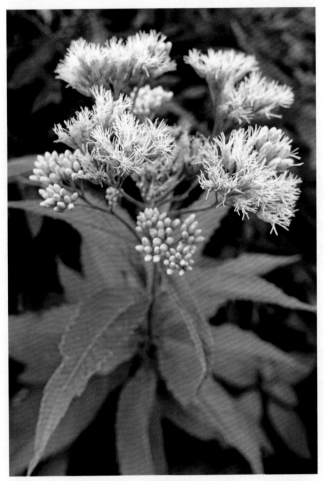

The mystery of how Joe Pye weeds got their name is a testament to the detrimental effects of colonialism. One of the more thoroughly researched accounts has it that the plant was named for Shauquethqueat, a Mohican sachem whose Christian name was Joseph Pye.

How to Identify

A perennial aster family plant, spotted Joe Pye weed is among a handful of *Eutrochium* species native to North America. Whorls of three- to six-toothed, lanceolate leaves up to 8 inches in length spiral up a purple-spotted, green to purple, unbranching stem. Joe Pye weed can form dense stands with several plants growing side by side in a shrubby-looking clump or plants can grow singly and reach up to 8 feet tall. The mass of thin, tan-brown roots are tangled looking.

In midsummer to fall, tiny pink to purple flowers bloom in clusters (inflorescences) at the top of the stem. Each flower in the inflorescence is made up of 10–16 even tinier florets. Butterflies and bees often visit the blooms.

I've highlighted spotted Joe Pye weed because it is the most widespread species in the Northeast. It's sometimes difficult to distinguish between the Joe Pye weeds. A key characteristic of spotted Joe Pye weed is its solid spotted stem and flat-topped inflorescence, compared with the more dome-shaped inflorescence of hollow (*E. fistulosum*) and purple or sweet-scented Joe Pye weed (*E. purpureum*), which is the Joe Pye weed named most often in older herbal accounts. Hollow Joe Pye weed has a—*guess what?*—stem that's hollow throughout and usually spot-free and more uniformly purple. Purple or sweet-scented Joe Pye weed may or may not be more fragrant than the others, only has purple splotches at the nodes, and is generally found in drier soil. Coastal plain Joe Pye weed (*E. dubium*) is like a squatter, smaller, narrower version of spotted Joe Pye weed.

Where, When, and How to Wildcraft
Sunny or partially shaded moist habitats are the domain of spotted Joe Pye weed. Look in marshes, riparian zones, the edges of lakes and wetlands, or where water gathers in fields and meadows.

In midsummer, collect stems, leaves, and flowers either before or just as the flowers open. Tincture them fresh or dry them for tea. From midsummer to late summer, gather flowers just as they open to use in flower essence.

In fall, when the plant goes to seed, dig the roots from individual plants in abundant stands. Tincture fresh.

Medicinal Uses
Diuretic and anti-inflammatory, spotted Joe Pye weed is a primary medicine for the urinary tract. Use it to treat cystitis, either alone or in combination with barberry, goldenrod, and plantain tinctures.

Another common name for Joe Pye weed is gravel root, which speaks to the tendency

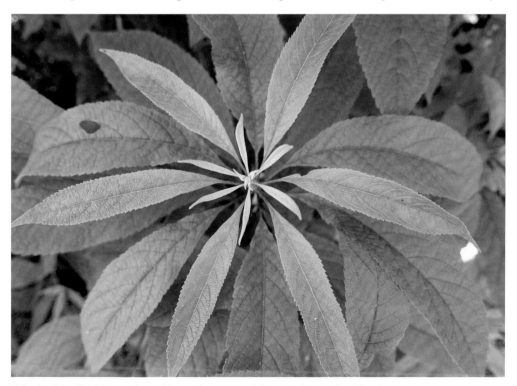

Whorls of toothed, lance-shaped leaves in groups of three to six spiral up the stem.

for the thin roots to be enmeshed in gravel and the ability of this root to break up kidney stones, also called gravel. In cases where kidney stones are present, the tincture or infusion of spotted Joe Pye weed roots, leaves, stems, and flowers along with other stone-breaking diuretics such as birch bark, wild carrot leaf and root, and dandelion root can bring relief.

The fluid-clearing nature of spotted Joe Pye weed facilitates the reduction of swelling in the joints, relieving painful symptoms of bursitis, arthritis, and gout. Use with crampbark, burdock, and Japanese knotweed infusion or tincture for greater effect.

A traditional use of this native herb is as a fever reducer. Used alone or with yarrow, boneset, and catnip in a hot infusion, spotted Joe Pye weed will get you sweating to release toxins and break the fever. Drink this tea and slip under the covers for a good sweat, followed by a long nap to speed recovery from acute illness.

Algonquin and Haudenosaunee people employ spotted Joe Pye weed for women's health concerns, particularly for its ability to relieve soreness in the uterus after childbirth.

The flower essence helps those who feel overwhelmed by choices or the energy of other people. It helps one realize they are not alone or separate from the universe and aids the development of healthier relationships.

Future Harvests

Other Joe Pye weeds are threatened in parts of the range—coastal plain Joe Pye weed in New York, Maine, and Nova Scotia; hollow Joe Pye weed in Maine and New Hampshire; sweet-scented Joe Pye weed in Vermont.

Leave plenty behind for the native bees and butterflies. One rule of thumb is to take no more than 20% from one stand. To encourage future harvests, collect the seeds in fall to directly sow in nearby soil. Plants can also be divided by cuttings in late spring.

HERBAL PREPARATIONS

Tea
Standard decoction of dried roots
Drink 1 cup 3 times per day.

Tincture
1 part fresh flowers, leaves, roots, and/or stems
2 parts menstruum (50% alcohol, 50% water)
Take 20–40 drops 3 times per day.

Flower essence
Follow instructions for making flower essences on page 54. Take 3 drops on the tongue up to 4 times per day or as needed.

Picea species

black spruce (*P. mariana*), blue spruce (*P. pungens*),
Norway spruce (*P. abies*), red spruce (*P. rubens*), white spruce (*P. glauca*)
PARTS USED bark, needles, resin, tips, twigs

*Spruce offers an abundance of medicine with healing benefits for lungs,
skin, and kidneys, as well as the immune and musculoskeletal systems.*

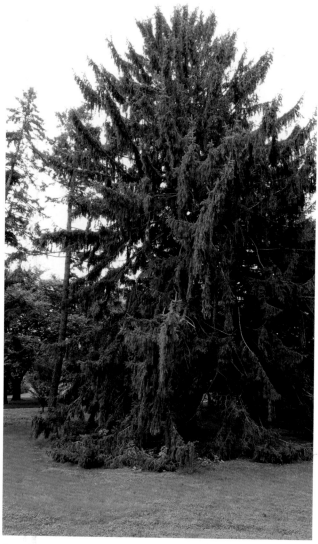

A mature spruce can grow up to 200 feet tall.

How to Identify

Spruce stands out from other evergreens with its four-sided needles, which are attached singly to the branch by what look like tiny tan petioles or stems called pulvini. These pulvini remain on the branch after the needles fall off, leaving behind little bumps or pegs.

Spruce trees can grow 60–200 feet tall, depending on the species and conditions. The branches are whorled like other pine family relatives and the tree has a cone-shaped habit, or what many would call a Christmas or yule tree shape. The bark is scaly and ranges from light to dark gray-brown.

Long narrow female cones, generally tan to brown in color with thin flexible scales, house seeds that birds like to eat.

In the Northeast there are five key species of spruce—three species native to the Northeast (black, red, and white), one introduced from western North America (blue), and one introduced from Europe (Norway).

Where, When, and How to Wildcraft

Norway spruce—commonly planted as an ornamental, border tree, or windscreen—has naturalized in parts of the Northeast. White spruce is found most often in inland forests and at higher latitudes with some coastal distribution in Massachusetts, Maine, New Brunswick, and Nova Scotia. Black and red spruce are fairly widespread north of Massachusetts, commonly found in bogs and swampy areas or mountainous regions. Blue spruce has a fairly spotty distribution and similarly to Norway spruce is found in yards and gardens as an ornamental.

Spring is the best time to gather bark from branches, twigs, resin, tips, and needles, though needles and resin can be gathered year-round as needed. Gather the tips or new spring growth from inner and lower branches, keeping in mind that you are pruning the tree as you do this. Gently remove resin from the bark with a knife and scrape it into a jar for use in tincture or oil.

You may want to wear long sleeves and gloves when harvesting, as spruce needles are quite sharp.

Medicinal Uses

The bark, needles, resin, and young tips of spruce are antimicrobial, diuretic, expectorant, pain-relieving, and wound-healing.

To alleviate stiff arthritic joints, brew a big batch of the needle infusion to add to a hot bath—save some to sip as well. Stay in for 15–20 minutes then follow the bath with a spruce-infused oil massage. The warming, circulatory-stimulating effects of spruce melt away tension and repair wear and tear on muscles and joints.

Like its pine relatives, spruce oozes resin or pitch to seal its wounds. Following its example, we can use spruce resin to seal and heal our wounds, too. Use the resin directly on wounds to draw out infectious material, stimulate blood flow, and speed the healing

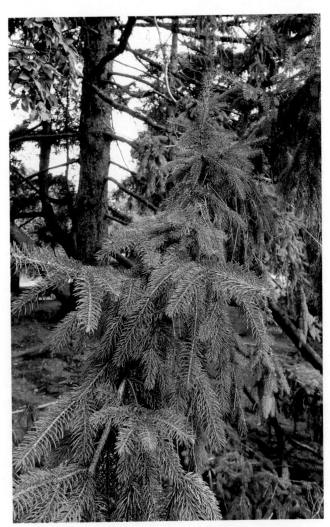

Single needles attach to the branch on little pegs called pulvini.

process. It can also be infused in oil and crafted into a salve.

High in vitamin C and with aromatic expectorating qualities, spruce infusion or tincture hastens recovery from respiratory ailments; the inner bark, needles, cones, and tips were traditionally used to treat tuberculosis and prevent scurvy. Drink an infusion of the young tips, needles, or cones to relieve mucousy coughs. A steam inhalation of the needles is another way to experience the congestion-relieving benefits of spruce.

Add spruce tips to a tincture with birch twigs, hawthorn berries, spicebush fruit, and chamomile flowers to use as a digestive aid before or after meals.

Future Harvests

When gathering young tips from spruce, gather only one or two from each branch and focus on the inner and lower branches.

While wildcrafting mindfully from spruce will not put the tree at risk, it's useful to know which species are plentiful and which are not. Favor harvests from introduced Norway spruce and tread lightly on native species. Black spruce is imperiled in Rhode Island, and red spruce is critically imperiled in New Jersey and vulnerable in Connecticut and Ontario.

HERBAL PREPARATIONS

Tea
Standard or cold infusion of fresh or dried needles and/or tips
Drink 4 ounces as needed. Makes a great bath tea, steam inhalation, or wash for wounds.

Tincture
1 part fresh needles, resin, and/or tips
2 parts menstruum (95% alcohol, 5% water)
Take 10–20 drops as needed.

Infused oil
1 part fresh needles, resin, and/or twigs
2 parts oil
Use for massage or add to a wound-healing salve.

stinging nettle

Urtica dioica

American stinging nettle (*U. dioica* ssp. *gracilis*), European stinging nettle (*U. dioica* ssp. *dioica*)

PARTS USED leaves, roots, seeds

Stinging nettle is a foundational herb that deserves a place in every apothecary. It is deeply nourishing and restorative to the entire body, especially the kidneys.

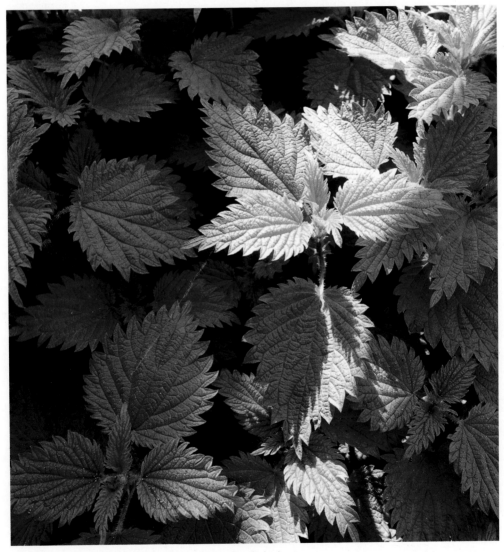

Look for stinging nettle in full shade or the sun-dappled edge.

How to Identify

Stinging nettle is an herbaceous perennial with square angular stems and opposite triangular toothed leaves. Veins appear sunken on the top of the leaf but protrude on its underside. The whole plant is covered in little stingers or prickly hairs filled with a mixture of compounds, including formic acid. There is one native and one introduced subspecies prevalent in the Northeast. If you're interested in distinguishing between them, the American subspecies has fewer stinging hairs on the stem than its European counterpart.

In late spring through summer—about late May to September—it goes into flower and by late summer to fall has gone to seed. The inflorescence emerges from the axils, a branched cluster of tiny light green flowers. Female flowers have an overall fuzzier appearance than the rounder male flowers. Sometimes a plant will have both male and female flowers (monoecious) but usually the plant is dioecious (has one or the other), hence the species name *dioica*, meaning "two houses." It's the fertilized female flowers you'll want to dry for the seeds.

The plant grows 3–4 feet high, sometimes higher, by summertime. Roots are tan to bright yellow rhizomes with long, thin stolons or runners.

A variety of native butterflies and moths, like the red admiral butterfly (*Vanessa atalanta*), depend upon stinging nettle.

Where, When, and How to Wildcraft

Stinging nettle is found in a variety of habitats—moist valleys, lake and riversides, at the edges of forests, and in areas disrupted by human activity. In general, stinging nettle likes moisture- and nutrient-rich soil and is likely to be in the shade or sun-dappled edge.

Harvesting stinging nettle is a good practice in mindfulness. First, put on gloves to avoid being stung, and long sleeves if you want extra protection. In spring just as the plants emerge, collect the top 4–6 inches of the tender leaves and stems, just above the leaf node, with clippers or scissors. It's likely you'll get stung despite precautionary measures, but that's part of the fun.

In late summer to fall, if the plants have been previously trimmed, there will be a second flush of young leaves to harvest. Use these tender leaves in broths, infusion, tincture, vinegar, or culinary preparations. Cooking the leaves removes the sting. I like to quickly blanch a whole batch, shock it in an ice bath, and freeze it for use in pesto and soup. I also dry a batch for later use in infusions and tea blends.

When the plant is in seed, cut the stalks from the top third of the plant, seeds and all. Keep those gloves handy! Strip the fresh seeds to tincture or dry the stalks in bundles with bags tied around them to catch anything that falls. After the seeds dry, strip them off the stalk. Gloves are still useful at this stage—while the sting has reduced considerably the dried hairs still pose an itch factor. The remainder of the dried plant material is a great addition to compost.

Dig roots when the plants die back in fall. Again, remember your gloves. Tincture or dry the roots.

Medicinal Uses

As a nourishing tonic drunk as an infusion daily (or so), stinging nettle leaf is restorative to pretty much all systems of the body. Am I calling it a panacea? Not quite. It's more like a tune-up for the body.

Stinging nettle leaf builds the blood with plentiful chlorophyll—the plant's version of heme, a component of hemoglobin. Make a syrup with other blood-enriching herbs, such as blackberry fruit and leaf, yellow dock root, and rosehips to take daily to recover from or prevent mild iron-deficient anemia.

It's full of nutrients, including vitamins A and C, iron, potassium, manganese, calcium, and trace minerals. It's incredibly protein-rich and makes a nice addition to soups. Blend with field garlic, garlic mustard, basil, olive oil, and toasted pumpkin or sunflower seeds for a delicious pesto. Infuse stinging nettle in vinegar to extract the minerals and take a spoonful a day as a dietary supplement.

Antihistaminic and anti-inflammatory, stinging nettle supports the immune system to lessen reactions to allergens. Start drinking a daily infusion about 1 month before allergy season for best results.

Stinging nettle strengthens hair, skin, and bones. Combine it in an infusion with other bone-building herbs like horsetail, elder leaves and stems, red clover, and raspberry leaf. The infusion makes a great rinse for the hair or a wash to balance skin pH.

Use stinging nettle with dandelion leaf to improve kidney function, reduce edema, and relieve gout—the herbs act as a diuretic that not only won't deplete minerals, but will supply them. Some herbalists use the seed tincture to restore function to the kidneys in cases of glomerulonephritis and as a protective to reduce kidney dysfunction from nephrotoxic medications. The seeds are also considered adaptogenic and are used specifically for adrenal exhaustion. They can be added to smoothies, salads, and soups.

Stinging nettle is great for expecting or new moms, providing daily nourishment and improving breastmilk production. Children usually like the taste of the tea and incorporating it into their diets is a good way to boost health.

Some folks with arthritis or rheumatism purposefully sting themselves with the nettles in a process called urtification.

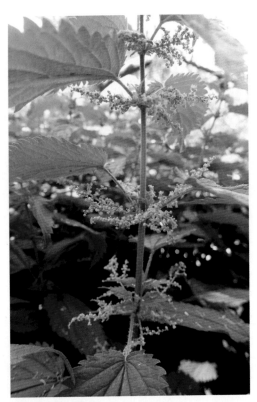

Stinging nettle flowers from late spring through summer.

This stimulates blood flow to the affected area, promotes a temporary inflammatory response, and when the swelling abates, the pain and swelling of the original condition are also reduced.

A tincture of the root is useful for alleviating swelling that makes urination difficult in cases of benign prostatic hyperplasia. The root increases vitality and is used in combination with other restorative tonic herbs to remedy erectile dysfunction and increase virility.

⚠ Precautions

Stinging nettle can be too drying for some folks. Add moistening herbs such as evening primrose, Solomon's seal, and mallow to prevent this drying effect.

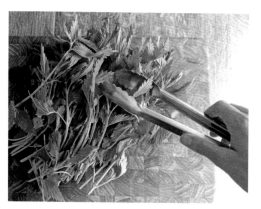

If you want to avoid the sting, handle fresh stinging nettle with tongs or gloves. I've come to like the sting for its unique medicine, a reminder of the plant's potency and energy.

The seeds may be too stimulating, even keeping some people up all night. Using the dried seeds and taking them early in the day could resolve this issue.

If you get stung by the hairs, follow this old adage: "nettle in, dock out." Use a fresh poultice of crushed dock (*Rumex* spp.) leaf to relieve the sting. These two plants often grow near each other, which is rather convenient. If you can't find dock, plantain will do. If you can't find either, bathing the affected part in cold water helps. Even without intervention, most people find that the prickly feeling abates within a few minutes to an hour.

Future Harvests

You don't have to worry about stinging nettle, it will persist. Just be sure to leave enough behind for the butterflies and moths who depend on it.

HERBAL PREPARATIONS

Tea
Standard decoction or long infusion (overnight) of dried leaves
Drink 1 cup 3 times per day.

Leaf tincture
1 part fresh leaves
2 parts menstruum (60% alcohol, 40% water)
or
1 part dried leaves
2 parts menstruum (50% alcohol, 50% water)
Take 15–30 drops 3 times per day.

Root tincture
1 part fresh roots
2 parts menstruum (50% alcohol, 50% water)
or
1 part dried roots
2 parts menstruum (50% alcohol, 50% water)
Take 40–60 drops 3 times per day.

Seed tincture
1 part fresh seeds
2 parts menstruum (75% alcohol, 25% water)
or
1 part dried seeds
2 parts menstruum (60% alcohol, 40% water)
Take 30–40 drops 4 times per day.

Infused vinegar
1 part fresh leaves
2 parts apple cider vinegar
or
1 part dried nettles
4 parts apple cider vinegar
Take 1–2 tablespoons daily. Makes a great salad dressing.

sumac

Rhus species

staghorn sumac (*R. typhina*), smooth sumac (*R. glabra*), winged or shining sumac (*R. copallinum*), fragrant sumac (*R. aromatica*)

PARTS USED bark, fruit, leaves

Tart, astringent sumac stanches bleeding, tightens tissues, and has a strengthening effect on the urinary tract. On a hot summer's day, sumac-ade (cold-infused sumac tea) makes a delicious, thirst-quenching lemonade substitute.

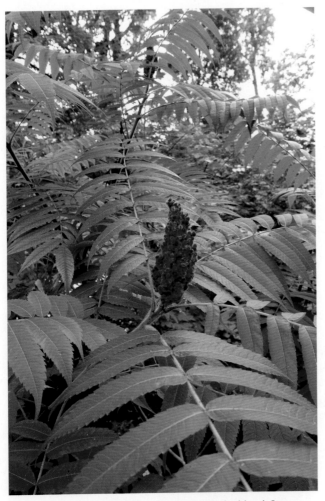

Bright red fruit of sumac indicates a link with the blood. Sumac halts internal bleeding and reduces hypertension and blood sugar spikes in those with type 2 diabetes.

How to Identify

Sumac is a deciduous shrub in the cashew family. Its compound leaves grow in a spiral pattern up the stem. In the four featured species, the leaves are pinnately compound with seven to thirty-one lanceolate to elliptical toothed leaflets. Winged sumac has wings between each pair of leaflets. Staghorn sumac features fuzzy stems—green when young and brown with age—resembling the antlers of a stag.

Cone- or pyramid-shaped clusters of tiny yellow-green flowers with five-pointed petals bloom in summer, male and female on different plants. Male flowers have five yellow-tipped stamens tucked in the corners between the petals. Female flowers have a three-pointed yellow style at the center. Female flowers, once pollinated, develop into clusters of fuzzy bright to deep red berries (drupes) that are very tart.

These species of sumac can grow 20–30 feet tall. A host

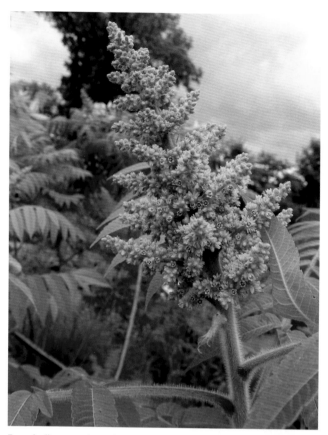

Female flowers of staghorn sumac in bloom, late spring. Once pollinated these will ripen into bright red, fuzzy berries (drupes) with a tart taste. In the Middle East, the berries are a key ingredient in za'atar, a delicious spice blend.

tincture or dry for later. Gather leaves just before or during the flowers' bloom. On a summer day collect a cone of the fruit when all the drupes are uniformly bright red. Touch a drupe to your tongue to check if it's sour. If so, proceed with the harvest.

Medicinal Uses

The bark, leaves, and fruit of sumac provide astringency to tone lax tissues and temper profuse discharges. Use an infusion or tincture of the bark, leaves, or fruit to halt excessive bleeding after childbirth and during menstruation and to reduce vaginal discharges. This can be applied externally as a wash to speed the drying effects. A wash is also useful for clearing up weeping sores or wounds on the skin.

Sumac has a strengthening effect on the kidneys and bladder, helping to resolve mild urinary incontinence and prevent bedwetting due to weakness in the urinary tract. It is toning to the intestines and drinking a sumac leaf, bark, or berry infusion can abate bouts of diarrhea.

Sumac leaf and bark infusion or tincture dries up a wet cough, soothes sore throat, and brings relief to mouth sores. Use the berry infusion or tincture diluted in water as a gargle for tonsillitis or a wash for bleeding gums or ulcers.

Sip a cold brew of sumac berries, rose, and sassafras to cool the blood, reduce excessive sweating, and cope with sweltering summer days.

of wild creatures depend on sumac for food and shelter, including bees, moths, butterflies, wild turkeys, mourning doves, rabbits, and deer.

Where, When, and How to Wildcraft

Sumac grows in the edges of roadways and waterways pretty much up, down, and across the entire continent. Winged sumac tends toward drier soil. Sumac is fairly abundant and, in some cases, considered weedy.

In spring find an abundant thicket and harvest a branch or two for the bark. Use the inner and outer bark together, fresh in

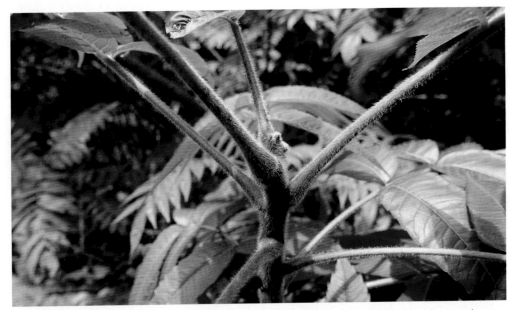

Sumac has a strong association with deer, the stems looking like their fuzzy antlers. Deer browse the leaves and the cover of the foliage protects their young.

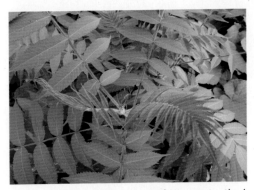

Compound leaves with seven to thirty-one toothed leaflets grow alternately in a spiraling fashion up the stem.

⚠ Precautions

Avoid sumac if you are allergic to cashews, pistachios, or mangoes.

Distinguish *Rhus* species from similar-looking poison sumac (*Toxicodendron vernix*) by its smooth stems and smooth-edged leaves.

Future Harvests

Most sumacs are in good conservation status in our area. The only exception is fragrant sumac, which is at risk in Connecticut and Vermont.

HERBAL PREPARATIONS

Tea
Cold infusion of fresh or dried berries
Strain well to avoid the scratchy hairs. Drink 4 ounces as needed. Makes a lovely cooling summer beverage with a touch of maple syrup or honey.

sunflower

Helianthus annuus

PARTS USED flowers, leaves, seeds

Native to the Americas and cultivated here for centuries, sunflower is prized around the world for its healthful oil, nutritious seeds, radiant flowers, and ability to cleanse toxic soil. The seeds and flower petals are useful for clearing dry, irritated cough.

How to Identify

Sunflower is an herbaceous annual plant growing 2–10 feet or more. Stemmed, coarsely toothed, ovate to cordate leaves with pointed tips grow alternately up a stiff, upright stem covered in small, bristly hairs. The flower grabs our attention with its large central disc and ray of golden to red petals. Wild sunflowers tend to have smaller inflorescences than cultivated varieties, around 3–6 inches in diameter. Composed of numerous small, tightly packed, tubular blooms forming a pattern of overlapping spirals, the flower disc beckons us to meditate on its geometry and symmetry.

Sunflower buds follow the sun in its arc across the sky.

Where, When, and How to Wildcraft

Look for sunflowers growing in old farm fields, meadows, roadsides, and disturbed habitats.

Collect petals from flowerheads in summer to dry for use in tea. I can't get enough of the subtly sweet scent of the dried petals. Harvest the whole flowerhead to make flower essence. In late summer to early fall, harvest the bowing flowerhead, keeping a few inches of stem as a handle. Hang to dry in a cool, dry place out of the sunlight. Use seeds fresh (in the soft shell) or dry for later. Keep seeds in the freezer to prolong shelf life.

The genus name *Helianthus* comes from the Greek words for "sun" (*helios*) and "flower" (*anthos*).

Medicinal Uses

Sunflower has been used as food and medicine for thousands of years in the Americas. Modern scientific studies have determined its antioxidant, anti-inflammatory, antimicrobial, antidiabetic, and anti-hypertensive virtues.

Its golden petals make a soothing infusion for dry, irritated lung conditions, such as bronchitis and whooping cough. The seeds can be used to the same effect, either eaten, brewed into a tea, or made into a syrup. Rich in vitamin E, the seeds are nutritive and moistening. Eat them raw, roasted, or sprouted for a heart-healthy snack.

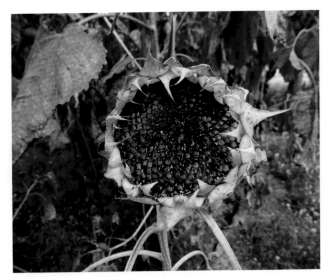

Sunflower seeds are fatty and moistening, a good source of vitamin E and fatty acids.

Sunflower petals make a lovely addition to skin care creations, and they can be infused in oil (*how about sunflower oil?*) to use in salves and lotions. Craft a salve with oils infused with sunflower petals, goldenrod, and dandelion blossoms to massage into the solar plexus to instill confidence and strengthen will. This blend also helps reduce pain and distention in the upper abdomen.

Like the sunflower traces the path of the sun, the flower essence helps us orient to the direction and energy of the sun. It infuses us with radiance, balances the solar plexus, and helps us relate to healthy solar (paternal, masculine, or authoritative) influences in our lives.

⚠ Precautions

Sunflower provides a great service by taking up heavy metals from the soil. Because they're such good accumulators, it's important to know the soil or the land-use history where you are harvesting.

Future Harvests

Sunflower is easily cultivated by seed. Leave plenty of seeds so the plant can self-seed for next year's harvest. And leave some behind for the birds, too.

HERBAL PREPARATIONS

Tea
Standard infusion of dried flower petals
Drink 4 ounces as needed.

Tincture
1 part fresh flower petals and seeds
2 parts menstruum (70% alcohol,
  30% water)
Take 20–30 drops as needed.

Syrup
Using the seeds, follow instructions for making herbal syrups on page 52.
Take 1 tablespoon 4 times per day.

Flower essence
Follow instructions for making flower essences on page 54. Take 3 drops on the tongue up to 4 times per day or as needed.

Melilotus species

white sweet clover (*M. alba*), tall yellow sweet clover (*M. altissimus*),
Indian sweet clover (*M. indicus*), yellow sweet clover (*M. officinalis*)

PARTS USED flowering tops

*Deliciously fragrant sweet clover used externally tones the skin, varicosities,
hemorrhoids, and connective tissue. When burned or used as a hydrosol,
its sweet scent shifts energy and soothes the spirit.*

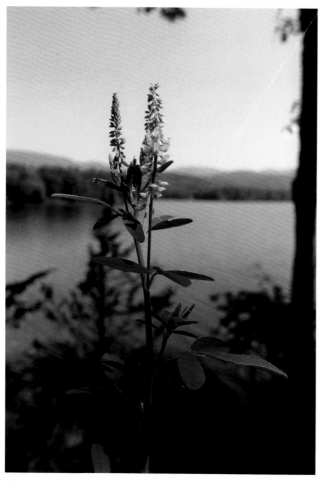

The genus name *Melilotus* is derived from the Greek words for
"honey," *meli*, and *lotus* (as in the flower). The scent of sweet
clover reveals the presence of coumarin, which is responsible for
its blood-thinning properties.

How to Identify

Sweet clover is a biennial or
perennial herbaceous plant in
the bean family. Tall and lanky
branching stems—about 3–5
feet high—are graced with
alternate compound leaves
composed of three finely
toothed leaflets. It's not called
sweet clover for nothing. From
late spring through fall, racemes
of strongly sweet-smelling,
small pea-like flowers of yellow
(*M. officinalis*) or white (*M. alba*)
bloom. The leaves give off the
same fragrance when crushed.
The aroma of the plant reminds
some folks of vanilla. To me
it smells a lot like sweetgrass
(*Hierochloe odorata*) and flowering cleavers, and all of these
plants contain blood-thinning
coumarins.

Sweet clover is a favorite
forage of honeybees.

Where, When, and
How to Wildcraft

Sweet clover is often found
in poor soils, at roadsides
and along paths, most often

in full sun. Sometimes you'll find it near waterways and in meadows. It was once popular as a cover crop for its soil-enriching, nitrogen-fixing powers, but it has become less common over the years.

Collect the top third of the plant when in bloom, through summer. Use fresh or dry completely for use in oils, salves, compresses, and poultices.

Medicinal Uses

Used externally, sweet clover is a versatile remedy for the skin, connective tissue, and lymph. Apply a poultice or fomentation, or add the infusion to a bath, to reduce swelling and congestion in the lymph and lessen dampness and aching in arthritic joints. Use a compress to relieve tension headache brought on by exposure to cold.

Infuse vinegar with sweet clover, grape leaf, plantain, and witch hazel twigs to apply to varicose or spider veins. These herbs powdered and added to cocoa butter or shea butter can be shaped into a suppository to shrink hemorrhoids.

Sweet clover, dandelion blossom, and violet leaf and flower infused in oil makes a stimulating massage oil to move stagnant lymphatics or to use in a Mayan abdominal massage to alleviate pelvic congestion and pain.

Sweet clover makes a beautiful hydrosol to use as a mood-lifting room spray or facial toner.

Dry sweet clover alone or with mugwort or cedar in a tightly tied bundle to burn for shifting the energy of a space.

⚠ Precautions

Use sweet clover fresh or fully dried. If the plant ferments or isn't fully dried, high concentrations of dicoumarol, a potent anti-coagulant, develop.

Sweet clover should not be taking internally by people taking blood-thinning medication or during pregnancy or breastfeeding.

Future Harvests

Sweet clover is a fairly prevalent farm escapee that can easily be propagated by seed. Harvest aplenty, just leave enough behind for the bees.

HERBAL PREPARATIONS

Tea
Standard infusion of dried flowering tops
Use as a bath tea, compress, poultice, or fomentation.

Infused vinegar
1 part fresh flowering tops
2 parts apple cider vinegar
or
1 part dried flowering tops
4 parts apple cider vinegar
Use as a liniment for varicosities.

Infused oil
1 part fresh flowering tops
2 parts oil
or
1 part fresh flowering tops
4 parts oil
Use as a lymphatic or pelvic massage oil.

Hydrosol
Follow instructions for making distilled floral water on page 300.

sweetfern

Comptonia peregrina
PARTS USED leaves

Sweetfern leaf applied externally alleviates inflammation from injury and rheumatism and relieves itchy, inflamed skin. Internally, it's used as a remedy for debilitated conditions and discharges.

How to Identify

Sweetfern is a deciduous shrub in the bayberry family. So, it's not actually a fern as the name suggests. The fern-like leaves inspired the common epithet—simple leaves (about 4 inches long) are waxy, green, narrow, and deeply notched in the margins. They emerge alternately from the reddish brown stem,

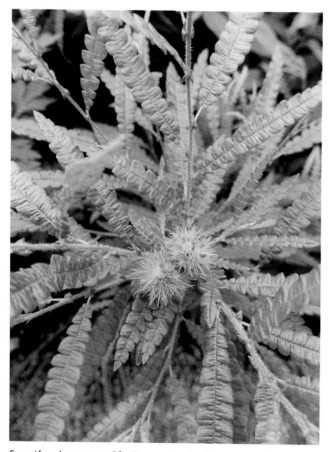

softly draped like feathers that give the shrub a shaggy appearance. Rub the leaves to release the pungent-sweet scent.

The flowers are male and female catkins, most often borne on the same plant (monoecious), emerging in spring. Male catkins are drooping cylinders, starting hairy and reddish brown and yielding to a pale yellow-green, eventually looking a bit like caterpillars. Female catkins are fairly inconspicuous and red, growing upright from the stem just beneath the male catkins on monoecious plants. Pollinated female flowers develop into a globular, pale green, bur-covered fruit, like a fuzzy ball, less than 1 inch in diameter. The shrub reaches 2–4 feet tall.

Sweetfern plays host to several butterflies and moths, including the gray hairstreak butterfly (*Strymon melinus*) and Io moth (*Automeris io*).

Sweetfern is so named for its sweet-spicy fragrance and fern-like leaves.

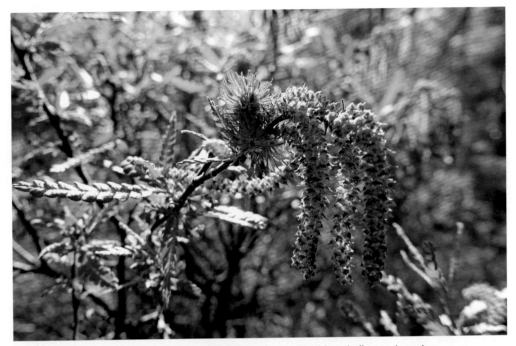

Drooping male catkins and fruit that developed from the fertilized female flowers in spring.

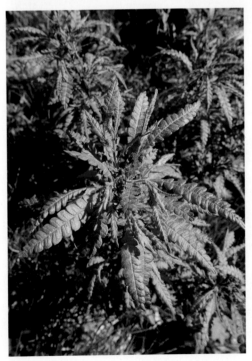

Alternate fern-like leaves have a spicy-sweet fragrance.

Where, When, and How to Wildcraft

Sweetfern is a pioneer that occupies barren sandy or gravelly soil. The roots of sweetfern house nitrogen-fixing bacteria, allowing the plant to grow in poor soil conditions. Look for it at the edges of meadows, forests, or coastal ranges in full sun to partial shade. Harvest mature leaves in midsummer to fall. Tincture or infuse in oil fresh or dry for later use.

Medicinal Uses

Partner with warming, astringent sweetfern for conditions of debility and wasting where there is leaking of fluids from the body. In other words, chronic diarrhea, leucorrhea, excessive sweating, and coughing up blood. Sweetfern improves assimilation of nutrients and bolsters the immune system, especially in those who are in a weakened state or who are convalescing. Combine sweetfern with Solomon's seal, burdock, and elderberry to build strength after illness.

Apply sweetfern externally as a fomentation or liniment to relieve swelling, bruising, and rheumatic conditions. Add yarrow and comfrey for added effect.

Infuse sweetfern in oil to apply to itchy, inflamed skin conditions. Pair with plantain in a salve to treat wounds and insect bites. Make a cold infusion of sweetfern to apply as a wash for poison ivy rash.

⚠ Precautions
If you find sweetfern too drying, adding moistening herbs like linden, mallow, or violet leaf may help.

Future Harvests
Carefully grazing the leaves from a healthy stand of sweetfern will not put the plant at risk. Check the leaves for butterfly or moth eggs or larva before harvesting.

HERBAL PREPARATIONS

Tea
Cold infusion, standard infusion, or standard decoction of fresh or dried leaves
Take 1–4 ounces up to 4 times per day. Use the cold infusion externally for itching or poison ivy rash.

Tincture
1 part fresh leaves
2 parts menstruum (50% alcohol, 50% water)
Take 10–15 drops as needed, up to 4 times per day. Use as a liniment for bruising and inflammation.

Infused oil
1 part fresh leaves
2 parts oil
Add to a salve for wound healing.

Acorus calamus

calamus

PARTS USED rhizomes

Sweet flag has been employed around the world as a rejuvenative tonic for the nervous and digestive systems. It promotes mental clarity, improves self-expression, and treats indigestion.

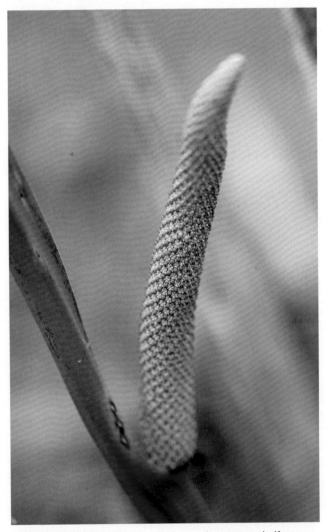

A semi-upright inflorescence called a spadix emerges halfway up the length of some leaves in colonies of sweet flag.

How to Identify

Sweet flag is a perennial herbaceous plant with long lanceolate leaves emerging from a fleshy rhizome that's strongly fragrant and brown on the outside and white on the inside. The plants can form dense colonies, spreading by rhizome in watery or muddy soil. Leaves are fragrant and often have an indentation up the length, and some have an upright to drooping, cylindrical inflorescence called a spadix that's 2–4 inches long. The spadix looks a bit like an ear of corn with a cross-hatch or diamond pattern of flowers. Tiny, six-tepaled, green-yellow flowers bloom on the spadix from late spring through summer.

Distinguish American sweet flag (*A. americanus*), also called several-veined sweet flag, by its many prominent veins on the leaf. The introduced species featured here (*A. calamus*) has a single-veined leaf. American sweet flag can also reproduce by seed, unlike the introduced species, which is sterile and reproduces only by rhizomes.

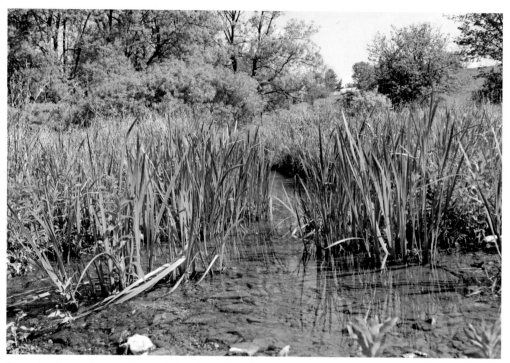

Sweet flag forms dense colonies at the edges of or directly in wetlands, spreading by rhizome.

Where, When, and How to Wildcraft

Sweet flag is a wetland grower, thriving in marshes, and the edges of ponds, lakes, and rivers. Harvest the rhizomes of plants that are 2–3 years old in early spring or fall before the first frost. They can be chewed fresh or dried; added to oil, tincture, infusion, or decoction; or candied. The flavor and aroma intensify as the roots dry.

Medicinal Uses

Sweet flag has a long history of use around the world, in Chinese medicine, Ayurveda, Native American herbalism, and the Western herbal tradition. Bitter, acrid, pungent, and aromatic, sweet flag stimulates digestion, normalizes appetite, and clears congestion from the sinuses and digestive tract. It improves symptoms of gastrointestinal imbalance, including gastric reflux, nausea, diarrhea, and dysentery. Chew a bit of the root (rhizome), about 1 teaspoon at a time, to quell motion sickness or nervous stomach.

Performers, teachers, and other people who use their voices for prolonged periods of time also benefit from chewing a bit of the root. In Ayurvedic medicine, it is known as "vacha" translated literally as "speaking" for its ability to encourage clear thinking, self-expression, and speech. It is traditionally prepared in ghee, oil, or milk decoction, or taken as a paste or powder.

In Chinese medicine, sweet flag is indicated for "wind" conditions of the nervous system, such as seizures, attention deficit, tremors, and forgetfulness.

Massage sweet flag-infused oil into arthritic joints to alleviate pain and inflammation.

Burn pieces of the dried root on charcoal to enjoy the grounding and focusing effects of sweet flag while studying or during meditation.

⚠ Precautions

Internal use of sweet flag is not recommended during pregnancy.

Large doses may be over-stimulating or induce nausea, vomiting, and mind-altering effects in the form of strange thoughts. Stick to the recommended doses to avoid these effects. In Ayurveda, gotu kola (*Centella asiatica*) is traditionally added to counter the stimulating properties of sweet flag.

The U.S. Food and Drug Administration has deemed sweet flag a carcinogen based on studies in mice that isolated one compound, asarone. In the long history of use of this herb, literally thousands of years, there have been no reported cases of cancer in humans.

Future Harvests

American sweet flag is critically imperiled in Pennsylvania, New Jersey, and Newfoundland, and is vulnerable in Vermont. Choose the European species whenever possible and propagate the American species by seed or rhizome in a rain garden to help prevent its eradication.

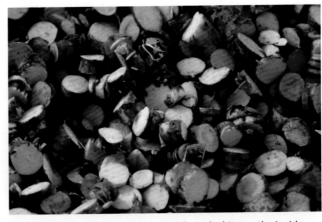

Fleshy rhizomes, brown on the outside and white on the inside, sliced and ready for drying.

HERBAL PREPARATIONS

Tea

Standard decoction or long cold infusion (overnight) of dried roots
Drink 2–4 ounces as needed.

Infused milk

Milk decoction of roots
Choose 1 cup of your favorite milk to infuse with 1 tablespoon of dried root. Simmer for 15 minutes on low heat. Add a spot of honey if desired. Drink 2–4 ounces as needed.

Tincture

1 part fresh rhizomes
2 parts menstruum (75% alcohol, 25% water)
or
1 part dried rhizomes
5 parts menstruum (50% alcohol, 50% water)
Take 10–30 drops 3 times per day.

sweetgum

Liquidambar styraciflua
PARTS USED fruit, leaves, resin, twigs

Found in the southern range of the Northeast, sweetgum resin, twigs, and fruit are antiviral, antispasmodic, and carminative. They're often recognized by the spiky seedballs that persist on the branches and ground through winter.

How to Identify

Sweetgum is a deciduous tree native to North America that commonly grows 50–70 feet tall. Some specimens have been found that were over 100 feet in height. The habit ranges from conical to spreading. Bark is deeply ridged and dark gray. Twigs and branches often have platy, winged protuberances of bark. Simple, palmate, toothed, star-shaped leaves are shiny green through summer, turning deep red to purple in fall. Male flowers, yellow-green with a red tinge, bloom on upright conical racemes in spring. Globular female flowers hang down below the leaves and, once pollinated, develop into spiky green fruit or seedballs. In fall, these spiky seedballs turn brown and either fall to the ground or remain on the tree, like ornaments. This is one tree you might happen upon by accidentally stepping on these spiky balls barefoot.

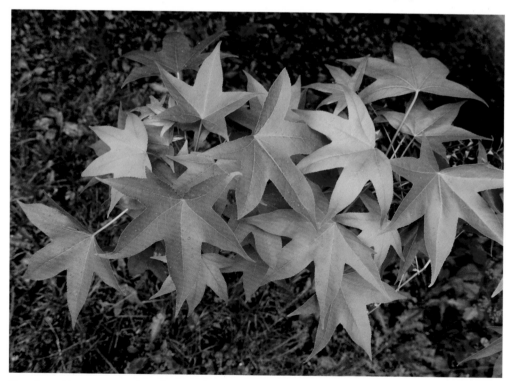

Star-shaped leaves are a unique feature of sweetgum.

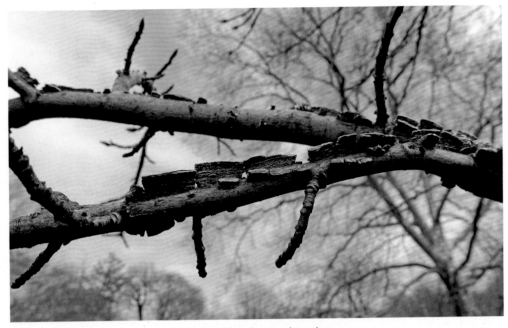

The platy, winged protuberances of bark that often form on branches.

Aromatic sticky resin or "sweet gum," also known as storax, exudes from wounds in the bark. The genus name *Liquidambar* comes from Latin for liquid (*liquidus*) and amber (*ambar*) describing the tree's fragrant resin. The species name *styraciflua* means "flowing with resin." Another species of *Liquidambar* native to the eastern Mediterranean called Turkish sweetgum (*L. orientalis*) has similar properties but it is rarely planted as an ornamental or street tree.

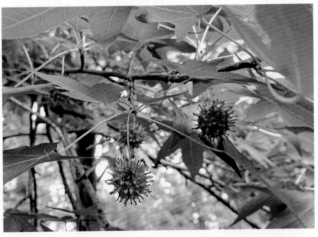

Collect the spiky fruit while it is still green in summer. You'll often find them still fresh on the ground after a storm or windy day.

Where, When, and How to Wildcraft

Sweetgum is a tree of marshes, parks, and wetland edges in Eastern Pennsylvania, New Jersey, and Southern New York. It reaches its northern range with spotty distribution in Connecticut and Massachusetts.

Collect the green fruit in summer before it ripens. An easy way to harvest is to wait for a summer storm or windy day and then gather the fruit from the ground. Slice the fruit open before tincturing. Gather leaves in summer as well. Collect fallen twigs to add to the tincture you make with the fruit.

Look for wounds in the trunk of the tree for golden to red amber droplets of resin. Alternately, make a small notch in the tree, 2 inches or so across, on a late winter to early spring day. Come back a few days later to harvest the sticky yet firm resin. If it's too runny it's not ready. You should be able to easily pull it away with your fingers or the edge of a knife.

Medicinal Uses

The green fruit of sweetgum resembles the influenza virus under a microscope and, interestingly enough, sweetgum is used to treat the flu. The seeds contain shikimic acid, a derivative that serves as the basis for an antiviral pharmaceutical for influenza A and B. Use the tincture of the unripe seedballs to reduce the severity of cold and flu. Add elderberry syrup or tincture for more antiviral power. Chew a piece of the resin to relieve cough and sore throat. This warming, aromatic resin is also carminative, relieving gastrointestinal distress and diarrhea.

Infuse oil with the resin, twigs, and leaves to use on muscle spasms and stiff joints. Craft the infused oil into salve for wound care, with the optional addition of pine, sweetfern, and self-heal.

Dried, hardened resin can be burned as incense on charcoal to cleanse a space.

⚠ Precautions

Sweetgum is not recommended for use in pregnancy.

Future Harvests

Collecting fruit, leaves, and twigs from mature trees will not put sweetgum at risk. Harvest resin in small amounts from individual trees. Overharvesting through cuts in the bark compromises the health of the tree.

Sweetgum is considered vulnerable in Connecticut.

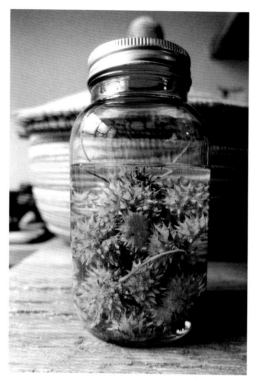

Slice the fruit in half before tincturing. Seeds contain shikimic acid, a precursor to pharmaceutical medications for influenza virus.

HERBAL PREPARATIONS

Tea
Standard decoction of fresh or dried twigs
Drink 4–8 ounces as needed.

Tincture
1 part fresh fruit, resin, and/or twigs
2 parts menstruum (95% alcohol,
   5% water)
Take 10–20 drops 4 times per day.

Infused oil
1 part fresh leaves, resin, and/or twigs
2 parts oil
Gently warm the oil to incorporate the resin then add the twigs and leaves. Steep for 2 weeks then strain. Massage into aching muscles and joints or apply to sores and wounds.

Dipsacus fullonum (syn. *D. sylvestris*)

Fuller's teasel

PARTS USED flowers, roots

Teasel root drives out toxicity in the body through the liver and kidneys. It relieves injury to connective tissue and, in some cases, is useful as a Lyme disease treatment.

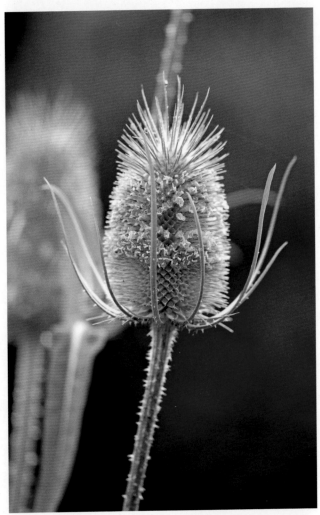

The concentric rings of flowers surrounding teasel's flowerhead are a signature for the bullseye rash some people experience after a tick bite carrying *Borrelia burgdorferi*.

How to Identify

Teasel is an introduced herbaceous biennial with a thin, tan-brown taproot. First-year plants appear as a basal rosette of oblong, lanceolate, light green leaves with prickly margins. In the second year, the stem emerges ranging from light green to green tinged with red and lined with flat ridges and random white prickles. Opposite lance-shaped leaves appear every few inches up the stem in pairs, each with prickles lining the underside of the midrib. Upper leaves clasp the stem. The genus name *Dipsacus* is derived from Greek for "thirsty" (*dipsan*), referring to the perfoliate leaves that collect water like a cup.

At the top of this stiff stem sits a prickly oblong flower spike up to 4 inches long and 1½ inches across. Tiny tubular pink to purple flowers ring this spiky inflorescence, blooming first in the center, then separating into rings at the top and bottom. Curving up from beneath the inflorescence are

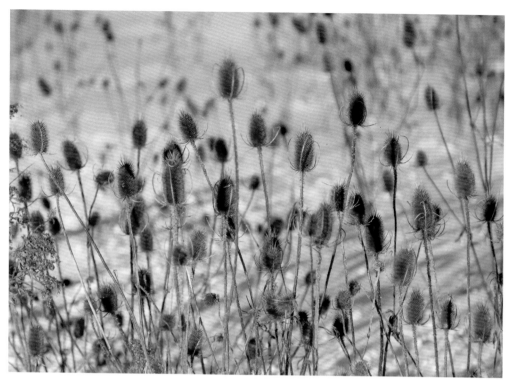
The spiky flowerheads, looking like hedgehogs, persist through winter.

several long thin prickly bracts. In winter, the flower spike looks like a dark brown hedgehog or a pin cushion covered with way too many pins.

Teasel can grow up to 6 feet tall, a slender lanky thing that stands out in the middle of a field.

Where, When, and How to Wildcraft
Look for teasel growing in full sun in disturbed habitats, in the middle of old farm fields, and in meadows. It's frequently seen growing along roadsides, too.

Collect flowers in midsummer for crafting a flower essence.

Wearing gloves and armed with a garden or hand fork, dig the roots in fall, before frost. Tincture or infuse in oil fresh. Dry roots in a warm, dry place or on a very low setting in a dehydrator.

Medicinal Uses
Teasel root is liver cleansing, kidney strengthening, and blood purifying. It works similarly to thistle, burdock, and dandelion roots to detoxify the body. Through these actions, it's able to drive out dampness in the body, which manifests as stiff aching joints and mental fog. These symptoms are also characteristic of Lyme disease. The flowers blooming in rings around the inflorescence are reminiscent of the bullseye rash that appears on some people with Lyme disease. Used alongside or following a prescribed antibiotic protocol, teasel has been known to heal some cases of Lyme. Doses are small, 1–10 drops 3 times per day, for 6 weeks.

The stem-clasping leaves are akin to connective tissue clasping muscle and bone and teasel is known for its ability to repair damaged tendons, ligaments, and muscles.

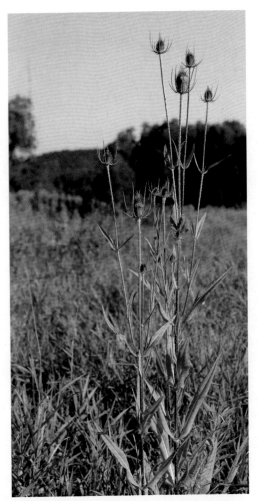

Stiff, tall, lanky teasel stands out in the middle of a field.

Take the tea or tincture internally and apply a poultice, oil, or liniment of the root tincture to the affected area to speed healing of injury to soft and connective tissue.

Teasel flower essence helps one maintain balanced energy especially through emotionally draining situations such as long-term illness.

Future Harvests

No need to worry about the future of this introduced plant that easily spreads by seed.

HERBAL PREPARATIONS

Tea
Standard decoction of dried roots
Drink 4 ounces up to 3 times per day.

Tincture
1 part fresh roots
2 parts menstruum (70% alcohol, 30% water)
Take 1–10 drops 3 times per day. Start with smaller doses and increase as needed. Use as a liniment for stiff joints.

Infused oil
1 part fresh roots
2 parts oil
Massage into aching muscles and joints.

Flower essence
Follow instructions for making flower essences on page 54. Take 3 drops on the tongue up to 4 times per day or as needed.

Liriodendron tulipifera
tuliptree, yellow poplar
PARTS USED branch tips, flowers, inner bark, leaves, twigs

Warming, bitter, and acrid, tulip poplar is helpful for relieving flu-like symptoms and restoring strength to the body after illness. It's also an appetite-stimulating digestive aid.

How to Identify

Despite its common name, tulip poplar is not related to poplar trees. Towering, majestic tulip poplar is a member of the magnolia family, native to eastern North America. Mature trees have thick, straight trunks with

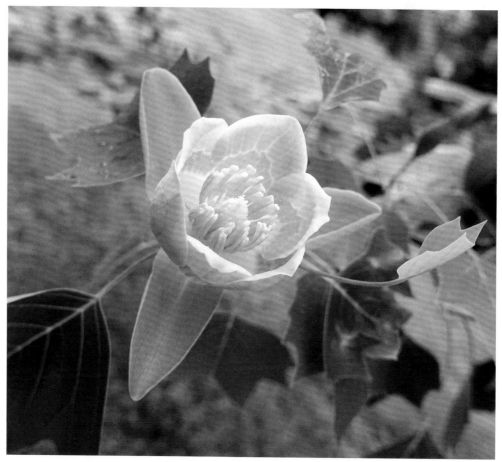

Flowers feature a flame-like orange band, a signature for its use in intermittent fever. The dried inner bark is also used as tinder for lighting fires.

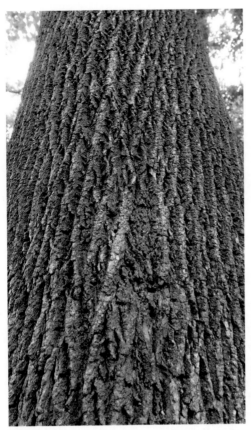

Thick straight trunks of tulip poplar were a staple material for canoe making.

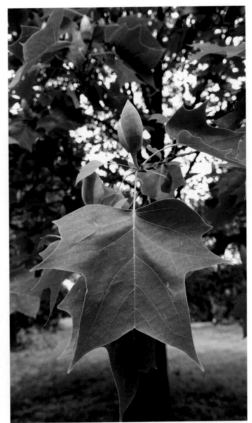

Leaves resemble the tulip flowers that are sewn onto Pennsylvania Dutch quilts.

furrowed gray-brown outer bark and fragrant yellow inner bark. Depending on age and conditions, a mature tree can be in the 60- to 90-foot range or reach as high as 150–200 feet. Older trees often lack low branches.

Vibrant green, smooth-margined leaves have six pointed lobes. In spring, blooming upright from the branch tips are six-petaled, three-sepaled, pale yellow-green flowers with an orange flame-like strip at the center. Flowers are perfect (having male and female parts) and cup-shaped like a tulip. The fruit is a slender tan-brown cone made up of several overlapping samaras. Looking up into the tree in winter, the dried brown fruit stand open and upright like little crowns.

Where, When, and How to Wildcraft

Deep, rich, moist soils in full to partial sun are home to tulip poplar. Find mature trees towering in or at the edge of forests; saplings emerge in dappled sun in clearings of the understory. Tulip poplar is an attractive shade tree planted in parks and gardens. In the Northeast, tulip poplar reaches as far north as Massachusetts and New York, creeping a bit into Vermont and northwest into Ontario.

Gather fallen twigs and branches in late winter to spring. Infuse twigs in oil or tincture and peel away the outer bark to reveal the fragrant inner yellow bark to tincture or dry for later use. If you happen upon lower-growing branches, collect just-opened blossoms for tea, tincture, or flower essence in mid to late spring. Prune branch tips and pluck newly emerged leaves for tincture or tea at this time as well.

Medicinal Uses

Traditionally used as a remedy for malaria, cholera, and intermittent fever, tulip poplar is suited for conditions leaving you feverish and achy, clammy with chills, and extremely worn down. All parts are strengthening and warming after debility or illness, even more so when combined with nutritive herbs like burdock root, sweetfern, and Solomon's seal. It has also been used for expelling intestinal parasites and would work well with black walnut hull tincture for this purpose.

The pungent bitterness and appetite-stimulating quality of tulip poplar lends itself well to a pre- or post-meal elixir to get the digestive juices flowing. Try it blended with other aromatic bitter herbs such as black walnut hulls, spicebush, sassafras, chicory root, lemon balm, and sweet flag and infused in mezcal or brandy and honey.

Tulip poplar is toning to the heart and vasculature and calming to the nervous system. It brings strength where there is tension due to weakness. Drink a tea with linden, hawthorn, and anise hyssop to fortify the physical and energetic heart and soothe nervous tension.

Use an infused oil for abdominal massage to bring warmth and relaxation to tension held in the uterus.

With an affinity to the sacral, solar plexus, and heart chakras, the flower essence helps us protect our inner fire and safely express our deepest selves in creative pursuits.

Future Harvests

The most sustainable way to wildcraft tulip poplar is to collect freshly fallen branches, twigs, leaves, and flowers. Pruning branch tips, leaves, and flowers from low branches is also not damaging to the tree. Check leaves for tiny butterfly eggs before harvesting—tulip poplar is a host to tiger swallowtail butterflies (*Papilio glaucus*).

Propagate trees by branch cuttings or seed to ensure future harvests.

Tulip poplar is critically imperiled in Vermont.

HERBAL PREPARATIONS

Tea
Standard infusion of dried branch tips, inner bark, and/or twigs
Drink 2–4 ounces 3 times per day or as needed.

Tincture
1 part fresh branch tips, flowers, inner bark, leaves, and/or twigs
2 parts menstruum (95% alcohol, 5% water)
Take 20–30 drops 3 times per day or as needed.

Infused oil
1 part fresh branch tips, inner bark, leaves, and/or twigs
2 parts oil
Use for massage.

Flower essence
Follow instructions for making flower essences on page 54. Take 3 drops on the tongue up to 4 times per day or as needed.

Valeriana officinalis

PARTS USED flowering tops, leaves, roots

This introduced garden escapee, weedy in some places, serves as a calming remedy for nervous exhaustion and tension.

How to Identify

Valerian is an herbaceous perennial in the honeysuckle family introduced from Eurasia. It starts in spring as a basal rosette with odd-pinnate compound leaves with five to fifteen toothed, lanceolate leaflets. At its apex, it reaches 3–5 feet tall. Feathery compound leaves—like the basal ones—grace the ridged, hollow stem in opposite pairs like wings. Tracing up the stem, you'll notice the sparse pairs of leaves get smaller as you reach the top. Tiny, fragrant, white to pale pink,

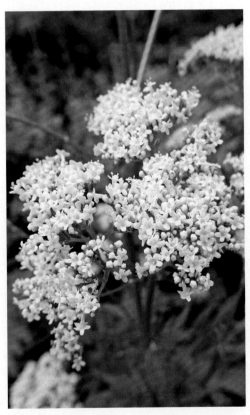

Cats are enticed by the strong smell of valerian. Stuff their toys with a bit of valerian and catnip and watch them go wild. This combo would also work well in a dream pillow or sachet for humans.

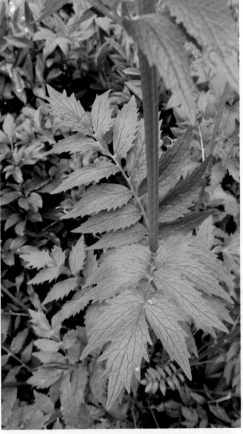

The name "valerian" likely derives from the Latin herb *valere* meaning "to rule, to be strong."

tubular flowers bloom in branched panicles at the top of the plant in late spring through summer. Long tan fibrous roots grow from the small rhizome.

All parts of the plant are aromatic, with the strongest scent award going to the roots. Some folks like the smell, others can't stand it. It certainly fits the description of pungent, as in ripe or perhaps a tad bit stinky. The scent concentrates as it dries so if it isn't hitting you fresh, just wait.

Distinguish introduced valerian from endangered native mountain valerian (*V. uliginosa*), which has a smaller inflorescence and smaller leaves and grows in wetter habitats, primarily in eastern white cedar (*Thuja occidentalis*) swamps.

Where, When, and How to Wildcraft

In its native Eurasia, valerian is most prevalent in damp grasslands. Here in the Northeast it seems less particular, choosing moist to dry soil in roadsides, vacant lots, and other human-disturbed habitats; coastal areas; open fields; and edges of forests.

Collect the flowering tops in late spring to early summer to infuse in tincture or craft in an elixir. Harvesting the flowering tops also promotes root growth. They can be dried for later use in tea. Gather the leaves in spring and summer for tea or tincture.

The root is the most potent part of the plant and is best tinctured fresh after harvesting in the fall, though the dried root has plenty of medicine, too. Harvest from plants that are 2–3 years old. Gently clean the fresh roots with a soft toothbrush to remove soil. Chop them up to dry or infuse fresh in alcohol, honey, or vegetable glycerin.

Medicinal Uses

With hypnotic, antispasmodic, nervine powers, valerian root is a beloved sleep aid

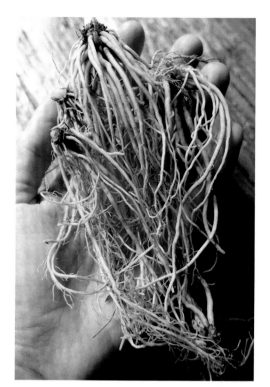

Fresh valerian root consists of a tangle of tan rootlets emerging from a small rhizome.

that relaxes nervous tension, for some. In a small percentage of people, this warming root promotes agitation and excitation. For those folks or people who tend to have hotter constitutions, the flower tea or tincture may be a gentler choice.

Wild lettuce, rose, lemon balm, hops, and passionflower are all nice additions to valerian root in sleep tincture blends. This blend may stimulate vivid dreams, so proceed with caution if that isn't your thing.

Quell a spasmodic cough and get some shut-eye with valerian, wild cherry, wild lettuce, and crampbark in tincture. Start with small doses of this mixture, about 10 drops, as it can be quite potent.

Use alone or pair with motherwort to ease hot flashes, menstrual cramps, and abdominal tension.

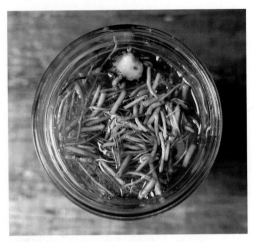

Taking honey infused with pungent valerian root is a sweet way to relieve spasmodic cough.

Prepare a liniment with valerian, Saint John's wort, and crampbark to alleviate muscle spasms and loosen stiff, cold creaky joints.

⚠ Precautions

Do not use valerian in pregnancy as it is used as an emmenagogue or uterine stimulant. Valerian should not be given to children under 3 years old.

Some herbalists say valerian is habit forming. For that reason, it may be prudent to cycle on and off every few weeks.

It's best to avoid using pharmaceutical sedative medications with valerian. And don't drive or operate heavy machinery after taking a dose of valerian as it may impair alertness.

For some folks, valerian has the opposite than desired effect, meaning it is stimulating and agitating. Take 1 drop of the tincture to feel its effects before continuing its use. Start with small doses and use only as much as you need to experience relaxation.

Future Harvests

Introduced valerian is considered a noxious weed in some parts of the Northeast. Gathering leaves and flowers will not put the plant's future at risk and harvesting the roots would be most welcomed by native plant lovers.

HERBAL PREPARATIONS

Tea
Standard decoction of dried roots
Drink 2–4 ounces as needed, up to 3 times per day. The root decoction, especially if from the dried root, may be an acquired taste.

Tincture
1 part fresh roots
2 parts menstruum (95% alcohol, 5% water)
or
1 part dried roots
5 parts menstruum (75% alcohol, 25% water)
Take 10–30 drops as needed. Use as a liniment for cold, stiff joints.

Infused honey
1 part fresh roots
2 parts honey
Take by the spoonful to relieve spasmodic cough.

Elixir
1 part fresh flowers
1 part honey
1 part spirit of choice
Follow instructions for making elixirs on page 51. Add a splash of the finished elixir to sparkling water to take the edge off after a stressful day.

Viola species

PARTS USED flowers, leaves

This down-to-earth plant is nourishing, moistening, and cooling to hot, dry conditions. It is mildly pain relieving and is traditionally employed as a poultice for heat-induced headache.

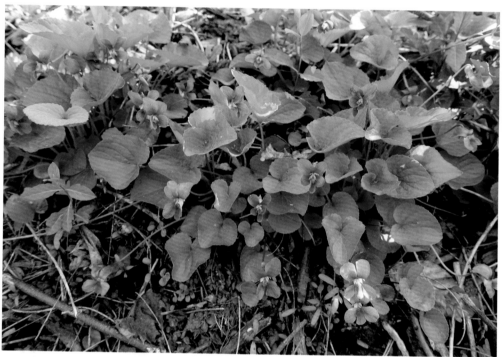

Of the many *Viola* species growing in the Northeast, *V. sororia* is the most widespread native species.

How to Identify

There are numerous species of violets worldwide with at least 30 (to possibly 50) growing in the Northeast. It's often difficult to distinguish individual species as they hybridize in the wild. The ones we are looking for generally fit the description outlined here.

The prominently veined, toothed leaves start tightly curled in, unfurl a bit to be just curled in at the base, and finally open up to reveal their heart shape. Leaves emerge from the root on individual leaf stalks in a rosette pattern. They form clumping colonies so parsing out individual plants takes getting down to the ground level.

Violets produce two kinds of flowers. The first type of flower is sterile but showy and blooms in spring. It's delicate and uniformly deep purple, or white or yellow with purple striations with five petals and five sepals. At the base of the flower where it meets the stem it nods a little. The second type of

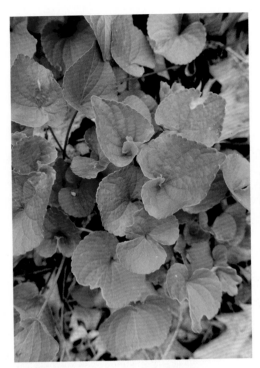

The leaves of violet unfurl at the base in a spiral pattern.

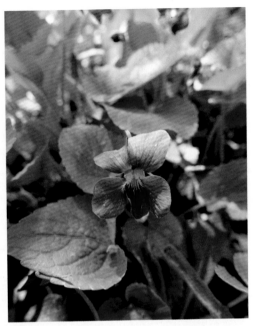

The delicate, sterile flowers of violet emerge in spring. Infused in honey with the leaves they make a soothing cough syrup. They're also pretty tossed into salads.

flower is an inconspicuous petal-less reproductive body that self-pollinates. It hides under the leaves so few people notice it. Once pollinated it develops into a little green seed capsule. Violet spreads by seed and by a creeping tan-colored rhizome.

Where, When, and How to Wildcraft

Violet happily and humbly exists in the cool dappled shade of forest edges and in partially shaded fields and lawns. Gather the leaves and flowers together in spring to infuse in honey, alcohol, vinegar, or oil. You can continue to gather leaves throughout summer to dry for tea.

Medicinal Uses

Violet is a nourishing, blood-purifying, tonic herb containing vitamins A and C, calcium, magnesium, bioflavonoids, and beta-carotenes. Eating violet leaves and flowers is a good way to benefit from this spring green. Another way to take in the goodness of violet is infused in vinegar, which extracts the minerals and makes a bone-building tonic, especially combined with red clover, stinging nettle, chickweed, and horsetail.

Cooling, moistening violet eases hot, dry conditions like constipation, dry coughs, and inflamed skin. Infuse the flowers and leaves in honey for a cough-calming syrup to enjoy by the spoonful. Take a tea of violet with burdock root and plantain for dry constipation. Use a tincture of the leaves and flowers or roots to relieve cough and reduce fever.

Violet is mildly pain relieving and with its cooling nature is useful as a leaf poultice for headache brought on by heat or anger. The infused oil can be used similarly.

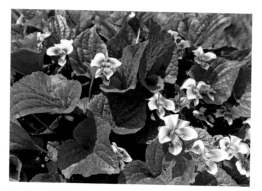
Violet appears in a variety of colors, from pure purple to pure white and somewhere in between.

Massage oil infused with violet, chickweed, and dandelion blossoms into swollen glands to move lymphatic fluids and into breast tissue to help resolve mastitis and dissolve cysts. Add a small amount of poke root–infused oil to this blend if things aren't moving along.

Violet flower essence is for highly sensitive types who have a hard time fully and authentically opening up in social or group situations.

Future Harvests

While native blue violet (*V. sororia*) is plentiful in the Northeast, several species are at risk, including hookedspur or dog violet (*V. adunca*), sand violet (*V. affinis*), northern coastal violet (*V. brittoniana*), and Canadian white violet (*V. canadensis*). Be sure you've identified the abundant species before harvesting.

HERBAL PREPARATIONS

Tea
Standard or cold infusion of dried leaves
Drink 4–8 ounces as needed.

Tincture
1 part fresh leaves and flowers
2 parts menstruum (50% alcohol, 50% water)
Take 10–30 drops as needed.

Infused honey
1 part fresh leaves and flowers, chopped
2 parts honey
Enjoy by the spoonful as a way to quiet dry, irritated coughs.

Infused vinegar
1 part fresh leaves and flowers, chopped
2 parts apple cider vinegar
Add to salad dressings or take a tablespoon in water with a splash of maple syrup for a cooling summer beverage.

Infused oil
1 part fresh leaves and flowers, chopped
2 parts oil
Use for massage, especially for the breasts and heart center.

Flower essence
Follow instructions for making flower essences on page 54. Take 3 drops on the tongue up to 4 times per day or as needed.

white horehound

Marrubium vulgare

PARTS USED flowering tops

Coughs of all kinds are calmed by bitter, antispasmodic, expectorant white horehound. This introduced plant also stimulates the appetite and encourages stagnant digestive processes.

How to Identify

Native to Eurasia and North Africa, white horehound is a perennial mint that grows in small clumping colonies, 12–18 inches in height. Wrinkly, soft, ragged leaves are borne in opposite pairs up the square stem. Tiny white flowers bloom in clusters in the axils just above the wings of leaves. The entire plant is covered in a soft white down. The taste of the leaves is markedly bitter, followed by a subtle minty-ness.

Where, When, and How to Wildcraft

White horehound is found in neglected areas, abandoned lots, and other human-disturbed terrain. Harvest the just-blooming flowering tops, about one-third of the way down from the top of the plant, in summer. Use fresh in tincture, syrup, or infusion, or dry for use in tea and electuary.

Medicinal Uses

Bitter white horehound is more palatable with a little sweetness and is traditionally made into candy or syrup. It thins mucus and eases spasms, reducing wheezing coughs from respiratory infections and asthma. An infusion with the addition of anise hyssop and licorice would benefit the respiratory system

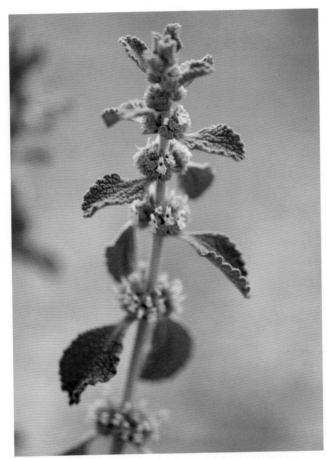

Little tufts of flowers emerge from the axils above the wrinkled, fuzzy leaves.

while improving the taste. Combine white horehound, mullein leaf, wild cherry bark, mallow root, and elderberry in a syrup to help resolve thick, wet coughs. These herbs can also be powdered and mixed with honey to make tasty electuaries.

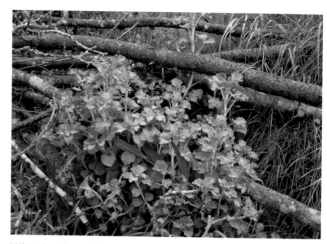

White horehound forms dense clustering colonies in human-disturbed areas.

The extreme bitterness of this herb points to its effectiveness in the digestive and nervous systems. It stimulates digestive juices to flow and encourages peristalsis by warming and stimulating the digestive tract. A few drops of white horehound tincture taken on the tongue restores the senses in case of shock and can help bring about focus when the mind is scattered.

 Precautions

The bitter taste of white horehound (*did I mention that it's bitter?*) is usually enough to keep people from taking too much. In high doses the herb is emetic and in prolonged courses it may affect heart rhythm, blood pressure, and blood sugar so those with arrhythmia, hypertension, and diabetes may want to stick to short courses, small doses, or choose a different herb altogether.

Avoid use of white horehound in pregnancy as it may be too stimulating to the uterus.

Future Harvests

Collecting the aerial portions of this plant will not be detrimental to future populations. Like other introduced mints, white horehound is doing just fine proliferating in areas that we humans disrupt or neglect.

HERBAL PREPARATIONS

Tea
Standard or cold infusion of dried flowering tops
Drink 2–4 ounces up to 3 times per day.

Tincture
1 part fresh flowering tops
2 parts menstruum (50% alcohol, 50% water)
or
1 part dried flowering tops
5 parts menstruum (50% alcohol, 50% water)
Take 10–15 drops 3 times per day.

Syrup
Follow instructions for making herbal syrups on page 52. Take 1 teaspoon as needed.

Electuary
2 parts dried flowering tops, powdered
1 part honey
Mix honey and powdered herb in a small bowl. Eat by the teaspoonful or refrigerate then roll the mixture into little balls. Coat with mallow root powder and store in the refrigerator or a cool, dry place.

white water lily

Nymphaea odorata
fragrant water lily
PARTS USED flowers, rhizomes

This native aquatic perennial is a balance of energies—simultaneously relaxing and strengthening, moistening and astringent, improving cold and damp conditions of the mucosa.

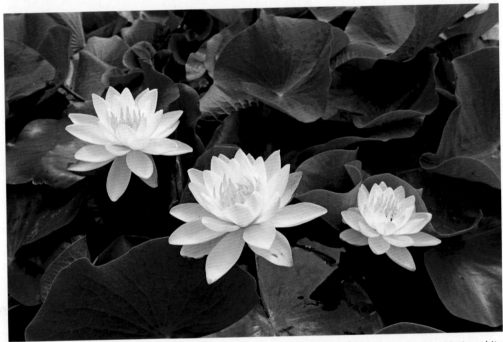

Water lilies are used as medicine around the world for their moistening and astringent powers. Native white water lilies have a long history of use in the Northeast, being employed for discharges, sores, and debility.

How to Identify

Floating in waterways throughout the Northeast, perennial white water lily is comprised of a creeping rhizome, long hollow stems, large round floating leaves, and many-petaled fragrant white flowers. The rhizome is fleshy and branching with long fibrous roots. Leaves are 4–12 inches in diameter, smooth-edged, and round with a triangular notch in one section, like a missing piece of pie. Sometimes the leaves float flat but when they are young and bunched together, they are curled in a bit and overlap each other. Veins radiate from the center where the stem is attached. Connecting the leaves to the rhizome is a long, hollow, red-green stem with four air chambers running up the length.

Flowers bloom throughout the summer, many-petaled and white with abundant, prominent stamens and a four-sepaled calyx.

Insects pollinate the flowers, bumbling around inside, bumping against the stamens and releasing pollen into the fragrant nectar at the center of the flower. Once pollinated, the flower curls up and is pulled down into the water by the tightening, coiling stem to develop into the fruit, which is a spongy green capsule that will eventually disperse the seeds into the water.

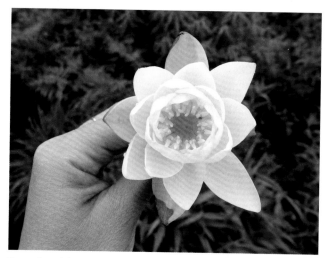

Bees dive right into the yellow centers of this bloom to gather pollen.

White water lily is an important source of food and shelter to insects, amphibians, reptiles, fish, and mammals. Muskrats and beavers eat the rhizomes. Dragonflies and damselflies rest on the leaves, fish rest under them. Several bird species consume the seeds.

Where, When, and How to Wildcraft

White water lily is at home in lakes and ponds, and calm rivers and streams throughout the Northeast.

Collect flowers when in bloom from late spring through mid- to late summer, depending on your locale.

Harvest the rhizome in late summer to fall before it gets too cold to get in the water. Get your waders on! And tie a bucket to your waist if you plan on harvesting more than one rhizome. Dig down with your feet to loosen the rhizomes from the mud. If it isn't deeper than a couple of feet you may be able to reach down and pull up the rhizome. Tugging on the stem might help, but it also might just break loose. If you have a shovel or long stick handy you might be able to pry it up and coax it to your hand. If you're feeling really adventurous you can wear a wetsuit and dive down (visibility might be an issue).

Clean off the roots and slice the rhizome. Air dry it in a warm dry place or in a dehydrator on a low setting. Infuse in tea or tincture.

Medicinal Uses

White water lily is a plant of balance and opposing forces, fertile darkness and light, with roots deeply submerged in muddy soil and flowers and leaves gently floating on the surface. It is simultaneously relaxing and strengthening. The rhizome is both moistening and astringent, balancing to cold and damp conditions of the mucosa.

It is traditionally used for tuberculosis, gonorrhea, mouth sores, and tooth pain. Taken internally and used as a douche, the infusion clears up leukorrhea. The infusion used externally as a wash and tincture taken internally together check discharges from wounds and infections. Take the tincture to resolve candida or thrush where there is a pale white coating on the tongue.

White water lily flower essence helps us feel our way through transformative processes with self-sufficiency and confidence. It deepens our intuition and enhances our

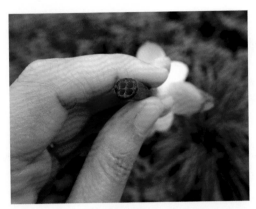

The stem is a four-chambered straw that acts as a sort of breathing tube for the mud-covered roots.

sensuality, allowing us to have a greater perception of and connection to the world within and around us.

Future Harvests

White water lily is considered pretty weedy in most places in the Northeast. Harvesting a couple of plants each year from abundant colonies should be just fine, so long as you leave plenty for all of the wild creatures who depend on this native aquatic plant.

wild bergamot

Monarda fistulosa
beebalm, sweet leaf
PARTS USED flowers, leaves, stems

Enjoyably spicy and aromatic, wild bergamot is a warming mint family plant that helps resolve acute respiratory infections, chronic yeast infections, and digestive upset. It's drawing and healing to insect bites, bee stings, and wounds, too.

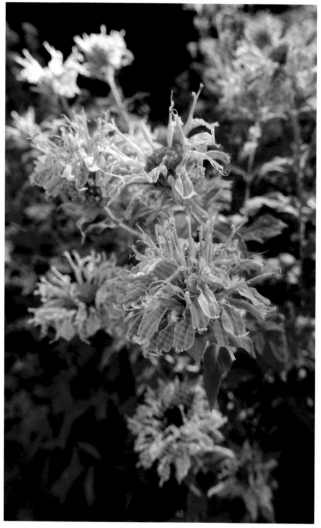

Wild bergamot is one of the most valuable and versatile medicine plants native to North America.

How to Identify

Lovingly dubbed "pizza plant" by some folks I know, wild bergamot is a mint family perennial that smells a lot like its relative oregano. It forms clumping colonies, with individuals reaching 2–4 feet tall. Leaves are toothed, ovate to broad-lanceolate, gray-green, and arranged oppositely on the square stem. Blooming at the top of the stem in summer sits a dense, round inflorescence with several tubular, two-lipped flowers ranging from lavender to red-lavender in color. Under the inflorescence is a whorl of leaf-like bracts ranging from green to lavender to reddish. Blooming begins at the center of the flowerhead, expanding outward as the season continues, ending with a ring of florets around the periphery, and giving the flower a sort of shaggy appearance.

As the common name beebalm suggests, bees are frequent visitors of the blooms, as are a variety of butterflies and moths.

There are three varieties of wild bergamot in the Northeast: *M. fistulosa* ssp. *fistulosa* var. *fistulosa*, *M. fistulosa* ssp. *fistulosa* var. *mollis*, and *M. fistulosa* ssp. *fistulosa* var. *rubra* (an escaped cultivar).

Where, When, and How to Wildcraft

Basking in full to partial sun in moist to slightly dry soil conditions, wild bergamot thrives in gardens, parks, fields, meadows, and by the wayside in disturbed habitats.

The time to harvest is in early to midsummer, just before or while the flowers are in peak bloom. Harvest before powdery mildew (noticeable as light gray spots on the leaves) is likely to set in later in the season. Gather the leaves separately before blooming, if you fancy, or gather the top third of the plant when flowering. The scent should be strongly oregano-like. Tincture fresh in alcohol or vegetable glycerin; infuse in vinegar, honey, or oil; or just hang the flowering tops upside down to dry out of sunlight. A bag tied loosely around the blooms will keep them from dropping too many florets or seeds on your floor. Use the leaves and flowers as a pungent, aromatic herb—akin to oregano—in the kitchen.

Medicinal Uses

Wild bergamot is an extremely handy herb to have on hand for its nerve-relaxing, antispasmodic, digestive-calming, antiviral, fever-reducing, drawing, and wound-healing medicine. It especially benefits conditions where the exterior of the body is cool and damp with deeper interior heat, for example fever with cold, clammy skin.

Like its mint family relatives oregano and thyme, wild bergamot is antimicrobial, antispasmodic, and carminative. It can be used in place of oil of oregano to prevent full-blown illness and remedy cold- and flu-related symptoms, including sore throat, cough, and congestion. Take the tincture in frequent doses throughout the day. Combine with elderberry and yarrow tinctures for added effect. Gargle with wild bergamot, echinacea, and/or prickly ash tincture diluted in water to soothe a raw sore throat. Wild bergamot–infused honey is a delicious way to relieve cough. Steam with wild bergamot, mint, spruce, and New England aster to clear congestion from the sinuses.

Drink a warm infusion or a few drops of the tincture in water to settle stomach upset, tame dyspepsia, resolve diarrhea, or relieve constipation.

Wild bergamot is used in small doses over days to treat chronic candida infections and gut dysbiosis. It has been used to treat cystitis and bladder infection, particularly where

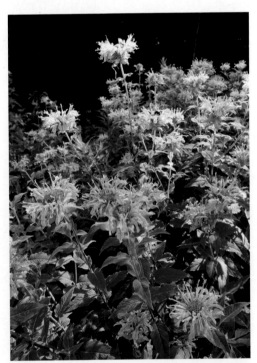

The frazzled look of the flowerheads is a signature for nervousness and anxiety. Wild bergamot is a nervine that calms and lifts the mood.

there is burning and inflammation, and it can be combined with barberry, goldenrod, or uva-ursi in these conditions.

Used as a spit poultice, wild bergamot draws out bee stings, insect bites, and alleviates poison ivy rash. Chewing the leaves and flowers also has a calming effect on the nerves, to take away the shock or anger of receiving the affliction. The spit poultice, cool compress, or infused vinegar draws out the heat of burns, including sunburns—refresh the cloth or poultice every 2–3 minutes to continue the cooling effect. Wild bergamot–infused oil or salve is healing to wounds and eases sore muscles. Craft a wound-healing salve with the addition of self-heal and plantain. The infused oil makes a lovely abdominal massage oil for stagnation in the uterus.

If you work with compost and can't stand the stink that pervades the sinuses, crush up a few wild bergamot leaves and sniff to neutralize the odor.

Future Harvests
M. fistulosa is a vulnerable species in Québec. Related spotted beebalm (*M. punctata*) is endangered in Vermont and Pennsylvania and scarlet beebalm (*M. didyma*), with its brilliant red blossoms, is vulnerable to exploitation in New York and imperiled in New Jersey.

⚠ Precautions
Strong preparations, such as infusions or tinctures, should be avoided during the first trimester of pregnancy due to the emmenagogic properties of wild bergamot.

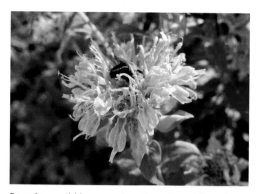

Bees love wild bergamot and a spit poultice of the leaves draws out their sting while calming the nerves.

HERBAL PREPARATIONS

Tea
Standard infusion of dried flowers, leaves, and stems
Drink 6–8 ounces as needed, up to 4 times per day.

Tincture
1 part fresh flowers, leaves, and stems
2 parts menstruum (50% alcohol, 50% water)
or
1 part dried flowers, leaves, and stems
5 parts menstruum (50% alcohol, 50% water)
Take 10–20 drops up to 5 times per day in acute infection. For digestive upset, take as needed.

Infused honey
1 part fresh flowers, leaves, and stems
2 parts honey
Enjoy by the spoonful or infuse in hot water for a deliciously sweet and spicy tea.

Infused oil
1 part fresh flowers, leaves, and stems
2 parts oil
Use for massage or add to salves for wounds.

Daucus carota

Queen Anne's lace

PARTS USED flowers, leaves, roots, seeds

Those lovely white-flowering plants we see along roadsides in summer are chock-full of medicine for the digestive, urinary, and reproductive systems.

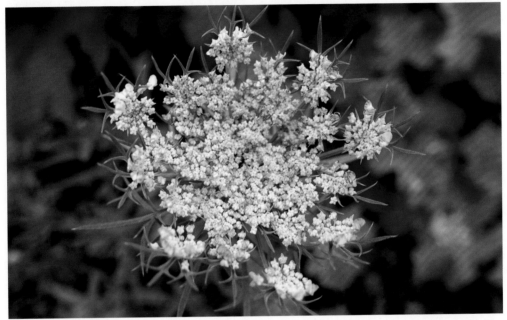

Wild carrot blossoms are white, sometimes tinged pink, and often have a dark red dot at the center of the inflorescence. Could there be a more obvious plant signature for the menstrual "period" than that?

How to Identify

This biennial herbaceous plant is the wild cousin to the domesticated carrot. In the first year of its lifecycle wild carrot appears as a rosette of lacy leaves with hairs on the underside. The second year, it blooms with flattish umbels of tiny white to white-pink florets. Sometimes you'll find a red to purple dot at the center of the inflorescence (sometimes not). Below the umbels are long, thin, curved, three-forked bracts like a collar surrounding the base of the blooms. The stems and leaf stalks of wild carrot are hairy, which distinguishes them from poisonous lookalikes.

Once the flowerhead develops into a seedhead, the whole umbel goes concave like a bird's nest of little oval-shaped, hairy seeds.

Picture the domestic carrot root you get from the farm stand or grocery store and then shrink it and fade the color to creamy yellow-white—that's your wild carrot. The root and the rest of the plant's parts have a distinctive carroty smell.

Where, When, and How to Wildcraft

Originally hailing from the Mediterranean, wild carrot is found throughout the entire Northeast in well-drained soil. It's pretty easy to spot by the roadside, along the edges of woods, in fields, meadows, and anywhere else that is mowed only a couple of times in the summer.

Wild carrot presents a two-year harvesting window, with roots and leaves being viable in the first year and flowers and seeds in the second.

Collect the leaves from spring through fall to use as a culinary seasoning, for tea, or to infuse in vinegar. Dig up the roots with a trowel or shovel from fall of the first year through early spring of the second. After this, they'll be too woody and lacking potency as they send their energy up to the flowering stalks. Tincture fresh or dry for infusions.

Blooming time is through the summer, from June to August. Gather the flowers as they just open to make flower essence or enjoy them dredged in flour and fried as fritters. When the flowerheads become concave and heavy with seed, they're ready to harvest. The seeds should be pungent and diffusive to the taste. Crushing the seeds just before tincturing or making infusions releases their medicinal compounds.

Medicinal Uses

Like other wild medicinal taproots—burdock, dandelion, chicory—wild carrot is gently detoxifying, supporting the liver to eliminate toxins. Through its mild diuretic actions, the root or seed decoction aids in removal of waste through the kidneys, even breaking down stones in some cases. Wild carrot roots, leaves, and seeds can be used as tea or tincture to help reduce water weight or fluid retention in the abdomen and the extremities.

Add the crushed seeds to food or take the tincture or tea as an aromatic digestive to encourage the breakdown of hard-to-digest meals or in cases where sluggish digestion is hindering absorption and assimilation of nutrients.

Wild carrot stimulates the pituitary gland to release reproductive hormones and the seeds are used as both an agent to prepare the uterus for implantation and as a natural contraceptive. If conception is your goal, first set a clear intention for a healthy pregnancy and birth. Then in the days leading up to ovulation, take 15–30 drops of the seed tincture up to 4 times per day. Stop taking before ovulating. For ongoing contraception, take 1 tablespoon of the freshly crushed seeds in water or juice or 15–30 drops of the seed tincture every 8 hours on the days during and after ovulation. For a "morning after" form of contraception, take 1 tablespoon of the freshly crushed seeds in water or juice or 15–30 drops of the tincture 8 hours after intercourse and for 3 days afterward as a means to prevent implantation.

The flower essence is used for improving psychic insight, helping one let go of psychic projection and see objective reality more clearly. It helps one integrate spiritual experiences into the physical plane of sense perception.

⚠ Precautions

Do not use wild carrot in pregnancy as it is stimulating to the uterus.

Before choosing wild carrot as a partner for contraception or conception, know your cycle well and consult additional resources. Herbalist Robin Rose Bennett has a good amount to share about this plant's gifts for conscious reproduction.

Some folks might confuse wild carrot with its deadly relative, poison hemlock (*Conium maculatum*), which can grow side by side. Fortunately, they are easy to distinguish from one another. Poison hemlock has a hollow, hairless stem with reddish or purplish splotches. Wild carrot has a solid, hairy stem that is fairly uniform in color. Poison hemlock's leaves and leaf stalks lack hairs; while wild carrot's leaves and leaf stalks are hairy. Unlike the prominent three-pronged bracts present on wild carrot, the bracts beneath the flower umbel of poison hemlock resemble tiny, simple leaves. They are not forked and are barely noticeable. Also, only wild carrot produces a bird's nest of seeds. Finally, you can try using your sense of smell if you have a pair of gloves to wear to protect your hands while crushing the plant. We'd expect the parts of a carrot plant to have a carroty scent, and it's said that poison hemlock ought to smell musty. However, it's possible that you might not be able to distinguish these scents, so go with the visual cues before using smell as the identifying factor.

Future Harvests

This weedy introduced plant is doing just fine on its own, but if you want to encourage abundant future harvests you can collect some seeds in fall to sow in spring in well-drained soil.

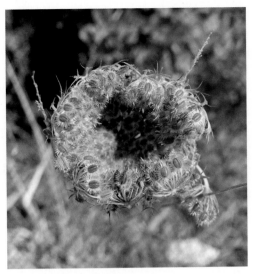

The nest or basket of seeds formed by the mature plant is likened to the shape of the uterus and the idea of fertility and nesting.

HERBAL PREPARATIONS

Tea
Standard infusion of dried seeds
or
Standard decoction of dried roots
Drink 4 ounces up to 4 times per day, or as needed.

Tincture
1 part fresh seeds
2 parts menstruum (95% alcohol, 5% water)
Take 15–30 drops up to 4 times per day, or as needed. Follow the instructions previously noted for use in conception and contraception.

Infused vinegar
1 part fresh leaves
2 parts apple cider vinegar
Add to salads, smoothies, or sparkling water.

Flower essence
Follow instructions for making flower essences on page 54. Take 3 drops on the tongue up to 4 times per day or as needed.

wild geranium

Geranium species

Carolina crane's-bill (*G. carolinianum*), spotted geranium or American crane's-bill (*G. maculatum*), herb Robert (*G. robertianum*)

PARTS USED flowers, leaves, rhizomes

Markedly astringent wild geranium is most often used to treat acute or chronic diarrhea and check bleeding and discharges from the delicate mucosa of the body.

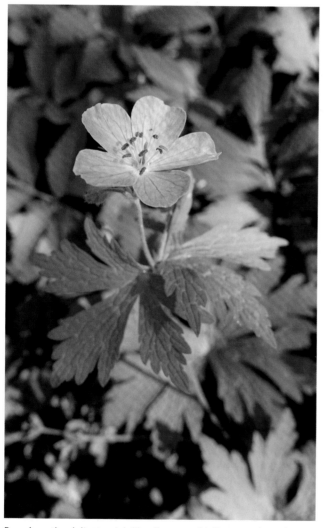

Bees love the delicate pink-lilac flowers with five round petals that bloom in midspring.

How to Identify

Of the fourteen *Geranium* species present in the Northeast, the most common are Carolina crane's-bill and spotted geranium or American crane's-bill, both native to North America.

Spotted geranium or American crane's-bill is a clumping perennial that grows 1–2½ feet tall. At the base of the plant, emerging from the rhizomes are pairs of toothed leaves with five deeply cut lobes, prominent veins, and hairs beneath. Someone with a good imagination likened the shape of the leaf to a crow's foot, and this is one of the plant's common names. Gracing the middle of the delicate hairy stems is another pair of leaves, growing opposite one another. Atop this is a loose cluster of two to five ethereal, pink-lilac, five-petaled flowers. The otherworldly beauty and graceful fragility of the blooms is enrapturing.

The flowers of Carolina crane's-bill are smaller, more tightly packed, and usually paler in color than those of

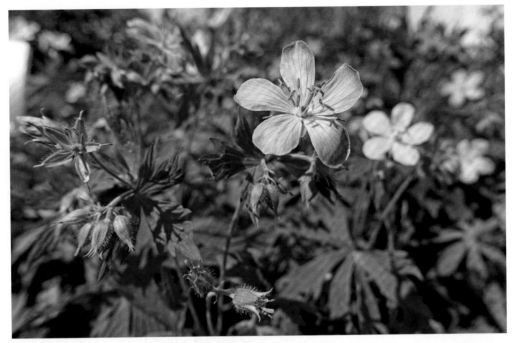
Drooping clusters of buds dangle beneath the blooms.

spotted geranium. The petals are also slightly notched at the tip. The leaves are similarly divided but with deeper divisions and narrower lobes. Herb Robert is another wild geranium with flowers resembling those of Carolina crane's-bill's in size yet they are typically a slightly deeper pink and the petals are not notched. The five lobes of the leaves of herb Robert have a rounded appearance and are even further divided than other *Geranium* species giving them a more feathery look.

The fruiting body of all wild geraniums is a splitting capsule resembling a crane's bill. *Geranium* derives from the Greek word for "crane," *geranos*. When the fruit is ready to expel the seeds, the carpels curl back to launch the seeds several yards from the plant.

The ruddy brown rhizome with white fleshy insides is 2–4 inches long with many long, thin rootlets. Tasting it reveals the tannin content with marked dryness and astringency in the mouth.

Where, When, and How to Wildcraft

Wild geranium is at home in dappled sun at the edges of forests, in meadows, and in disturbed soils throughout the Northeast.

Gather the rhizome in spring just before the plant goes into flower. Gather a few leaves at this time, too, or when the plant is just flowering. Tincture them fresh or dry them for infusions. Collect flowers for making flower essence just as they bloom, in midspring.

Medicinal Uses

The rhizomes, leaves, and flowers of wild geranium are astringent, diuretic, styptic, and antiseptic, with the rhizomes being the most potent. A tincture or decoction of the rhizome is helpful for cases of diarrhea or dysentery, whether it is an acute bout, a constitutional tendency, or a symptom of irritable bowel syndrome. Add yellow dock root and barberry if there is liver involvement or infection. Wild geranium is a good ally to have on hand when venturing to places where the water may contain parasites and traveler's diarrhea is a likelihood. Combine with catnip, chamomile, or lemon balm if the stomach and intestines are gurgling due to jittery nerves.

Having a toning influence on the mucosa and circulatory system, wild geranium stanches discharges and long-standing hemorrhages from internal ulceration or abscess, whether they are in the respiratory, gastrointestinal, or urinary tract.

Apply wild geranium leaf infusion externally as a wash to clear up pus-filled wounds or poison ivy rash.

Wild geranium flower essence lifts us out of feelings of unworthiness, self-doubt, and overwhelm, bringing lightness to the heart and nervous system. When we are trapped in a loop of old stories or trauma, wild geranium instills security. It allows us to let go of control and perfectionism to follow through with tasks, unburdened by the past.

Future Harvests
Harvest a few rhizomes from an abundant colony with respect and care. Mindfully gathering no more than about 10–15% of the leaves from a large stand is reasonable. Only a few flowers are needed to make flower essence, so leave plenty for the bees and the birds, who eat the fruit. Wild geranium is easily propagated by rhizome and seed.

Herb Robert is considered critically imperiled in Rhode Island. Avoid gathering Bicknell's crane's-bill (*G. bicknellii*), which is at risk in Connecticut, Massachusetts, Pennsylvania, Rhode Island, and Vermont.

HERBAL PREPARATIONS

Tea
Standard decoction of fresh or dried rhizomes
Drink 2–4 ounces as needed, up to 5 times per day.
or
Standard infusion of leaves
Drink 4 ounces as needed. Use as a wash for wounds or poison ivy rash.

Tincture
1 part fresh rhizomes
2 parts menstruum (60% alcohol, 40% water)
Take 15–30 drops as needed, up to 5 times per day.

Flower essence
Follow instructions for making flower essences on page 54. Take 3 drops on the tongue up to 4 times per day or as needed.

Vitis species
fox grape (*V. labrusca*), riverbank
grape (*V. riparia*), wine grape (*V. vinifera*)
PARTS USED flowers, fruit, leaves, seeds

*Cheers to this wild climber for its antioxidant, anti-inflammatory,
and cardioprotective powers!*

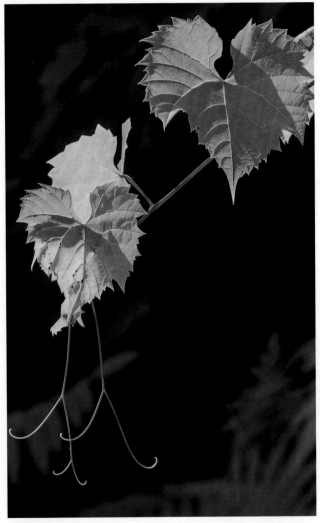

The long tendrils of wild grape tenaciously grip onto whatever is within reach.

How to Identify

Aside from the introduced and cultivated wine grape, which is isolated to areas where it has escaped cultivation, all of the species of grape found in the Northeast are native. Wild grapes are vines 50–60 feet in length, climbing up trees, across shrubs, around fences, and anywhere they can get a tendril hold. The leaves of most species have a maple-like look to them, but tend to be fairly large, up to 6 inches long and 4 inches across in wild species. Clusters of tiny white flowers bloom in early summer, developing into bright green grapes by midsummer.

It's probably safe to say you know what a grape looks like—globular deep purple to blackish fruit growing in drooping clusters. The thing is, wild grapes aren't always like the kind you'd find at the market; they have a higher concentration of tartaric acid and are therefore tarter.

Riverbank grape with its nearly hairless and coarsely toothed leaves grows extremely

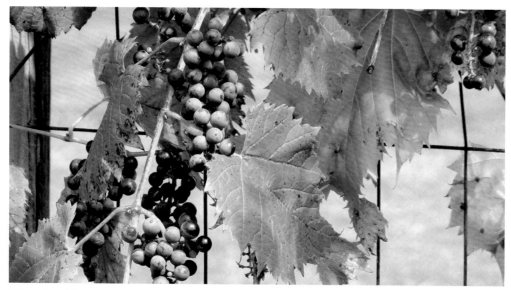

Vitis is the old Latin word for "vine," specifically the grape vine.

sour grapes, the sourness being its own particular medicine. Birds like them anyway. Fox grape leaves are woolly with smaller teeth and the plant produces tendrils from almost all of its nodes, unlike its relatives with fewer tendrils; this species is the wild ancestor of Concord grape.

Be on the lookout for a couple of grape lookalikes. Canada moonseed (*Menispermum canadense*) bears a strong resemblance to grape. The key differences are that Canada moonseed lacks tendrils, has smooth leaf margins, and each piece of fruit (a berry-like drupe) contains one crescent moon–shaped seed (hence the name) versus grape's multiple roughly heart-shaped seeds. The root of Canada moonseed was once used medicinally in small doses. It probably fell out of favor for its strong purgative and emetic effects and is currently considered poisonous.

Porcelain berry or Amur peppervine (*Ampelopsis brevipedunculata*) has deeply divided grape-like leaves that can sometimes resemble the leaves of summer grape (*V. aestivalis*). The biggest difference is in the berries. Porcelain berry has the prettiest pastel blue and purple berries that look like bird eggs. The good news is that the berries are not poisonous (but not tasty either), and the leaves can be used externally in the same way as grape leaves.

Where, When, and How to Wildcraft

Wild grape is a fairly common roadside inhabitant. It's also found in and at the edge of wooded areas or twining its way around shrubs near waterways. It likes well-drained sandy to gravelly soil in full to partial sun.

Gather the leaves for medicine whenever they are green to use fresh as a poultice, infuse in vinegar, or dry for later. If you plan to collect the leaves for food, gather them before fruiting when they aren't too tough. Use fresh or blanch and freeze them for later. Harvest flowers in midsummer to craft into flower essence. Collect fruit when it's ripe in late summer to early fall, depending on the species. Juice the grapes fresh, make your own wine or vinegar, chomp a few along with their seeds, or dry them to make raisins.

Medicinal Uses

From the time of ancient Greece or even earlier, grapes have been praised for their healing powers. Today grapes, grape juice, and wine are touted (and marketed) for their resveratrol content, one of the compounds that contributes to their antioxidant and cardioprotective benefits. Taken over time the fruit and seeds improve blood cholesterol and reduce high blood pressure.

Grapes are rich in vitamins C and E, iron, and niacin, and they're a good source of dietary fiber. Eaten fresh or as raisins, grapes have a laxative effect—soak a handful of raisins in water and eat them to relieve constipation.

Wild grapes are very tart compared to their cultivated family members due to the higher presence of tartaric acid. One way to get an abundance of fruit medicine while not suffering is to juice the grapes and let the juice sit for a few days. Potassium in the juice will react with the tartaric acid, and form potassium bitartrate (cream of tartar), a gritty, grayish white precipitate. Once everything has settled, strain off the juice, and dispose of the sediment.

Apply the leaf poultice to injuries to reduce swelling and inflammation and prevent bruising. Vinegar infused with grape leaf and applied externally on a daily basis promotes circulation and tones lax veins and capillaries, in cases of varicose or spider veins. The infused vinegar makes a nice facial toner as well. Make a sitz bath with an infusion of grape leaf, plantain, and witch hazel to heal hemorrhoids or fissures.

The flower essence is used to encourage loving leadership in those with domineering personalities.

⚠ Precautions

Be sure to correctly identify wild grape from its lookalikes.

Future Harvests

Despite the tenacious and weedy characteristics of most grape species, two native species are at risk in the Northeast. Summer grape (*V. aestivalis*) is endangered in Maine and frost or winter grape (*V. vulpina*), which reaches its northerly range in New Jersey and Pennsylvania, is considered endangered in New York.

Gather a few leaves from each plant, rather than stripping them off the branches. Leave plenty of grapes for the birds and other wild creatures.

HERBAL PREPARATIONS

Infused vinegar

1 part fresh leaves

2 parts vinegar

Apply with a cotton ball to varicose or spider veins or use as a toner. Use in salad dressing or take a couple of tablespoons in water.

Flower essence

Follow instructions for making flower essences on page 54. Take 3 drops on the tongue up to 4 times per day or as needed.

Lactuca species

wild or bitter lettuce (*L. virosa*), prickly lettuce (*L. serriola*), Canada or tall lettuce (*L. canadensis*), tall blue or bitter lettuce (*L. biennis*)

PARTS USED aerial parts in flower, latex, leaves, roots, stems

Wild lettuce is a potent ally that relaxes the nerves, calms spasmodic cough, and relieves pain. The entire plant, and especially the latex, are used in infusions and tinctures, or smoked for their medicinal benefits.

How to Identify

This biennial herbaceous plant in the aster family starts out as a basal rosette of lanceolate leaves that is 5–10 inches in length. Depending on the species, the leaves are either entire and toothed, have deep rounded sinuses, or are deeply divided. Those new to wild lettuce might mistake it as dandelion or chicory in its first year. The likeness ends in the second year when wild lettuce sends up a branching stalk with alternate leaves that clasp the stem. In summer, the plant blooms in clusters of small flowers that look like tiny chicory or dandelion blooms. Depending on the species the flowers are pale blue, white, or yellow. Tall blue lettuce can grow to over 13 feet while other species tend to be in the 4- to 7-foot range.

Sow-thistles (*Sonchus* spp.) are a potential lookalike, with the major difference being wild lettuce leaves have prickly hairs that line the underside of the midrib, unlike sow thistle.

Look for wild lettuce in recently disturbed habitats or in the dappled edge of woodlands.

Where, When, and How to Wildcraft

Prickly lettuce occupies newly cleared land, abandoned lots, and cracks in sidewalks, or you might see it smack dab in the middle of a field. Canada and bitter lettuces are typically found at the edge of woodlands in diffuse or dappled light.

In spring, the young leaves of wild lettuce are edible, with Canada lettuce being the most palatable. If gathering for medicine, harvest a few leaves from individual second-year plants, in the middle of summer before they go to seed. You can dry these leaves for tea. Alternately, harvest the entire plant for the leaves, stems, and roots to decoct and tincture.

Introduced wild lettuce (*L. virosa*) is the officinal species that reportedly contains the highest concentrations of latex or lactucarium versus other species.

If you have access to plants that you can spend a good amount of time with, a sustainable way to harvest the latex without uprooting the plant is to cut the tops of the second-year stalks above the top leaf node. The latex will ooze out of the stalk. Let it dry and then collect the hardened latex in a small container. Continue to cut down the length of the stalks just above the nodes to gather more latex. Tincture the latex, use it directly, or save it for smoking.

Medicinal Uses

Bitter and cooling, wild lettuce is a nonaddictive, pain-relieving hypnotic useful for insomnia caused by anxiety or hyperactivity. For difficulty falling asleep, combine wild lettuce, hops, chamomile, and lemon balm in a tea or tincture to take 30 minutes before bedtime. For trouble staying asleep, try a tincture of wild lettuce, skullcap, and rose petals upon waking in the middle of the night.

A tincture of the leaves works well in cough blends for a dry tickling or hacking cough that disturbs sleep. Combine with wild cherry, violet, and linden tinctures for this purpose.

Wild lettuce alleviates pain, and the tincture can be used to ease menstrual cramps and lower back pain and stiffness. The herb

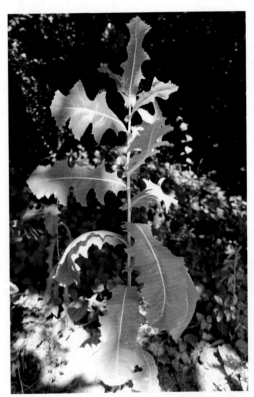

In the second year of its lifecycle, wild lettuce sends up a stalk decorated with alternate prickly edged leaves and flowers that bloom in midsummer.

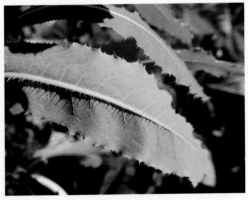

The prickly midrib under the leaf distinguishes wild lettuce from lookalikes.

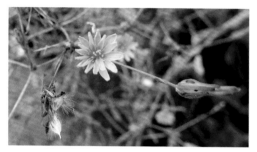
Mini dandelion-like flowers ranging from yellow to white to light blue bloom in midsummer.

is bitter and warm and relaxes the parasympathetic nervous system, easing digestive processes and allowing the body to release tension in the gastrointestinal tract.

Mix the leaves into a smoking blend with mugwort, rose, and passionflower for a pre-bedtime dream-enhancing ritual.

⚠ Precautions

Start with small doses—1 drop of the concentrate and up to 3 drops of the tincture—to determine your therapeutic threshold, especially if pain relief (not sleep) is the primary intention. Higher doses of wild lettuce preparations will induce sleep. Do not drive or operate heavy machinery after taking wild lettuce.

Do not use wild lettuce in pregnancy.

Future Harvests

While most wild lettuces are considered weeds, two native species in this genus are considered at risk in the Northeast—tall hairy lettuce (*L. hirsuta*) and woodland lettuce (*L. floridana*).

The most sustainable way to harvest wild lettuce is to gather latex and leaves, rather than uprooting the plant. If the species you are harvesting is considered a weed in your state or province then feel free to gather the whole plant with respect and thanks to this wild and weedy being.

HERBAL PREPARATIONS

Tea
Standard infusion of dried leaves
Drink 4 ounces as needed.

Tincture
1 part fresh aerial parts in flower, leaves, roots, and/or latex
2 parts menstruum (95% alcohol, 5% water)
Chop the plant material, then blend with the menstruum at high speed in a blender and let macerate for 4–6 weeks. Take 5–10 drops as needed.
or
1 part fresh latex
4 parts menstruum (95% alcohol, 5% water)
Take 10 drops as needed.

Concentrate tincture
1 part fresh leaves, roots, and stalks
4 parts water
Menstruum (80–95% alcohol, 5–20% water)
Chop the plant material, then gently steam or barely simmer for 30 minutes. Cover and let cool. Strain liquid and compost the marc. Decoct this liquid by reducing it to a thick, molasses like consistency. Use a slow cooker set on low or keep a pot on the stove at the lowest point so that the decoction just steams. To this concentrate add an equal part of high-proof alcohol (80–95%). Take 3 drops as needed.

wild sarsaparilla

Aralia nudicaulis
rabbit root
PARTS USED rhizomes

This wild understory native smells and tastes like root beer, in which it was originally an ingredient. It nourishes and detoxifies the body after illness, stress, or long winters have taken their toll.

How to Identify

This native, herbaceous, shrub-like perennial is in the ginseng family. Its single stalk graced with three branches reaches 1–2 feet tall and spreads by runners. So, what seems like several plants may be one, interconnected beneath the ground. Its compound leaves contain five toothed, ovate leaflets that are 2–5 inches long. The veins underneath may be hairy on some plants.

In late spring, tiny white-greenish flowers bloom in round clusters of twelve to thirty flowers. The flowers ripen to purple-black drupes midsummer. Birds and bears eat the drupes, and deer and moose browse the foliage. Apparently rabbits like to eat the roots, inspiring one of its common names, rabbit root. The yellowish brown rhizomes are sweet, spicy, and aromatic reminding soda drinkers of root beer.

Where, When, and How to Wildcraft

Wild sarsaparilla is a common understory plant throughout the Northeast. Look for it in rich soil in forests and woodlands.

Find a large colony and dig the rhizome in late summer to fall to tincture fresh. The rhizomes are fairly close to the surface and it's possible to dig with your hands and trace a runner along under the ground until you reach another plant. The root should be sweet and spicy smelling and tasting.

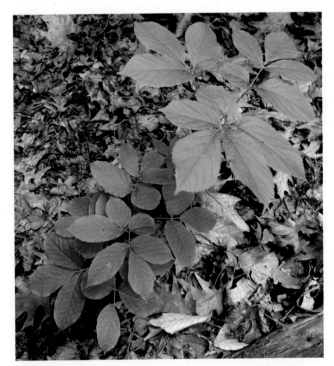

A single stalk branches out in three directions with compound leaves of five leaflets. The species name *nudicaulis* refers to the "naked" or hairless stem.

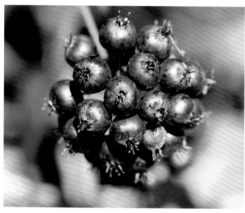

Globular bunches of plump purple-black fruit ripen in mid- to late summer.

Medicinal Uses

Sweet, nourishing, and blood-cleansing, wild sarsaparilla supports the body through detoxification and renews strength after the sedentariness of winter. Like its relatives ginseng and American spikenard, wild sarsaparilla builds up energy after illness, stress, or debility, restoring a sense of well-being.

The tincture or decoction promotes sweating to help break a fever or sweat out the toxins left in the body by infection. Its warming and stimulating nature benefits sluggish digestion, slow-to-go coughs, and achy joints from arthritis or rheumatism.

Future Harvests

Collecting just one or two rhizomes from large stands of wild sarsaparilla will yield enough for a batch of tincture to last through a season. Always rebury portions of the root that are unearthed and harvest carefully so as not to disturb neighboring plants.

A related and somewhat analogous plant, bristly sarsaparilla (*A. hispida*) can be used in place of wild sarsaparilla. However, this plant is a bit less common.

HERBAL PREPARATIONS

Tincture
1 part fresh rhizomes
2 parts menstruum (50% alcohol, 50% water)
Take 5-15 drops as needed.

wild strawberry

Fragaria species
Virginia strawberry (*F. virginiana*), woodland strawberry (*F. vesca*)
PARTS USED flowers, fruit, leaves

You know—and maybe love—the delicious red fruit of this plant, but did you know that it's also medicinal? The leaves and fruit are nourishing, astringent, diuretic, wound healing, and more.

How to Identify

Just like the cultivated strawberry, the wild type has a compound leaf of three-toothed, roughly ovate leaflets with fine hairs on the undersides. It also has five-petaled, white blossoms with yellow centers borne in clusters on hairy stems. The juicy, red, heart-shaped berries even look the same, but in miniature.

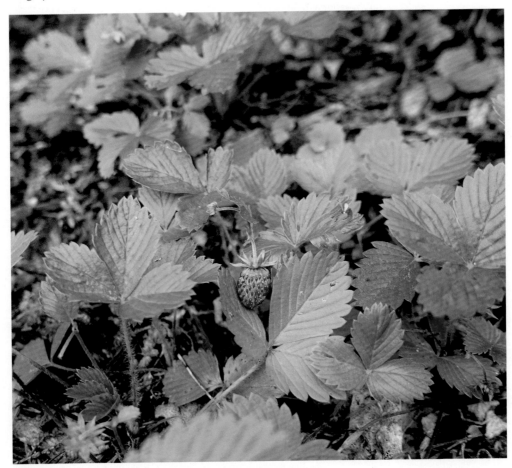

Wild strawberry fruit is smaller than what you'd find at the market.

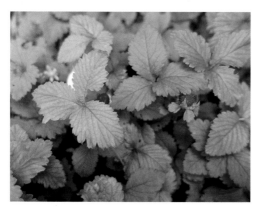

This is not true wild strawberry, but mock strawberry (*Potentilla indica*).

Be on the lookout for the lookalike plant mock strawberry (*Potentilla indica*). It's not poisonous, it just isn't strawberry. You'll know by tasting (or not tasting) the similar-looking aggregate fruits—they are pretty bland. The flowers are yellow, the fruit grow more upright than dangling strawberry and have a more prominent "collar" of leafy bracts beneath the fruit. An easy-to-spot difference is that the seeds on real wild strawberry are sunken into the surface, while the seeds of mock strawberry protrude above the surface.

Where, When, and How to Wildcraft

Wild strawberries like damp soil in full to partial sun. They are often pioneers of recently disturbed soil at the edges of woodlands, along trails, or at the margins of fields.

Gather leaves through spring and summer and nibble a couple of the berries around that time, depending on when they ripen in your neck of the woods. Collect flowers in spring to make a flower essence.

Medicinal Uses

Strawberry is a mild diuretic, laxative, and astringent herb that has been used traditionally in North America to treat diarrhea, dysentery, and stomachache in children. The fruit and fresh leaves are high in vitamin C and contain a range of nutrients, including iron, calcium, and trace minerals.

Drink the leaf tea as a daily tonic along with other rose family relatives, raspberry leaf, rose petals, and rosehips to build the blood and regulate the menstrual cycle.

Strawberry leaf is sometimes used in place of raspberry leaf in herbal blends for prenatal support and as a galactagogue to encourage healthy flow of breastmilk.

The juicy red berry has been used as a tooth cleanser and whitener; rub the fruit over the teeth for a few minutes to remove plaque, then rinse with warm water.

Make a poultice or wash of the leaves to treat sores, wounds, or ulcers on the skin.

The flower essence is connected with the root chakra and feelings of self-worth and self-confidence. It helps us approach life with embodied presence and grace.

Future Harvests

Wild strawberry is pretty good at spreading. Still, mindfully gather only what you need. Leave plenty of fruit for the birds and other creatures who enjoy it as much as we do. If you want to encourage more harvests, sow some seeds of wild strawberry indoors and transplant into an edible forest garden landscape.

HERBAL PREPARATIONS

Tea
Standard infusion of dried leaves
Drink 4–8 ounces as needed.

Flower essence
Follow instructions for making flower essences on page 54. Take 3 drops on the tongue up to 4 times per day or as needed.

Salix species
white willow (*S. alba*), black willow (*S. nigra*)
PARTS USED bark, catkins, leaves

Willow is valued for its pain-relieving, anti-inflammatory, and fever-reducing effects. The salicylates present in willow also benefit the skin, helping to clear acne, eczema, and wounds.

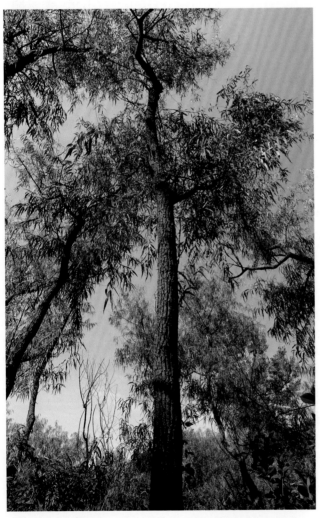

Willows vary greatly in size, color, and habit. Their appearance depends on the conditions they grow in, and their variation makes it sometimes challenging to determine the species.

How to Identify

There are around four hundred species of willow worldwide, with at least thirty of them present in the Northeast. Great variation exists between and within species due to local habitat, climate, and other environmental factors, sometimes making it difficult to identify individual species.

In general, the willows here are deciduous trees with slender pliable branches and lanceolate to long, ovate leaves that are finely serrated. Male and female flowers or catkins appear on separate trees in early spring, before the leaves. Leaf buds have a single scale and the leaves begin to emerge as the catkins are ripening with seed in midspring.

Willow tends to form dense thickets in wetland areas, spreading by a tenacious root system. Willow easily sheds and regrows branches and root shoots. It contains its own rooting hormone, so directly replanting cuttings in the soil will likely yield a new tree. The ability of willow to easily root and renew itself lends well to coppicing, an ancient practice of creating continual harvests by cutting back and harvesting the shoots down to the stump of the felled tree.

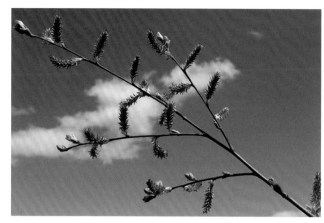

Fertilized catkins and just-unfurling leaf buds in spring.

Introduced white willow, the officinal species in Europe, and native black willow are both found in abundance throughout the Northeast.

Black willow features either one stout trunk or multiple slender ones with a wide shaggy habit. The gray-black bark of mature trees is coarse and furrowed. Long, lanceolate leaves, 3–5 inches long and about ½ inch across, are almost uniformly green and hairless, slightly darker on the surface than the undersides. Yellow-green catkins are 1–3 inches long. The tree reaches 30–90 feet tall.

White willow has an overall paler appearance, more in line with the term "sallow," another word for willow that also means gray-green-yellow in color. The usually singular trunk features yellow-brown, ridged bark. The 4-inch-long, lanceolate, finely toothed leaves are gray-green on top and downy white underneath. Male catkins (around 2 inches long) are a pale yellow-green and the smaller female catkins are pale green. This species reaches 50–80 feet tall.

Where, When, and How to Wildcraft

Most willows are happy in watery environs, in or at the edges of marshes, swamps, lakes, ponds, rivers, and streams.

Before harvesting, clip a small twig from a branch and chew on it. If it tastes bitter and astringent, you've found a good wildcrafting tree. In late winter to early spring when the sap is flowing, prune branches about ¾–1 inch in diameter. Trace a line with a knife down the length of the stick down to the heartwood. Peel away the inner green bark with the outer bark. If it pulls away easily, you'll have a curled-up sheet of bark. Slice that up into ½-inch pieces to tincture fresh or dry. For an immediate field medicine, chew the bark or twigs directly. Gather leaves from spring through fall to use fresh in infusion or dry for later. In early spring, collect male catkins to craft a flower essence.

Medicinal Uses

Like its derivative aspirin, salicylate-containing willow is pain relieving, anti-inflammatory, fever reducing, and blood thinning. The tincture or decoction is an excellent remedy for headaches, arthritis, and other pain-related ailments. It alleviates the pain and inflammation of bladder infections and cystitis as well. Taking a bath infused with willow bark and leaf decoction melts away muscular tension and alleviates dry, scaly skin conditions. A willow foot bath, in conjunction with the tincture or tea taken internally, helps mitigate a gout attack.

Drink or use the infusion of the leaves as a gargle for sore throat or a mouthwash for mouth sores and tooth pain. Externally the leaf or bark tea can be used as a wash to stanch bleeding or weeping wounds and as a toner to improve skin health.

Willow flower essence is useful for restoring flexibility and resilience to help one go with the flow.

⚠ Precautions

Willow is blood thinning so stop taking it 2 weeks before a planned surgery. Avoid concomitant use with pharmaceutical blood thinners.

Children under 16 with fever or recovering from viral infection should avoid willow for the risk of Reye's syndrome, a rare but serious condition induced by salicylates.

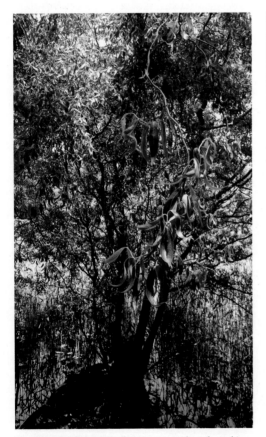

Flowing and flexible willow is most often found in or near water.

Future Harvests

One way to create a sustainable wildcrafting condition is to develop a relationship with and harvest from one or two trees. With mindful harvesting, you'll be able to come back year after year to the same tree for medicine.

Keep in mind that nineteeen of the thirty or so species of willow in the Northeast are at risk in one or more states or provinces due to changes in climate and human manipulation of wetland ecosystems. Most willow species easily root from cuttings, either planted directly in the soil or allowed to root in water indoors. Help secure the future of endangered willow species by propagating them in a rain garden.

HERBAL PREPARATIONS

Tea

Standard decoction of fresh or dried bark
Drink 2–4 ounces as needed, up to 4 times per day. Use as a bath tea to relieve aches and pains.
or
Standard infusion of fresh or dried leaves
Drink 2–4 ounces as needed, up to 4 times per day. Use as a gargle or mouthwash, or as a wash for injuries.

Tincture

1 part fresh bark
2 parts menstruum (75% alcohol, 25% water)
or
1 part dried bark
5 parts menstruum (50% alcohol, 50% water)
Take 15–30 drops as needed, up to 4 times per day.

Flower essence

Follow instructions for making flower essences on page 54. Take 3 drops on the tongue up to 4 times per day or as needed.

Gaultheria procumbens
teaberry, checkerberry
PARTS USED fruit, leaves

Distinctively aromatic wintergreen is well known as a flavoring agent for toothpaste, mouthwash, and gum. It also eases the aches and pains of rheumatism, soothes irritation in the urinary tract, and alleviates gas and cramping in the intestines.

How to Identify

Wintergreen is a diminutive evergreen ground cover shrub with a woody rhizome from which, in spring, red stalks emerge topped with a little red leaf bud. As the new leaves emerge, they change from bright red to reddish green to deep green by summertime. The young leaves feature fine, dark hairs along their margins. As the plant matures, the hairs drop, leaving miniscule indentations in their stead. The leaves are waxy or leathery in texture. Leaf shape ranges from elliptical to oblong, sometimes with a pointed tip. They are arranged alternately at the top of the woody stem. In winter, the leaves change from green to red-green to deep red, returning to green in spring and summer.

At the ends of branches and in the leaf axils a cluster of white urn or bell-shaped flowers with two bracts and five sepals develops. Once fertilized these ripen to round bright red berries, often with brown styles sticking out the bottom.

The whole plant has the distinct spicy-sweet-minty scent and taste of wintergreen that you might recognize from toothpaste, gum, or candy.

All kinds of wild creatures like the berries—including deer, bear, fox, and wild turkey.

Where, When, and How to Wildcraft

Wintergreen inhabits acidic soil in the understory of forests throughout the Northeast. You'll find it growing beneath a canopy of pines or oaks, interspersed between other heath family plants like rhododendrons and kalmias, along mountain trails or in barrens.

Gather leaves from spring through fall, while they are green. From late summer through winter, gently snap off

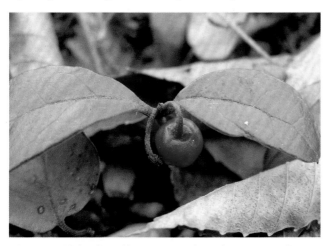

Wintergreen's bright red berries ripen through summer and often remain through winter. The young leaves start out red then turn green to red and back to green again as the seasons and temperatures shift.

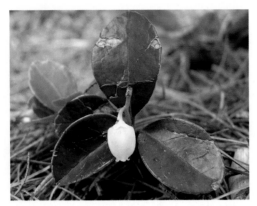
White urn or bell-shaped flowers bloom in spring.

the leaves and berries all together at the top of the stalk. If you are worried you might be too rough, use little scissors or pruners. Look for abundant patches and overlapping leaves. Think of it as lightly pruning a bit here and there, taking care not to strip entire sections or leave big bald patches. Tincture or infuse in oil directly or dry the berries and leaves for use in tea, syrup, or dental preparations.

Medicinal Uses

That characteristic taste and aroma of wintergreen gives away its methyl salicylate content. Like other plants that share this compound—willow, meadowsweet, cottonwood, birch—wintergreen has pain-relieving and anti-inflammatory effects. Use the tincture as a liniment or massage the infused oil into painful, inflamed joints and muscles.

Add the tincture to mouthwash formulas for its astringent, antiseptic powers. Powder the dried leaves and combine with baking soda, sea salt, and kaolin clay for a homemade toothpowder.

With a soothing effect on the digestive tract, relieving gas and cramping, wintergreen makes a flavorful addition to digestive or bitters blends. Make a syrup with the leaves and berries to add to sparkling water or tea for a refreshing pre- or post-meal beverage.

Wintergreen eases irritation and pain in the urethra, bladder, and kidneys. Use in combination with other anti-inflammatory herbs with an affinity for the urinary tract for relief of cystitis, urethritis, or interstitial nephritis.

⚠ Precautions

Do not use wintergreen in pregnancy as it is stimulating to the uterus.

The distilled oil of wintergreen is a potent medicine derived or synthesized based on this plant. While using the whole plant is generally safer than using the commercially extracted oil, proceed with caution if you have sensitivity to aspirin.

Future Harvests

Take care not to overharvest a patch of wintergreen by gently grazing rather than stripping a whole colony. Harvest only the aerial portions, leaving the roots intact. Save plenty of leaves and berries for our feathered and furred friends.

HERBAL PREPARATIONS

Tea
Standard infusion of dried berries and leaves
Drink 2 ounces as needed.

Tincture
1 part fresh berries and leaves
2 parts menstruum (50% alcohol,
  50% water)
Take 5–15 drops as needed.

Syrup
Follow instructions for making herbal syrups on page 52. Take 1 teaspoon as needed, or add to tea or sparkling water.

Infused oil
1 part fresh leaves
2 parts oil
Use for massage.

Hamamelis virginiana

PARTS USED bark, flowers, leaves, twigs

The consummate astringent, witch hazel is an important remedy for stopping internal and external bleeding and discharge, toning veins and mucous tissues, and promoting healthy skin.

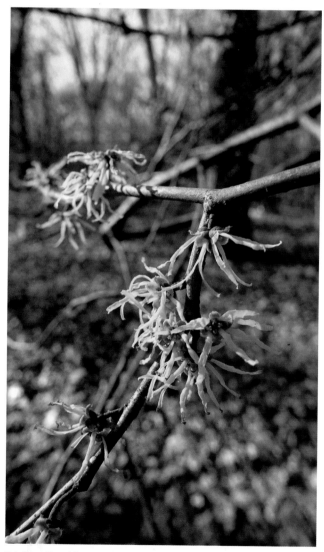

Bright yellow blooms glow like fireworks in the drab post-foliage autumn landscape.

How to Identify

Witch hazel is a deciduous shrub or tree that usually grows in small clumps or groves. It can reach 30 feet high, though it's typically somewhere between 12 and 15 feet and as broad as it is high. Its oblong to ovate leaves are wavy-edged and asymmetrical at the base and grow from spiral-shaped twigs. The numerous intertwining branches are smooth, gray, and flexible—the "witch" part of the name comes from *wiche*, the Middle English word for "bendable." The forked twigs of this plant were once commonly used as a divining rod to find underground springs. The genus name *Hamamelis* comes from an ancient Greek word for the medlar, a fruiting tree native to the eastern Mediterranean, Middle East, and Caucasus.

In the middle of fall when most of the trees have dropped their leaves, witch hazel adds color to the landscape with its twisting ribbon-like yellow flowers. They remind me of a celebration of confetti and fireworks, as do the explosive seed capsules, which propel the shiny black seeds several yards from the tree, popping and landing with a crash on crispy dry leaves in winter.

The leaves are sometimes host to the witch hazel cone gall aphid (*Hormaphis hamamelidis*). The galls, shaped like little cones or witch's hats, are protecting the aphids inside and not harmful to the plant.

In urban parks and botanic gardens you may encounter the introduced Chinese (*H. mollis*) or Japanese species (*H. japonica*), or a hybrid variety. These typically bloom in late winter before any other plants in the landscape.

Where, When, and How to Wildcraft

Witch hazel tends toward damp forests, swampy areas, or riparian habitats and is present throughout the Northeast.

Mindfully prune twigs and small branches for bark in spring before leafing. Gather leaves from spring through fall to use straight away as a poultice, infuse fresh in tincture or vinegar, or dry for later use. Fall-blooming flowers provide a harvest when most aerial parts of plants are dormant. Collect them as they bloom for use in flower essence.

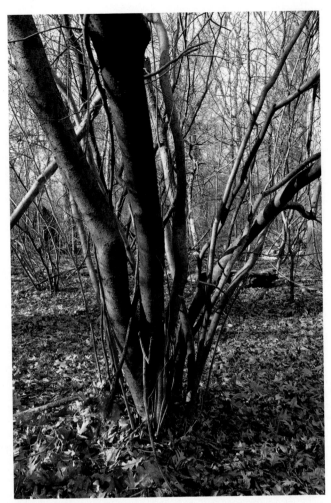

The overall appearance of witch hazel is twisting, turning, spiraling, and intertwining.

Medicinal Uses

Witch hazel has been utilized traditionally in North America as a decoction for a variety of internal and external ailments, mainly for injury to the soft tissues and mucous membranes. Scarlet fever, cholera, and dysentery have all been treated by witch hazel. It has been and is still used to alleviate sore throat, mouth ulcers, and internal hemorrhaging.

Most herbalists today stick to the external uses of witch hazel, for which there is no shortage of applications. The leaf poultice treats scratches, insect bites, and swollen, tired eyes. Make a decoction of the twigs and leaves to add to a bath or apply a hot compress for relief of bruises, sprains, sore muscles, breast inflammation, and postpartum abdominal pain.

Vinegar infused with witch hazel works well as a facial toner. It tones veins and makes a good treatment for varicose or spider veins. Keep some on hand in the kitchen for burns, or have a batch ready, with the optional addition of rose- or elderflower-infused vinegar, in the summer for sunburn.

Using the decoction, prepare a sitz bath to treat hemorrhoids or rectal prolapse. Add raspberry leaf, rose, plantain, and mugwort to a postpartum vaginal steam.

Another way to treat hemorrhoids is by making a suppository with the powdered leaves blended with shea or cocoa butter, or coconut oil. Alternately make a decoction of witch hazel, oak, and blackberry leaf, and blend it with coconut oil and beeswax to make a hemorrhoid cream.

Witch hazel flower essence lights the way through the dark winter months. It helps those who are feeling out of sorts and not able to see the end of the darkness.

⚠ Precautions

Witch hazel should not be used internally during pregnancy and should be reserved for short-term use due to its high tannin content.

Future Harvests

Wildcraft leaves and twigs from mature shrubs with care to ensure these valuable medicine plants stay healthy.

HERBAL PREPARATIONS

Tea

Standard decoction of fresh or dried leaves and twigs

Take 2 ounces as needed. Use as a wash to improve skin health, or as a sitz bath for hemorrhoids.

Tincture

1 part fresh bark, leaves, and twigs
2 parts menstruum (80% alcohol, 20% water)

or

1 part fresh bark, leaves, and twigs
5 parts menstruum (50% alcohol, 50% water)

Take 10–20 drops as needed. Use as a liniment for sore muscles.

Infused vinegar

1 part fresh bark, leaves, and twigs
2 parts apple cider vinegar

Use on burns, as a facial toner, or to diminish varicose and spider veins.

Flower essence

Follow instructions for making flower essences on page 54. Take 3 drops on the tongue up to 4 times per day or as needed.

yarrow

Achillea millefolium
PARTS USED aerial parts in flower, leaves

A versatile wild medicine ally, yarrow has an affinity with the blood being able to both stanch and promote blood flow. It's a good partner for cold and flu, especially with fever, and its bitter nature stimulates digestion.

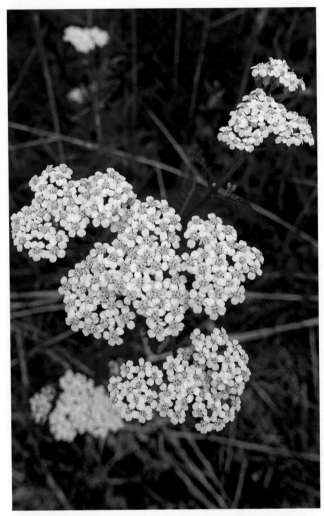

Achillea is named for Achilles, warrior hero of ancient Greece, who was dipped into a vat of yarrow tea by his mother at birth. The hand that held his ankle is to blame for his weak spot, or Achilles' heel.

How to Identify

This graceful aster family perennial is recognized by its deeply and finely divided feathery leaves and flat heads (corymbs) of tiny white to pink composite flowers. The specific name *millefolium* describes the "thousand leaves," or rather leaf parts, that make up the whole. The leaves can be downy pale green-gray or deep green. Basal leaves reach 3–4 inches long while the smaller upper leaves clasp alternately up the fuzzy stem. The flowers bloom through summer.

There are three native species in the Northeast, and one introduced. In garden varieties (usually *A. filipendula*), blooms vary greatly in color—including yellow, orange, red, and deep pink.

Where, When, and How to Wildcraft

Yarrow is at home in well-drained soil in a variety of habitats. You're just as likely to find it at roadsides, in meadows and fields, on stream banks, and near lakeshores as on rocky mountain ledges or summits.

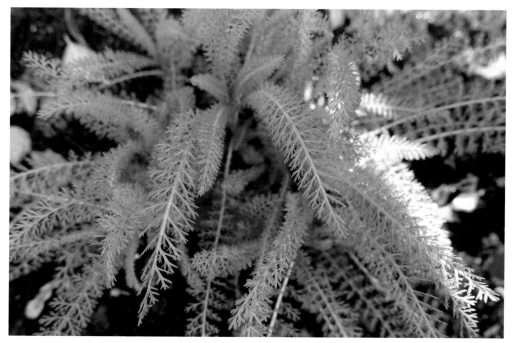

Deeply divided leaves are a signature for healing deep cuts or wounds.

The best time to harvest yarrow is in the summer when it's in flower, though if you're out in the field and need yarrow medicine in a pinch, the leaves can be collected anytime from spring through fall. Gather the aerial portions of the plant in flower, tracing about one-third of the way down the plant and cutting above the nearest leaf node. Tincture fresh, infuse in oil, or dry upside down in bundles in a cool, dry place for later use. Collect flowers separately for flower essence.

Medicinal Uses

A little pouch of dried yarrow or yarrow tincture is an essential component of a well-stocked first-aid kit. It stanches bleeding, provides antimicrobial protection, and reduces pain and inflammation. Keep it on hand in case of accidental cuts, scrapes, burns, or bruises. Use the infused oil to make a salve for bruises and minor skin injuries, or to add to lotion to moisturize dry skin.

Antiviral, decongestant, and sweat-inducing, yarrow is a great partner when you come down with a viral infection. A classic cold and flu tea blend includes yarrow, elderflower, and mint. Sip this blend then get under the covers to sweat out a fever, relieve the sniffles, and alleviate achy malaise.

In addition to its physical healing applications, this versatile herb has a long history of metaphysical use. Carrying yarrow in a medicine pouch or using the flower essence is said to enhance intuition, establish healthy boundaries, and provide protection. Add yarrow to the bath for a healing and protective self-care ritual. Hang a bundle of yarrow by your front door or burn some dried herb over coals to cast out negative energies. *The I Ching (Book of Changes)*, an ancient Chinese divination text, is most often cast using yarrow sticks.

Yarrow also works magic on the digestive tract. Its bitter properties make it a great digestif—it is commonly found in bitters formulas and was once used in beer brewing. Take a few drops of yarrow tincture after a meal to improve digestion and assimilation. Use the tea or tincture to reduce excessive menstrual bleeding and relieve cramps.

 Precautions

Yarrow is not recommended during pregnancy for its strong effects on the blood.

Future Harvests

As long as you don't uproot or completely cut down this perennial plant, it should return for future harvests.

HERBAL PREPARATIONS

Tea

10 minute infusion of dried aerial parts in flower

Drink 2 ounces as needed. It's pretty bitter so adding honey is a good idea.

Tincture

1 part fresh aerial parts in flower

2 parts menstruum (50% alcohol, 50% water)

or

1 part dried aerial parts in flower

5 parts menstruum (50% alcohol, 50% water)

Take 10–20 drops as needed.

Infused oil

1 part fresh aerial parts in flower

2 parts oil

Use for massage, in skin-healing salves, or lotions.

Flower essence

Follow instructions for making flower essences on page 54. Take 3 drops on the tongue up to 4 times per day or as needed.

yellow dock

Rumex crispus
curly dock
PARTS USED leaves, roots, seeds

Gently detoxifying and blood-building, yellow dock supports liver health and brings relief to arthritic and chronic skin conditions.

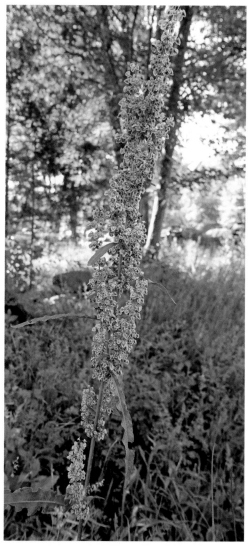

How to Identify

Yellow dock is a biennial herbaceous plant in the buckwheat family that starts as a basal rosette of lanceolate leaves with wavy edges. The leaves can get rather long, upward of 18 inches. In its second year of growth, the plant sends up an upright, hairless, grooved stem, green to reddish in color. Alternating sparsely up the stem are long, lanceolate, curly-edged leaves, like the basal ones, getting smaller as they reach the apex. Where

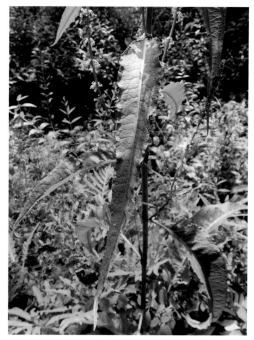

Seeds ripening in early summer. They'll be ready to harvest once they turn a deep rust color.

The long, lanceolate upper leaves of yellow dock sparsely decorate the stalks.

the leaves meet the stalk is a sheath that becomes papery with age.

In summer, inconspicuous green drooping flowers borne in whorls decorate the length of multiple branching offshoots that emerge about one-third to halfway up the main stalk. The flowers yield to densely packed, edible, papery, heart-shaped seeds which start out green and ripen to a deep rusty brown.

The root is a thick, fleshy taproot (about 8–12 inches long) that is reddish brown on the outside and whitish yellow on the inside.

A related species, broad-leaf dock (*R. obtusifolius*) has an overall broader appearance, with oblong-ovate to oblong-cordate leaves and sparser flowers that ripen to a lighter orange-brown. It can be used similarly, though yellow dock is considered the officinal species.

Where, When, and How to Wildcraft

You'll find yellow dock just about anywhere with moist soil and full sun—in ditches, puddles, next to ponds and streams, ocean beaches, and tidal zones. It's often found gracing abandoned lots, parks, and open farm fields.

Pick the young leaves in spring while they still taste lemony (and not super bitter) to add to salads or blanch and blend into pesto. You can also dehydrate and powder the leaves with other leafy green herbs like plantain, nettles, and violet to make a green smoothie powder. Harvest the brown seeds from summer through winter by cutting the seed stalks and stripping them off. Since it's difficult to separate the grain from the chaff and the papery bracts contain extra dietary fiber, you can keep them whole. Toast them gently in the oven until they are absolutely dry. You can grind the toasted seeds in a mortar and pestle, seed grinder, or food processer to use in baked goods, though some foragers aren't

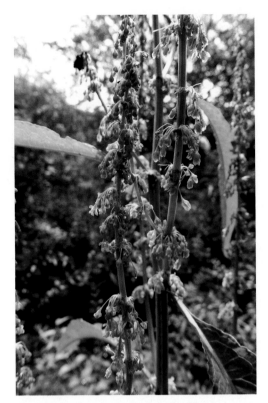

The just-developing seeds circle the ridged flower stalk.

fond of the strong taste it lends to them when ground. Alternately, add them whole as a fairly neutral bulking agent when baking cookies, crackers, and hearty breads.

A poultice of the leaves is helpful field medicine for bug bites and nettle stings, two things you might experience while wildcrafting.

Dig the roots in the fall of the first year or late winter to spring of the second before the plant sends its energy up into the flower stalk. Either tincture directly or slice the root into smaller pieces and dry in a dehydrator or on a screen.

Medicinal Uses

Yellow dock is rich in vitamin C and iron, and the roots are utilized in tincture and tonic to restore blood levels of iron in those with anemia. Take a daily tonic made with yellow dock, blackberry fruit and leaf, dandelion leaf, stinging nettle leaf, elderberry, hawthorn berry, and rosehips to boost and maintain iron levels.

The root is a gentle detoxifier that stimulates appetite, enhances digestion, improves liver function, and regulates elimination. Those with arthritic and rheumatic conditions, eczema, acne, and psoriasis may benefit from a daily decoction or tincture of yellow dock for its ability to clear stagnation and toxins from the body. Infuse the roots in oil to make a salve for alleviating dry, scaly, or itchy skin conditions.

Future Harvests
Don't worry about yellow dock, it'll come back.

HERBAL PREPARATIONS

Tea
Standard decoction of dried roots
Drink 2–4 ounces per day.

Tincture
1 part fresh roots
2 parts menstruum (65% alcohol,
   35% water)
or
1 part dried roots
5 parts menstruum (50% alcohol,
   50% water)
Take 20–30 drops up to 4 times per day.

Blood-building iron tonic
See the blackberry section on page 121 for the recipe.

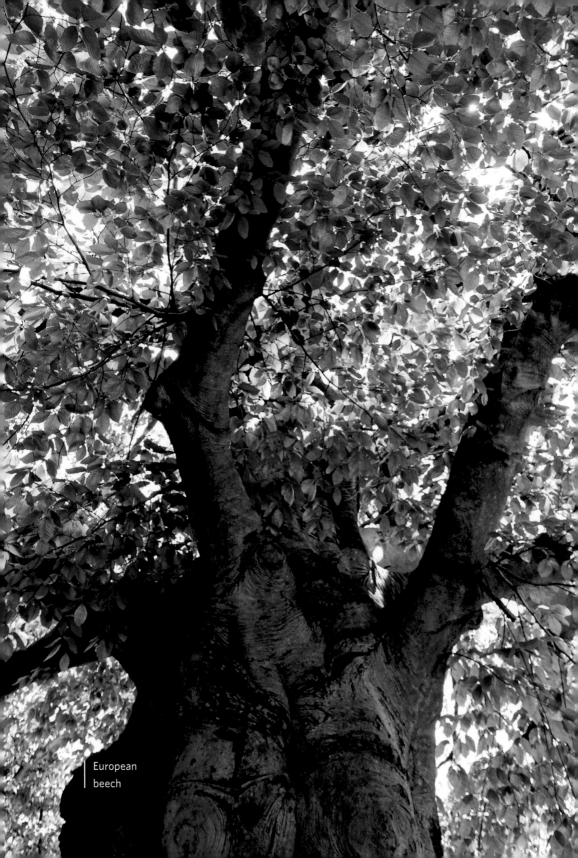

European
beech

METRIC CONVERSIONS

INCHES	CENTIMETERS
¼	0.6
⅜	1.0
½	1.3
¾	1.9
1	2.5
2	5.1
3	7.6
4	10.0
5	12.7
6	15.2
7	17.8
8	20.3
9	22.9
10	25.4

FEET	METERS
1	0.3
2	0.6
3	0.9
4	1.2
5	1.5
6	1.8
7	2.1
8	2.4
9	2.7
10	3

TO CONVERT LENGTH	MULTIPLY BY
Yards to meters	0.90
Inches to centimeters	2.54
Inches to millimeters	25.40
Feet to centimeters	30.50

TEMPERATURES

$$°C = 5/9 \times (°F - 32)$$

$$°F = (9/5 \times °C) + 32$$

ACKNOWLEDGMENTS

Knowledge is not gained in isolation and nothing is really the work of one person alone. It is the effort of a great community, a collaboration with all of life. I owe deep gratitude to the following members of my community for their generosity of words, guidance, encouragement, and love. Without them, this book would not be possible.

Leda Meredith, I'll never forget that first foraging tour I went on with you and how it lit me up and guided me to the path I follow today. Thank you for being my foraging fairy godmother and for dropping the opportunity to write this book in my lap with impeccable timing.

Will McKay, Mike Dempsey, and all the folks at Timber Press for believing in me and helping me along the way. I couldn't have asked for better partners for creating my first book. And thanks to the design team for making it all look so beautiful.

Mollie Firestone, thank you for your expert editing eye and thoughtful contributions. You made the process a breeze.

To my partner, Eric, for egging me on, for saying "just write!," for the "boys days" that made this book possible, and for your love. To Stellan, my sweet son and foraging buddy, your love and bold spirit have transformed my life and made me grow in ways I didn't know were possible.

Dearest Noe Venable, I love you, sister, and can't say it enough. I am so deeply grateful for our connection and for your unwavering support.

Mike Krebill, for your botanical prowess and foraging expertise. Thank you for improving this book with your corrections and suggestions, and for sharing your lovely photographs.

7Song, I am honored to include your photos in this book. Thank you for taking the time to contribute feedback before your busy season took hold.

Deep gratitude to the herbalists who've shared their knowledge with generosity and love: Karen Rose, Jacoby Ballard, Peeka Trenkle, Robin Rose Bennett, Julia Graves. Blessings to the herbalists whose perspectives I admire, I would not have been able to write this book without your wisdom: Rosemary Gladstar, Kiva Rose, Susun Weed, Matthew Wood, Jim McDonald, Tis Mal Crow, Stephen Harrod Buhner.

Miriam McBride, you are such an awesome cheerleader. Thank you for your generosity of time and wisdom. Zoya Baker, for your keen eye and thoughtfulness, and for being a passionate defender and steward of the land. And for your yarrow story! Pam Turczyn, for your loving connection to and communication with the trees.

Jordan Catherine Pagán, of Ostara Apothecary, for being my partner in mugwort magic and plant gathering escapades. Sokhna Heathyre Mabin, amazing human, feeling gratitude for your contribution to the partridgeberry section. And for your radiance, always. Lainie Love Dalby, for sparkling shamelessly and being a fierce warrior priestess for personal sovereignty. Sana, for braving Brooklyn traffic for our wildcrafting adventures. Emma Graves, for the beautiful and kind words on your most favorite chapters. Boris Bernadsky, for your Chinese medicine know-how. Megan Poe, for shaking things up with your special kind of magic. Milo, for your love of violets.

Susan Pincus, of Sawmill Herb Farm, thank you for growing medicine plants with love—their energy spills over onto these pages. To Vanessa Chakour for being a champion of the wild. To Adriana Magaña and Andrew Faust for sharing the joy and knowledge of permaculture with so many people.

Uli Lorimer, thank you for indulging my fantasy of jumping into the pond to get closer to the white water lilies. To Jenny and Maeve, for always inquiring and for the hard work you do to keep the garden looking beautiful.

The MINKA family for loving me and cheering me on. The Pachamama Alliance, and the NY/NJ and Brooklyn Communities for your vision and determination, and for understanding when I had to step away to dive into this book. Irma and the Dream Party, for believing the impossible and keeping the dream alive. To my students, for helping me become a better teacher and bridge between the human and plant realms.

Parental units, thank you for your love.

Mama friends, you know who you are. I love you.

To Prospect Park, my urban oasis, I couldn't live in the city without you.

Utmost gratitude to the plants and my guides for being the best partners on this journey. I'm ever-grateful to the creative universe for listening.

To the Lenape people whose land I inhabit. Waníshi for tending this land for many generations. To the wise women and cunning folk who've come before, from all over the world, for cross-pollinating knowledge and passing it down from generation to generation, against all odds. May the words and images presented in this book be worth the water, trees, petroleum, and energy used to print and distribute them.

RESOURCES AND REFERENCES

This book serves as a guide for quick and easy identification of many well-known medicinal plants in the Northeast and the basic ideas for medicine making. The following pages include resources containing in-depth identification parameters and botanical information about a broader range of plants in our region and beyond; websites with more information about the conservation status of plants in North America and what you can do to encourage the future of at-risk plants; well-loved resources for more herbal recipes, herb-to-menstruum ratios, and inspiration; as well as additional references that were of great help in the writing of this book. Thank you to all who made this knowledge available.

Plant Identification

Elpel, Thomas J. 2004. *Botany in a Day: The Patterns Method of Plant Identification.* 5th Ed. Pony, MT: HOPS Press.

Foster, Steven, and James A. Duke. 2000. *A Peterson Field Guide to Medicinal Plants and Herbs: Eastern and Central North America.* 2nd Ed. Boston: Houghton Mifflin Company.

Identify that Plant: identifythatplant.com.

Illinois Wildflowers: illinoiswildflowers.info.

Minnesota Wildflowers: minnesotawild flowers.info.

Newcomb, Lawrence. 1977. *Newcomb's Wildflower Guide.* New York: Little, Brown and Company.

Peterson, Roger Tory, and Margaret McKenny. 1996. *A Peterson Field Guide to Wildflowers: Northeastern/North-central North America.* Boston: Houghton Mifflin Company.

Plants for a Future Database: pfaf.org.

Plant Conservation and Mapping

Biota of North America Program (BONAP): bonap.org.

Cornell University, Department of Horticulture: hort.cals.cornell.edu.

International Union for Conservation of Nature (IUCN) Red List: iucnredlist.org.

Invasive Plant Atlas of New England (IPANE): eddmaps.org/ipane.

Native Plant Trust's Go Botany: gobotany. nativeplanttrust.org.

NatureServe Explorer, An Online Encyclopedia of Life: explorer.natureserve.org/index.htm.

Plant Native: plantnative.org.

Prairie Nursery: prairienursery.com.

United Plant Savers, Medicinal Plant Conservation: unitedplantsavers.org.

USDA Animal and Plant Health Inspection Service: aphis.usda.gov.

USDA PLANTS Database: plants.usda.gov.

Medicine Making

Bennett, Robin Rose. 2014. *The Gift of Healing Herbs: Plant Medicines and Home Remedies for a Vibrantly Healthy Life*. Berkeley, CA: North Atlantic Books.

Cech, Richo. 2000. *Making Plant Medicine*. Williams, OR: Horizon Herbs.

Easley, Thomas, and Steven Horne. 2016. *The Modern Herbal Dispensatory: A Medicine Making Guide*. Berkeley, CA: North Atlantic Books.

Gladstar, Rosemary. 2008. *Herbal Recipes for Vibrant Health*. North Adams, MA: Storey Publishing.

Green, James. 2000. *The Herbal Medicine-Maker's Handbook*. Berkeley, CA: Crossing Press.

Herbal Roots Zine: herbalrootszine.com.

Learning Herbs: learningherbs.com.

Additional References

7Song. 2012. The *Eupatorium* story—Joe Pye weed, boneset and white snakeroot, part two. 7song.com/the-eupatorium-story-joe-pye-weed-boneset-and-white-snakeroot-part-two/.

Alfs, Matthew. 2014. An herbal breakthrough in rheumatology: bull thistle (*Cirsium vulgare*) for spondyloarthropathy. *Journal of the American Herbalists Guild* 12(3). americanherbalistsguild.com/sites/default/files/sample-articles-pdfs/alfs_bull_thistle_for_spondyloarthropathy.pdf.

American Chemical Society. 2018. Maple leaf extract could nip skin wrinkles in the bud. acs.org/content/acs/en/pressroom/newsreleases/2018/august/maple-leaf-extract-could-nip-skin-wrinkles-in-the-bud.html.

Bensky, Dan, Steven Clavey, Andrew Gamble, and Erich Stöger. 2004. *Chinese Herbal Medicine Materia Medica*. 3rd Ed. Seattle, WA: Eastman Press.

Blair, Katrina. 2014. *The Wild Wisdom of Weeds: 13 Essential Plants for Human Survival*. White River Junction, VT: Chelsea Green Publishing.

Blankenspoor, Juliet. 2012. Partridgeberry materia medica. chestnutherbs.com/partridgeberry-materia-medica/.

Bone, Kerry, and Simon Mills. 2013. *Principles and Practice of Phytotherapy*. 2nd Ed. London: Churchill Livingstone.

Buhner, Stephen Harrod. 2012. *Herbal Antibiotics: Natural Alternatives for Drug-Resistant Bacteria*. North Adams, MA: Storey Publishing.

———. 2011. *Pine Pollen: Ancient Medicine for a Modern World*. Springvale, ME: SurThrival.

Committee on Herbal Medicinal Products (HMPC). 2017. Ivy leaf *Hedera helix* L., folium. ema.europa.eu/documents/herbal-summary/ivy-leaf-summary-public_en-0.pdf.

de la Forêt, Rosalee. 2013. Meadowsweet elixir: a home remedy for pain. learningherbs.com/remedies-recipes/home-remedy-for-pain.

———. 2008. What's chemistry got to do with it? methowvalleyherbs.com/2008/09/whats-chemistry-got-to-do-with-it.html.

Dharmananda, Subhuti. Safety issues affecting herbs: pyrrolizidine alkaloids. itmonline.org/arts/pas.htm.

Ellingwood, Finley. 1919. *American Materia Medica, Therapeutics and Pharmacognosy*. swsbm.com/Ellingwoods/Ellingwoods_plants_only.pdf.

Emerson, Ralph Waldo. 1904. *The Fortune of the Republic. The Complete Works of Ralph Waldo Emerson: Miscellanies*. Boston: Houghton, Mifflin and Company. The Riverside Press, Cambridge.

Falconi, Dina. 2013. *Foraging and Feasting: A Field Guide and Wild Food Cookbook*. Accord, NY: Botanical Arts Press.

Felter, Harvey Wickes, and John Uri Lloyd. 1898. *King's American Dispensatory*. 18th Ed. 3rd Rev. henriettes-herb.com/eclectic/kings/index.html.

Flower Essence Services: fesflowers.com.

Frawley, David, and Vasant Lad. 2001. *The Yoga of Herbs*. Twin Lakes, WI: Lotus Press.

Gladstar, Rosemary, and Pamela Hirsch. Eds. 2000. *Planting the Future: Saving Our Medicinal Herbs*. Rochester, VT: Healing Arts Press.

Graves, Julia. 2012. *The Language of Plants: A Guide to the Doctrine of Signatures*. Great Barrington, MA: Lindisfarne Books.

———. The lily circle. lilycircle.com/the-lily-circle/.

Grieve, Maud. 1931. *A Modern Herbal*. botanical.com/botanical/mgmh/mgmh.html.

Guo, Shuangshuang, Yan Ge, and Kriskamol Na Jom. 2017. A review of phytochemistry, metabolite changes, and medicinal uses of the common sunflower seed and sprouts (*Helianthus annuus* L.). *Chemistry Central Journal* 11:95. ncbi.nlm.nih.gov/pubmed/29086881.

Hardin, Kiva Rose. Monarda: honeyed spice of the canyons. wildlingsherbary.com/monarda?rq=monarda.

Harding, A. R. 1936. *Ginseng and Other Medicinal Plants*. swsbm.com/Ephemera/Ephemera.html.

Haudenosaunee Confederacy: haudenosauneeconfederacy.com.

Hawke, Richard. 2014. A comparative study of Joe-Pye weeds (*Eutrochium* spp.) and their relatives. *Chicago Botanic Garden Plant Evaluation Notes* 37. chicagobotanic. org/downloads/planteval_notes/no37_joepyeweed.pdf.

Henriette's Herbal: henriettes-herb.com.

Herrick, James. 1997. *Iroquois Medical Botany*. 1st Ed. Syracuse, NY: Syracuse University Press.

Hobbs, Christopher. Herbal medicine: constitutional herbalism and the herbal energetics of western herbs. healthy.net/Health/Article/Constitutional_Herbalism_and_The_Herbal_Energetics_of_Western_Herbs/958.

Kimmerer, Robin Wall. 2013. *Braiding Sweetgrass*. Minneapolis, MN: Milkweed Editions.

Lloyd, John Uri, and Curtis Gates Lloyd. 1930. *Drugs and Medicines of North America, 1884–1887*. henriettes-herb.com/eclectic/dmna/index.html.

Lutsenko, Yulia, Bylka Wieslawa, Irena Matlawska, and Roman Darmohray. 2010. Hedera helix as a medicinal plant. *Herba Polonica* 56(1): 83–96. researchgate.net/publication/266594470_Hedera_helix_as_a_medicinal_plant.

McDonald, Jim. New England aster. herbcraft.org/aster.html.

———. Wild sarsparilla. herbcraft.org/sarsparilla.html.

Meredith, Leda. 2014. *Northeast Foraging: 120 Wild and Flavorful Edibles from Beach Plums to Wineberries*. Portland, OR: Timber Press.

Meyn, Norman. 2014. Winter identification of Norway maple and sugar maple. *Journal Star*. blogs.pjstar.com/gardening/2014/01/31/winter-identification-of-norway-maple-and-sugar-maple.

Moazazi, Zolikha, and Durdi Qujeq. 2014. Berberis fruit extract and biochemical parameters in patients with type II diabetes. *Jundishapur Journal of Natural Pharmaceutical Products* 9(2): e13490. ncbi.nlm.nih.gov/pmc/articles/PMC4036375.

Moerman, Daniel. 2009. *Native American Medicinal Plants: An Ethnobotanical Dictionary*. Portland, OR: Timber Press.

Moore, Michael. *Herbal Materia Medica*. 1995. 5th Ed. Southwest School of Botanical Medicine. Bisbee, AZ. swsbm.com/ManualsMM/MatMed5.pdf.

National Center for Homeopathy: homeopathycenter.org.

Native American Ethnobotany Database: naeb.brit.org.

Native Tech, Native American Technology and Art: nativetech.org/plants/index.html.

Neto, Catherine C., and Joe A. Vinson. 2013. *Herbal Medicine: Biomolecular and Clinical Aspects*. 2nd ed. London: Churchill Livingstone.

Ostara Apothecary. Sunflower flower essence. ostaraapothecary.com/shop/sunflower-flower-essence.

Pareek, Anil, Manish Suthar, Garvendra S. Rathore, and Vijay Bansal. 2011. Feverfew (*Tanacetum parthenium* L.): a systematic review. *Pharmacognosy Reviews* 5(9): 103–110.

Popham, Sajah. 2017. The key to herbal energetics and constitutional systems. evolutionaryherbalism.com/2017/01/11/the-key-to-herbal-energetics-and-constitutional-systems/.

Razzaghi-Abyaneh, Mehdi, and Mahendra Rai. Eds. 2013. *Antifungal Metabolites from Plants*. Springer.

Sawandi, Tariq. Yorubic medicine: the art of divine herbology. planetherbs.com/research-center/theory-articles/yorubic-medicine-the-art-of-divine-herbology/.

Scott, Timothy Lee. 2010. *Invasive Plant Medicine: The Ecological Benefits and Healing Abilities of Invasives*. Rochester, VT: Healing Arts Press.

Srivastava, J. K., E. Shankar, and S. Gupta. 2010. Chamomile: a herbal medicine of the past with bright future. *Molecular Medicine Reports* 3(6): 895–901.

State University of New York College of Environmental Science and Forestry in Partnership with the New York State Department of Environmental Conservation. New York Natural Heritage Program. guides.nynhp.org/.

Thayer, Sam. 2006. *The Forager's Harvest: A Guide to Identifying, Harvesting, and Preparing Edible Wild Plants*. 1st Ed. Bruce, WI: Foragers Harvest Press.

Tierra, Michael. 1988. *Planetary Herbology*. Twin Lakes, WI: Lotus Press.

Tree Frog Farm: treefrogfarm.com.

University of Maine Cooperative Extension. Highbush cranberry. extension.umaine.edu/cranberries/highbush-cranberry/.

———. How to tap maple trees and make maple syrup. extension.umaine.edu/publications/7036e/.

USDA, US Forest Service. Fire Effects Information System (FEIS). *Pinus rigida*. https://www.fs.fed.us/database/feis/plants/tree/pinrig/all.html.

Weed, Susun. 1986. *Wise Women Herbal for the Childbearing Year*. Woodstock, NY: Ash Tree Publishing.

Winston, David, and Steven Maimes. 2007. *Adaptogens: Herbs for Strength, Stamina, and Stress Relief*. Rochester, VT: Healing Arts Press.

Wood, Matthew. 1997. *The Book of Herbal Wisdom*. Berkeley, CA: North Atlantic Books.

———. 2008. *Earthwise Herbal: A Complete Guide to Old World Medicinal Plants*. Berkeley, CA: North Atlantic Books.

———. 2009. *Earthwise Herbal: A Complete Guide to New World Medicinal Plants*. Berkeley, CA: North Atlantic Books.

———. 2016. *The Earthwise Herbal Repertory*. Berkeley, CA: North Atlantic Books.

Woodland Essence. Black cherry flower essence. woodlandessence.com/products/black-cherry-prunus-serotina.

———. Linden flower essence. woodlandessence.com/products/linden-tilia-americana.

PHOTOGRAPHY CREDITS

7Song, pages 100, 101, 102, 133, 134, 167, 168, 234, 242, 284, 295, 296, 338, 339, 340, 344, 345, 346, 356, 357, 377, 383, 384

Eric Bet, pages 63, 71

Andrew Faust and Adriana Magaña, page 238 (model Juniper Faust Magaña)

Mike Krebill, pages 135, 150, 188, 370, 371

Leda Meredith, pages 268, 316

Jordan Catherine Pagán, pages 36, 55

Flickr

Used under a CC Attribution 2.0 Generic license

Superior National Forest, page 237

Used under a CC Attribution-Share Alike 2.0 Generic license

Giles Watson, page 241

Wikimedia Commons

AnRo0002, page 31 (bottom)

Williammehlhorn, page 30 (top)

Used under a CC Attribution-Share Alike 2.5 Generic license

Andreas Trepte, www.photo-natur.net, page 159

Used under a CC Attribution-Share Alike 3.0 Unported license

Аимаина хикари, page 165

Eric Coombs, page 208

Christian Fischer, page 276

Jean-Pol Grandmont, page 30 (bottom right)

James H. Miller, Ted Bodner, page 31 (top right)

Mihael Simonic, page 228

André-Ph. D. Picard, page 277

All other photographs are by the author.

INDEX

C

Callirhytis species, 264

calm disposition, encouraging, 294

Camellia sinensis, 43

Canada goldenrod, 203, 204, 205

Canada lettuce, 373, 374

Canada moonseed, 371

Canadian white violet, 355

cancer remedies, 128, 309

cancer therapies, detoxifying from, 157

candelilla wax, 58–59

candida infections, 155, 205, 359

canker sore remedies, 101

Capsella bursa-pastoris, 311

cardiovascular system support

  blood cleansers for, 114

  combinations for, 233

  hawthorn for, 212

  restorative tonics for, 250

  stimulating herbs for, 190, 191–192

  tonics for, 325–326

  toning herbs for, 129, 166, 349

  treatments for multiple ailments, 296

carminative herbs, 343, 362

carnauba wax, 58–59

Carolina crane's-bill, 367–368

carpal tunnel syndrome, 205

castor oil, 56

catnip, 82, 146–147

cats, valerian and, 350

Ceanothus americanus, 295

cedar-apple rust, 175

cedar waxwing, 175

Celastrina ladon (butterfly), 295

Centella asiatica, 340

Cerastium species, 148

Cerastium fontanum, 148

Chamaemelum nobile, 199

chamomile, 62, 189

chamomile, German, 86, 198–199

checkerberry, 383

cheese mallow, 163

cheeseweed, 163

cherry birch, 116, 117

chest rubs, 173, 174, 176, 275

chickweed, 48, 62, 72, 82, 148–150

chicory, 12, 82, 151–153, 169, 373

childbirth, 267, 292

children, 68

  boosting health for, 326

  fever treatment for, 230

  precautions for, 173, 352, 382

  remedies for, 199

  remedies for multiple ailments, 147

  soothing herbs for, 164, 232

  stomachache treatments for, 248, 379

Chimaphila umbellata, 276

chokecherry, 123

cholera, 349

churchsteeples, 100

Cichorium intybus, 151

Cicuta maculata, 29

cinquefoil, 82, 84, 154–155

circulatory stimulants, 201, 271, 274, 312, 317

circulatory system. See cardiovascular system support

Cirsium vulgare, 141

Clark's rule, 68–69

cleavers, 72, 84, 156–157, 333

Clostridium infections, 215

coastal areas, Season by Season plant charts, 94–97

coastal plain Joe Pye weed, 319, 320

coconut oil, 56

coffee filters, use of, 258, 260

coffee substitutes, 152, 153, 170–171

cognitive function, improvement of, 201

cold and flu remedies. See also cough remedies

  boneset, 137–138

  combinations, 181, 192, 248, 299, 303, 362

  early treatment, 126, 178, 194, 197, 282

  infusions, 233, 279, 389

  pine for, 274

  sweetgum for, 343

cold infusions, 45

cold sores, 230

colitis, 215

coltsfoot, 74, 92, 158–159

comfrey, 84, 160–162

common barberry, 108

common blackberry, 120

common juniper, 175

common larch, 227

common mallow, 84, 163–164

common names, 13

common prickly ash, 284

common ragweed, 287

common selfheal, 308

common starwort, 148

common stitchwort, 148

compassion and empathy, increasing, 292

composite flower parts, 20

compound leaf types, 18

compresses, 62

Comptonia peregrina, 335

Concord grape, 371

coneflower, 177

confidence, herbs for, 141, 142, 184

congestion

  clearing, 150, 274, 296, 339

  decoctions or tinctures for, 173

  expectorants for, 210

  infused honey for, 192

  remedies for, 186, 334

  steams for, 62–63, 362

Conium maculatum, 29, 208, 365–366

connective tissue support, 246, 259, 334, 345. See also musculoskeletal health

conservation status of herbs, 32–33

constipation relief. See also laxative herbs

  bulking agents, 280, 372

  peach pit for, 269

  precautions, 271

  stimulating herbs, 210

  teas for, 354

  tinctures, 138

  tonics for, 152–153

constituent types, solubility of, 42, 44–45

contact dermatitis, 253

contraceptives, 365

convalescents, treatments for, 336

cooling herbs, 157

  blends for, 301

  and blood thinning, 307

  cinquefoil, 155

anti-inflammatory herbs for, 223
combinations for, 320
compresses for, 186
compresses or baths for, 150
dandelion root for, 171
liniments for, 346
pain relief for, 173
poultices for, 132, 259
tinctures for, 142
jojoba oil, 56
Juglans nigra, 128
Juniperus communis, 175
Juniperus virginiana, 175

K

keying out plant species, 32
kidney function, improving, 175, 176, 210, 326, 329
kidney stones, 119, 166, 205, 319–320
Kimmerer, Robin Wall, 26
knitbone, 160

L

Lactuca species, 373
Lactuca biennis, 373
Lactuca canadensis, 373
Lactuca floridana, 375
Lactuca hirsuta, 375
Lactuca serriola, 373
Lactuca virosa, 373, 374
lakesides, Season by Season plant charts, 90–95
landowners, permissions and, 27
land use history, 33–34
larch, 76, 227–228
large cranberry, 167
Larix species, 227
Larix decidua, 227
Larix laricina, 227
latex, harvesting and processing, 374
laxative herbs, 170, 181, 379. *See also* constipation relief
lead contamination, 219, 289
leaf types, 18–19
leaves and buds, harvest methods, 36–37
lemon balm, 86, 229–230
Leonurus cardiaca, 249
lesser periwinkle, 270

leukorrhea, 359, 360
light, and crafting flower essences, 54
lime tree, 231
linden, 37, 76, 231–233
Lindera benzoin, 316
Linnaeus, Carolus, 14
Linné, Carl von, 14
lip balms, 230
Liquidambar orientalis, 342
Liquidambar styraciflua, 341
Liriodendron tulipifera, 347
liver health
blends for, 368–369
burdock for, 145
dandelion for, 170
detoxification, 153
detoxifying plants for, 393
infusions or tinctures for, 129
precautions for, 159, 161–162
reducing inflammation, 310
rose for, 299
tonics for, 109, 136
lobelia, 86, 234–235
Lobelia inflata, 234
Lobelia siphilitica, 235
Lonicera japonica, 220
lotions and crèmes, 60–61
lozenges, making, 53
lung health, 176, 186, 201–202, 258, 259. *See also* respiratory system support
lupulin, 215
Lyme disease, 110, 126, 224, 345
lymphatic system support, 104, 157, 177, 282, 334, 355

M

mad-dog skullcap, 133
Mahonia aquifolium, 109
maidenhair tree, 200
malaria, 138, 349
Malva neglecta, 163
maple (tree), 76, 236–240
maple syrup, 52, 236, 237–239, 240
marcescence, 111, 263
Marrubium vulgare, 356
marshes/bogs, Season by Season plant charts, 90–95
massage oils
blends for, 355

infused with evening primrose, 188
infused with spruce, 322
for muscle soreness, 172, 174, 176
for pain relief, 173
for solar plexus region, 171, 205
for tension relief, 235
for warming extremities, 317
mastitis, 221, 267, 282, 355
Matricaria discoidea, 199
Matricaria recutita, 198
meadow dropwort, 241
meadowfoam seed oil, 56
meadow garlic, 192
meadowsweet, 86, 241–243
Medicinal Uses sections, 22
meditations, for harvesting, 34
Melilotus species, 333
Melilotus alba, 333
Melilotus altissimus, 333
Melilotus indicus, 333
Melilotus officinalis, 333
Melissa, 229
Melissa officinalis, 229
Menispermum canadense, 371
menopause, 140, 294
menstrual cramps, 199
compresses or baths for, 150
crampbark for, 166
herbs for, 351
remedies for, 147
soothing heat for, 221
stimulating herbs for, 252
tinctures for, 136, 250
menstrual support
emmenagogues for, 147, 297, 352
premenstrual symptoms, easing, 134, 299
stimulating herbs for, 107, 176, 252
tinctures for, 136
menstruums, 42, 44–45, 46
mental clarity, promoting, 339
Mentha species, 247
Mentha aquatica, 247
Mentha arvensis, 247
Mentha canadensis, 247
Mentha ×piperita, 247
Mentha spicata, 247
Mentha suaveolens, 247

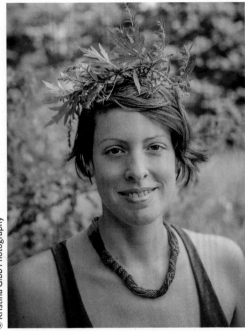

Liz Neves is an herbalist, mama, reiki practitioner, artist, dreamer, and meditator.

In 2005, Liz left her career as a copywriter in medical marketing with a yearning to spend more time outdoors, immersed in nature. Through her permaculture studies, she found her true calling in herbal medicine. Liz credits many teachers—plant, animal, mineral, and human—with guiding her on the path of healing and learning.

Her first foray into sharing plant medicine with her community was formulating and handcrafting a line of botanical home and body care products. Liz's passion for the plants deepened into a desire to restore the human-earth connection. In 2014, she founded Gathering Ground as a platform for herbal education, earth-based spirituality, meditation, and energy healing. Liz leads healing plant walks to introduce city dwellers to the myriad of medicinal flora in the urban environment.

When she's not teaching plant medicine–making workshops, Liz is wildcrafting and preparing herbal medicines for her family and community. She's also an avid dreamworker and introduces fellow dreamers to herbs that facilitate a more intentional and active dream experience.